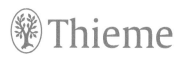

Ophthalmology Q&A Board Review

Lora R. Dagi Glass, MD
Assistant Professor
Department of Ophthalmology
Columbia University Irving Medical Center
New York, New York

400 Illustrations

Thieme
New York • Stuttgart • Delhi • Rio de Janeiro

Library of Congress Cataloging-in-Publication Data is available from the Publisher

Thieme Publishers New York
333 Seventh Avenue, New York, NY 10001 USA
+1 800 782 3488, customerservice@thieme.com

Georg Thieme Verlag KG
Rüdigerstrasse 14, 70469 Stuttgart, Germany
+49 [0]711 8931 421, customerservice@thieme.de

Thieme Publishers Delhi
A-12, Second Floor, Sector-2, Noida-201301
Uttar Pradesh, India
+91 120 45 566 00, customerservice@thieme.in

Thieme Publishers Rio de Janeiro,
Thieme Publicações Ltda.
Edifício Rodolpho de Paoli, 25º andar
Av. Nilo Peçanha, 50 – Sala 2508
Rio de Janeiro 20020-906 Brasil
+55 21 3172 2297

Cover design: Thieme Publishing Group
Typesetting by Thomson Digital, India

Printed in USA by King Printing Company, Inc.   5 4 3 2 1

ISBN 978-1-68420-066-5

Also available as an e-book:
e-ISBN 978-1-68420-067-2

Important note: Medicine is an ever-changing science undergoing continual development. Research and clinical experience are continually expanding our knowledge, in particular our knowledge of proper treatment and drug therapy. Insofar as this book mentions any dosage or application, readers may rest assured that the authors, editors, and publishers have made every effort to ensure that such references are in accordance with **the state of knowledge at the time of production of the book.**

Nevertheless, this does not involve, imply, or express any guarantee or responsibility on the part of the publishers in respect to any dosage instructions and forms of applications stated in the book. **Every user is requested to examine carefully** the manufacturers' leaflets accompanying each drug and to check, if necessary in consultation with a physician or specialist, whether the dosage schedules mentioned therein or the contraindications stated by the manufacturers differ from the statements made in the present book. Such examination is particularly important with drugs that are either rarely used or have been newly released on the market. Every dosage schedule or every form of application used is entirely at the user's own risk and responsibility. The authors and publishers request every user to report to the publishers any discrepancies or inaccuracies noticed. If errors in this work are found after publication, errata will be posted at www.thieme.com on the product description page.

Some of the product names, patents, and registered designs referred to in this book are in fact registered trademarks or proprietary names even though specific reference to this fact is not always made in the text. Therefore, the appearance of a name without designation as proprietary is not to be construed as a representation by the publisher that it is in the public domain.

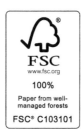

To Akiva, who taught me to study efficiently!

Contents

Preface

Studying for an exam can be challenging. Preparing while training or in practice can feel nearly impossible. Who has the time?

That's where this book comes in. The multiple-choice format is meant to mirror the test itself, but the questions also guide you through a thorough ophthalmology curriculum. If you understand what you are being asked—where the question stems are guiding you, and why the question choices are right or wrong—you have covered a huge range of knowledge.

Time is precious; use it wisely!

Lora R. Dagi Glass, MD

Contributors

Aliaa H. Abdelhakim, MD, PhD
Vitreoretinal Fellow
Department of Ophthalmology
Columbia University Irving Medical Center
New York, New York

Carolina Adams, MD
Department of Ophthalmology
NewYork-Presbyterian Hospital
Columbia University Irving Medical Center
New York, New York

Norimitsu Ban, MD
Vitreoretinal Fellow
Department of Ophthalmology
Columbia University Irving Medical Center
New York, New York

Anne Barmettler, MD
Director
Oculoplastic Surgery Division
Department of Ophthalmology and Visual Sciences
Assistant Professor
Department of Ophthalmology
Albert Einstein College of Medicine
Montefiore Medical Center
New York, New York

Michelle Trager Cabrera, MD
Associate Chief
Department of Ophthalmology
Seattle Children's Hospital
Associate Professor
Department of Pediatric Ophthalmology and Strabismus
University of Washington
Seattle, Washington

Ashley A. Campbell, MD
Assistant Professor
Department of Ophthalmology
Wilmer Eye Institute
Johns Hopkins University School of Medicine
Baltimore, Maryland

Catherine S. Choi, MD
Assistant Professor
Department of Ophthalmology
Tufts University School of Medicine
Boston, Massachusetts

Alberto Giuseppe Distefano, MD
Assistant Professor
Department of Ophthalmology
Boston University School of Medicine
Boston, Massachusetts

Richard M. France, MD
Cataract Surgeon
Ocular Immunology and Uveitis specialist
Department of Opththalmology
Eyecare Medical Group
Portland, Maine

Larissa Kadar Ghadiali, MD
Assistant Clinical Professor
Department of Ophthalmology
Loyola University Medical Center
Maywood, Illinois

Lora R. Dagi Glass, MD
Assistant Professor
Department of Ophthalmology
Columbia University Irving Medical Center
New York, New York

John Gorfinkel, MD, FRCS
Assistant Professor
Department of Ophthalmology and Vision Sciences
University of Toronto
Toronto, Ontario

Syed A. Hussnain, MD
Vitreoretinal Fellow
Department of Ophthalmology
Columbia University Irving Medical Center
New York, New York

Maanasa Indaram, MD
Assistant Professor
Department of Ophthalmology
University of California
San Francisco, California

Viral Juthani, MD
Assistant Professor
Department of Ophthalmology
Albert Einstein College of Medicine
New York, New York

Euna B. Koo, MD
Clinical Assistant Professor
Department of Ophthalmology
Stanford University School of Medicine
Palo Alto, California

Spencer Langevin, MD
Ocular Oncology Fellow
Department of Ophthalmology
Columbia University Irving Medical Center
New York, New York

John Lloyd, MD, FRCS
Director
Postgraduate Education
Department of Ophthalmology and Visual Sciences
University of Toronto
Toronto, Ontario

Allison R. Loh, MD
Assistant Professor
Department of Ophthalmology
Oregon Health and Science University
Portland, Oregon

Peter MacIntosh, MD
Assistant Professor
Department of Ophthalmology
Neuro-Ophthalmology Service
Oculoplastic and Reconstructive Surgery Service
University of Illinois College of Medicine
Peoria, Illinois

Brian P. Marr, MD
Director
Ocular Oncology Service
Professor
Department of Ophthalmology
Columbia University Irving Medical Center
New York, New York

Lisa Park, MD
Associate Professor
Department of Ophthalmology
Columbia University Irving Medical Center
New York, New York

Veena Rao, MD, MSc
Glaucoma Specialist
Charlotte Eye, Ear, Nose, and Throat Associates
Charlotte, North Carolina

Stephanie M. Llop Santiago, MD
Assistant Professor
Department of Ophthalmology
Icahn School of Medicine
New York Eye and Ear Infirmary of Mount Sinai
New York, New York

Craig W. See, MD
Associate Staff
Cole Eye Institute
Cleveland Clinic Foundation
Cleveland, Ohio

Tarun Sharma, MD, FRCSEd, MBA
Department of Ophthalmology
Columbia University Irving Medical Center
New York, New York

Christian Song, MD
Instructor
Department of Ophthalmology
Harvard Medical School
Boston, Massachusetts

Grace Sun, MD
Assistant Professor
Department of Ophthalmology
Weill Cornell Medical College
New York, New York

Tongalp H. Tezel, MD
Instructor
Chang Family Professor of Ophthalmology
Director of the Retina Service
Director of Vitreoretinal Fellowship Program
Columbia University College of Physicians and Surgeons
Department of Ophthalmology
Edward S. Harkness Eye Institute
Columbia University Irving Medical Center
New York, New York

Danielle Trief, MD, MSc
Assistant Professor
Department of Ophthalmology
Columbia University Irving Medical Center
New York, New York

Sylvia H. Yoo, MD
Assistant Professor
Department of Ophthalmology
Tufts University School of Medicine
Boston, Massachusetts

Study Tips

When it comes to studying, you are more of a pro than most people out there. At this point in your career, you have successfully crossed the hurdles of multiple lengthy and important tests for years. Grade school, high school, college, and medical school all brought you to this exam and to the career opportunities it allows for. Despite all this, studying for and taking a test that is so closely tied to your ultimate professional goal can be daunting. Let this chapter serve as a reminder of studying basics, as well as an opportunity to change ineffective study habits.

Life Basics

Nutrition: Healthy food leads to a healthy life. The stress of studying can cause some to lose their appetite, leading to an unhealthy, anorexia-like state, whereas others tend to over-eat. Eating well when studying means eating a balanced diet. Snacks can be a way to keep yourself awake when studying, but beware of the excess sugar, fat, and calories! If you need more snacking than usual, consider specifically choosing healthier options such as crunchy vegetables. If you tend to forget to eat, focus on making sure you actually eat something nutritious at mealtime.

Sleep: Very few people claim to sleep enough—how much more so does this apply when studying on top of everything else! But an awake mind is an alert mind, and an alert mind can process information more efficiently. Only you know how much sleep your body needs to feel rested, but try to be consistent. And if you need a nap, 15- to 20-minute mini naps can be easier to wake up from than multi-hour naps.

Exercise: Studying can make you tired and down, but exercise can wake you up and make you happy! Whether it is time at the gym or a walk, try to incorporate routine movement into your studying life. Some find studying while exercising easy and helpful. For example, you could listen to a recording or bring flashcards. Others find it better to keep the two separate. If you feel yourself getting sleepy or inefficient, you might walk to a coffee shop or library for both the exercise and the change in study environment.

Attitude: This is obviously an important test, so it is wise to take studying seriously. On the other hand, this is not everything in life. Be optimistic and keep things in perspective! A little stress helps fuel studying, but too much stress will paralyze you.

Study Basics

Study Pacing: If you cram, you will forget. You don't just need this study material for an exam, you need it for a lifetime. Try to create a paced schedule. Ideally, a curriculum of your choosing can be completed in the time period you have to implement it. If your study goals are impossible to attain from the get-go, your choice is not going to be a functional study method for you. Define beginning and end dates, and acknowledge days that will be impossible to use. When using a question book like this one, outline the number of questions you will do daily. If you can do more questions than planned one day, you can give yourself a break and do fewer on another. Two weeks before the exam, start to review difficult material. Perhaps you have taken notes on it, or underlined it in the Answer section. Mark the most particularly difficult material during this time, and then review it one last time in the last couple of days before the test.

Study Modalities: No-one said that you have to study everything in the same way. Using multiple modalities to study a single subject can be effective. Or, you might find that some subjects are better studied in one way, while others are better studied in another. As you begin to test yourself, try to be cognizant of what types of learning modalities best suit your needs. Is it photographs? Tables? Flash cards? Bullet point outline form? Full sentences? Books? Questions? And remember—what worked for you one year might not be so effective in another, and it may be because of time available or change in study style. And that's OK! You could try to have various methods of testing and integrating information. For example, take notes on your most difficult question answers and keep them in a small notebook or on your phone. When you have a minute between things, review a page to keep the information fresh.

Question Skills: At the end of the day, a smart question reader is a better test taker. When you read a question, pay special attention to words like "true," "false," or "except." When you read answer choices, cross out clearly incorrect ones—but if you are using the book version of these questions, do not waste time crossing out the whole answer. A little symbol suffices. Always select the best, or most correct, answer. Try not to second guess your original answer—your initial answer is more likely to be the correct one. Remember that incorrect answers do not count against your score, so it is always worth choosing something. If you feel a question is taking too much time, select an answer and mark the question so that you can spend time carefully rereading the question and answers at the end of the exam.

Cross-assimilation: Learn from the correct and incorrect answer explanations. Even though the majority of answer choices are typically incorrect, the answer explanations for incorrect answers are specifically built to help you learn more information. If a topic seems foreign to you, use the question as an opportunity to look up more information.

Timing: For those who need to work on timing, try to do a set number of questions in a timed manner, and then review answers in depth, rather than looking at the answers between each question. It is helpful to take a break every 45 minutes or so of studying. Your initial goal might be 25 questions in a 30-minute period. You might work up to 50 questions in an hour. Remember that the test itself is 250 questions over 5 hours.

Day of Stress Techniques: Certain stressors can be ameliorated by controlling them. If you are worried about getting to the test on time, ask a friend or family member to call you in case you snooze your alarm. Think about what you want available to eat or drink during your testing breaks and pack them the night before. Also, pack whatever you need for identification at the testing center. Maybe you have a favorite test sweater—that's another form of stress reduction, and it's OK! If you realize you are getting stressed or need a mental break during the exam, try a minute of meditation, deep breathing exercises, or picturing your favorite type of vacation. It may be a calm and empty beach with lapping waves and a lightly fluttering wind... A very short moment of brain and body relaxation might help you focus and finish the test more effectively and efficiently.

Good luck!

Chapter 1

Cornea, External Disease, and Anterior Segment

Carolina Adams, Danielle Trief

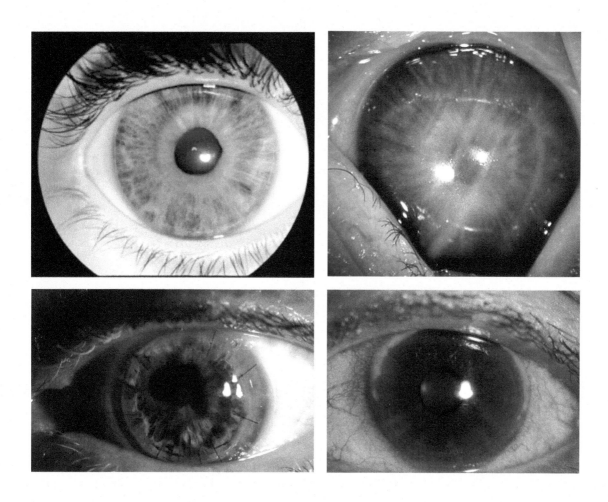

1.1 Questions

Easy	Medium	Hard

1. A 67-year-old female presents to the outpatient clinic with a history of recurrent nodules of the right upper eyelid for the past 5 years that were treated with multiple intralesional injections of triamcinolone. On exam, you notice two right upper lid nodules associated with madarosis and lid margin thickening. The left eyelids are unremarkable. What condition are you concerned about?

A. Recurrent chalazion

B. Sebaceous gland carcinoma

C. Basal cell carcinoma

D. Squamous cell carcinoma

2. A 47-year-old female presents with a history of chronic foreign body sensation and tearing associated with inferior punctate epithelial erosions. You decide to evaluate tear production without topical anesthetic. What is the name of this test?

A. Basic secretion test

B. Schirmer I test

C. Schirmer II test

D. Schirmer IV test

3. Which of the following is a quantitative test of tear production?

A. Lactoferrin

B. Immunoglobulin G

C. Schirmer testing

D. Meibography

4. A 45-year-old female with a history of seborrheic dermatitis complains of foreign body sensation and tearing. On exam, there is a rapid tear breakup time and foam in the tear meniscus. What would be the most likely cause of this patient's dry eye?

A. Sjogren's syndrome

B. Age-related dry eye

C. Trachoma

D. Meibomian gland dysfunction

5. A 19-year-old Caucasian female presents with a history of meibomian gland dysfunction for the past 2 years. On slit lamp exam, she has lid margin telangiectasias and anterior blepharitis in both eyes and corneal neovascularization of the right eye as shown in figure. What is the most likely underlying etiology of this patient's findings?

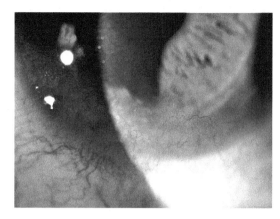

A. Rosacea

B. Staphylococcal blepharitis

C. Keratoconjunctivitis sicca

D. Chalazion

6. A 45-year-old female presents to your office due to persistent left eye foreign body sensation and pain. She visited the emergency room 5 months ago due to sudden left facial weakness including the forehead. On exam, she is noted to have interpalpebral fluorescein uptake. Which of the following findings on clinical exam would you expect to find?

A. Reduced sensation of the cornea on the affected side

B. History of ptosis surgery on the affected side

C. Failure to close the eye completely on the affected side

D. Uncontrolled high blood pressure

7. Which one of the following is not a cause of neurotrophic keratopathy?

A. Herpes simplex virus (HSV)

B. Riley–Day syndrome

C. Hansen's disease

D. Human immunodeficiency virus (HIV)

8. A 34-year-old obese male with obstructive sleep apnea presents to the cornea clinic due to progressive decline in visual acuity in the right eye. He visited a community optical shop and was told he had irregular astigmatism in the right eye. Clinical findings revealed laxity of the bilateral upper eyelid with severe tarsal papillary reaction. What is the most likely diagnosis?

A. Floppy eyelid syndrome

B. Superior limbic keratoconjunctivitis

C. Dermatochalasis

D. Ocular rosacea

9. A 57-year-old woman presents with a history of chronic ocular surface disease since a bilateral upper lid blepharoplasty 3 years ago. Clinical findings include a fine papillary reaction on the superior tarsal conjunctiva associated with hypertrophy of the superior limbus and fine punctate epithelial erosions in the superior one-third of the cornea. What would be the most likely diagnosis?

A. Floppy eyelid syndrome

B. Exposure keratopathy

C. Foreign body under superior eyelid

D. Superior limbic keratoconjunctivitis

10. A 25-year-old healthy female presents with a history of multiple episodes of sudden left eye pain upon awakening associated with photophobia and tearing. She has a remote history of a left eye corneal abrasion due to a fingernail trauma 3 years ago. Which of the following is not a potential therapy for this patient?

A. Lubricating ointment at night

B. Sodium chloride hypertonic ointment

C. Phototherapeutic keratectomy (PTK)

D. Laser-assisted in situ keratomileusis (LASIK)

11. A 29-year-old medical resident presents with a worsening corneal infiltrate and edema despite topical antibiotics. The resident had a corneal abrasion and was treated initially in the emergency department. Clinical exam findings include keratic precipitates, a necrotic ring opacity, and ciliary flush. The patient reports compliance and denies the use of contact lenses or history of trauma. Which of the following diagnoses should be considered?

A. Topical anesthetic abuse

B. Acanthamoeba keratitis

C. Fungal keratitis

D. Herpetic keratitis

12. A 12-year-old female with a history of a bone marrow transplant 2 months ago presents with dry eye not responding to standard lubrication management. On exam, she is noted to have a loss of the palisades of Vogt in two-thirds of the limbus and early corneal neovascularization. What would be the most likely diagnosis?

A. Toxic keratoconjunctivitis

B. Stem cell deficiency

C. Keratoconjunctivitis sicca

D. Rosacea

13. A 3-year-old boy is referred by his pediatrician due to progressive right eye corneal clouding since birth. On exam, he is noted to have opacification resembling sclera limited to the corneal periphery and 10 D of hyperopia in each eye. Which of the following corneal anomalies is most likely to be present?

A. Microcornea

B. Megalocornea

C. Cornea plana

D. Posterior embryotoxon

14. An 8-year-old boy with multiple craniofacial and dental abnormalities presents for follow-up. On anterior slit lamp examination, as shown in the figure, you notice one of the following. What is the most likely diagnosis?

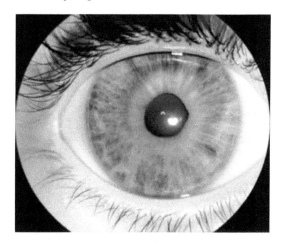

A. Peters anomaly

B. Keratoconus

C. Axenfeld–Rieger syndrome (ARS)

D. Sclerocornea

15. A 1-day-old premature male born at 30 weeks of gestation presents with multiple cardiac malformations, cleft lip, and skeletal abnormalities. On exam, bilateral corneal opacities are noted. You suspect a condition characterized by the findings on the provided figure. What is the most likely diagnosis?

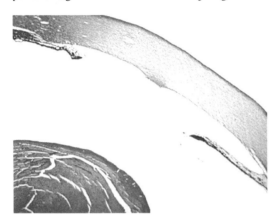

A. Corneal ulcer
B. Peters anomaly
C. Trauma
D. Dermoid

16. An 8-year-old male presents to clinic due to bilateral eye pain and redness. He has a history of premature delivery overseas. While interviewing the patient you note that the patient has a hearing deficit and dental abnormalities. On examination, as seen in the given figure, he is noted to have microcystic edema, intense stromal vascularization, and ghost vessels. Which of the following treatment would have prevented this corneal pathology?

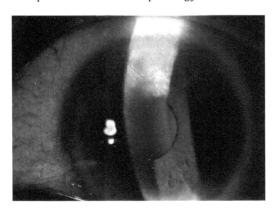

A. IV penicillin
B. IV ceftazidime
C. IV acyclovir
D. IV voriconazole

17. A 5-day-old female with no systemic abnormalities presents with left eye corneal opacities as shown in the given figure. What would the most likely cause of the findings?

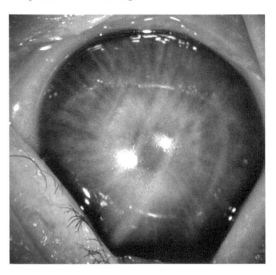

A. Forceps trauma
B. Congenital glaucoma
C. Cortical cataract
D. Corneal ulcer

18. A 35-year-old female complains of chronic progressive foreign body sensation in the left eye for the past 5 years. On exam, she is noted to have a nasal conjunctivalization with elastotic changes on pathology review. Which of the following is most likely to be present?

A. Stocker's line
B. Hudson–Stahli line
C. Fleischer's ring
D. Ferry's line

19. A 78-year-old woman with no past ocular history presents with progressive bilateral corneal opacity for the past 7 years associated with foreign body sensation and decreased visual acuity. She has a history of sun exposure and on examination she was found to have translucent, golden brown deposits in the superficial peripheral cornea. All of the following are potential therapies, except?

A. Lubricating ointment
B. Superficial keratectomy
C. Phototherapeutic keratectomy
D. Photorefractive keratectomy

20. A 45-year-old female with a history of diabetes mellitus type 2 and end-stage renal disease presents with recurrent episodes of eye pain and photophobia in the left eye. On examination, she is noted to have a horizontal white plaque at 3 and 9 o'clock on the right eye and a large one across the inferior visual axis in the left eye (see the figure provided). Which of the following is not advised as primary treatment of this condition?

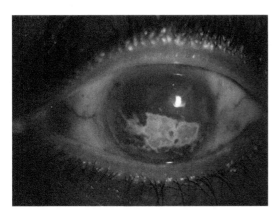

A. Ethylenediaminetetraacetic acid (EDTA) chelation

B. Phototherapeutic keratectomy (PTK)

C. Artificial tears

D. Bandage contact lens

21. A 65-year-old male presents to the clinic for an annual exam. He has no complaints and requests a new glasses prescription. On exam, he is noted to have unilateral arcus senilis. Which of the following test you should order next?

A. Renal function test

B. Hemoglobin A1C

C. Carotid doppler

D. Echocardiogram

22. A 45-year-old male with no systemic diseases presents complaining of decreased visual acuity. Two years ago, you had noted a mild superonasal pannus in the left eye. Today, the patient has high astigmatism in both eyes and bilateral painless superior deposits (see the figure provided) thinning with neovascularization. The rest of his exam appears within normal limits. Which is the most likely diagnosis?

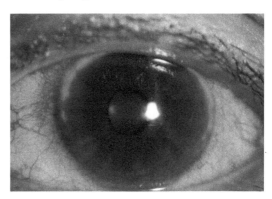

A. Peripheral ulcerative keratitis (PUK)

B. Mooren's ulcer

C. Staphylococcal marginal degeneration

D. Terrien's marginal degeneration

23. A 47-year-old healthy female with progressive bilateral superior corneal thinning, an intact epithelium, and neovascularization presents for refraction. On exam, there is marked thinning on the top one-third of cornea with a leading edge of lipid. Her conjunctiva is white and there are no signs of infection. Which of the following diagnostic procedures will help you make the diagnosis?

A. Corneal topography

B. Confocal microscopy

C. Anterior segment ocular coherence tomography

D. Corneal scraping

24. A 40-year-old Caucasian female presents to your office due to foreign body sensation of the right eye over several years. Slit lamp exam reveals the findings as shown in the figure. What is the most likely diagnosis?

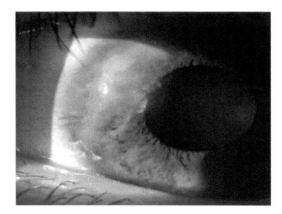

A. Phlyctenulosis
B. Band keratopathy
C. Salzmann's nodular degeneration
D. Corneal ulcer

25. A 56-year-old male presents with a bluish gray lesion in his paracentral cornea, foreign body sensation, and the following findings on anterior segment optical coherence tomography (OCT) (see the figure provided). The lesion is well demarcated and measures 2 mm. It is slightly raised. He is wondering if anything can be done about this lesion and what you recommend. You advise should be:

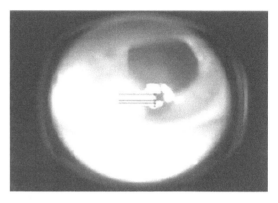

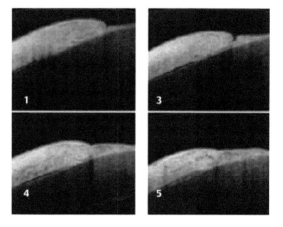

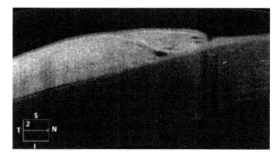

A. Penetrating keratoplasty
B. Deep anterior lamellar keratoplasty
C. Superficial keratectomy
D. Corneal biopsy with cryotherapy and adjuvant chemotherapy

26. A 35-year-old female presents with progressive loss of vision in the left eye over the past 7 years. On exam, she is noted to have a superonasally displaced pupil, intraocular pressure of 34 mm Hg, and mild corneal edema. Gonioscopy reveals posterior anterior synechiae to Schwalbe's line. Posterior exam reveals a cup-to-disc ratio of 0.8. Before referring the patient to a glaucoma specialist, you should perform which of the following definite diagnostic procedure?

A. Corneal topography

B. Specular microscopy

C. Anterior segment optical coherence tomography (OCT)

D. Ultrasound biomicroscopy

27. A 65-year-old male with atrial fibrillation presents for a routine eye exam. Slit lamp exam reveals a whorled pattern haze in the central cornea. Which of the following is the most likely inciting agent?

A. Metoprolol

B. Amiodarone

C. Diltiazem

D. Apixaban

28. A 4-year-old female is referred by her pediatrician for an eye exam. On anterior slit lamp exam, she is noted to have bilateral whorl-like corneal pattern. Which of the following conditions is associated with your exam findings?

A. Fabry disease

B. Hunter syndrome

C. Scheie syndrome

D. Hurler syndrome

29. A neonatology intensive care attending decides to request a consult for a patient who has persistent tearing without crying. At arrival you note obvious corneal enlargement. Which of the following is the normal corneal diameter in infants?

A. 9.5–10.5 mm

B. 13–15 mm

C. 8–9 mm

D. 14–15 mm

30. You have been following an 18-year-old male with keratoconus for the past 8 months. After multiple visits, you decide the patient is an excellent candidate for collagen cross-linking. Which of the following collagen types is the main target for collagen cross-linking?

A. Collagen type I

B. Collagen type II

C. Collagen type III

D. Collagen type IV

31. A 66-year-old male comes to your clinic for a second opinion. He underwent left eye cataract surgery 1 year ago and since then has experienced progressive decline in visual acuity. On exam, he is noted to have minimal corneal edema and an irregular appearance to his corneal endothelium on direct illumination. Which of the following would give you an endothelial cell count?

A. Specular microscopy

B. Pachymetry

C. Corneal topography

D. Anterior exam optical coherence tomography

32. A 34-year-old high myope man presents with a history of 3 days of progressive pain, light sensitivity, and tearing in the right eye. He has a history of chronic use of contact lenses and has recently been swimming in his lenses. On exam, he is noted to have a paracentral large infiltrate. Which of the following imaging modalities would help most with making this diagnosis?

A. Specular microscopy

B. Confocal microscopy

C. Anterior exam optical coherence tomography

D. Ultrasound biomicroscopy

33. A penetrating keratoplasty is planned for a 1-year-old patient with bilateral corneal opacities and iridocorneal adhesions. From which of the following embryological structures does the absent corneal layer in this patient originate?

A. Surface ectoderm

B. Neural crest

C. Mesoderm

D. Endoderm

34. A 55-year-old with history of recurrent bilateral eye pain upon awakening presents with following bilateral findings on slit lamp exam (see the figures provided). What is the most likely diagnosis?

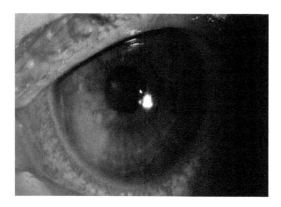

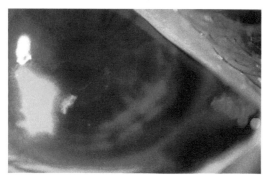

A. Reis–Bucklers corneal dystrophy (RBCD)
B. Thiel–Behnke corneal dystrophy (TBCD)
C. Epithelial basement membrane dystrophy (EBMD)
D. Meesmann epithelial corneal dystrophy

35. Recurrent corneal erosions present in all of the following corneal dystrophies, except?

A. Epithelial basement membrane dystrophy (EBMD)
B. Meesmann epithelial corneal dystrophy (MECD)
C. Lisch epithelial corneal dystrophy (LECD)
D. Reis–Bucklers corneal dystrophy (RBCD)

36. A 20-year-old female presents with progressive glare and light sensitivity. Histology review reveals the following (see the figures provided). What is the patient's most likely underlying diagnosis?

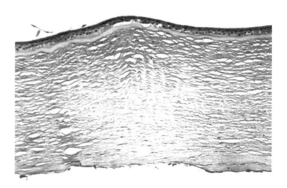

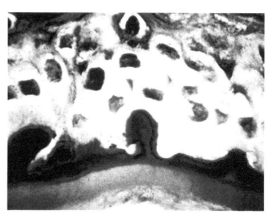

A. Epithelial basement membrane dystrophy (EBMD)
B. Meesmann epithelial corneal dystrophy (MECD)
C. Lisch epithelial corneal dystrophy (LECD)
D. Reis–Bucklers corneal dystrophy (RBCD)

37. A 50-year-old landscaper reports monocular diplopia in the left eye for the past 5 months. Exam findings revealed visual acuity 20/20 in the right eye and 20/40 in the left eye; you suspect a corneal dystrophy with Ki-67 positive staining. What is the most likely diagnosis?

A. Meesmann epithelial corneal dystrophy (MECD)
B. Epithelial basement membrane dystrophy (EBMD)
C. Lisch epithelial corneal dystrophy (LECD)
D. Thiel–Behnke corneal dystrophy (TBCD)

38. A 55-year-old man presents with chronic recurrent erosions and reports that he has suffered from this since the age of 5. Slit lamp exam reveals the findings as shown in the figure provided. Histopathology demonstrates granular deposits that stain with Masson trichrome stain. What is the most likely underlying diagnosis?

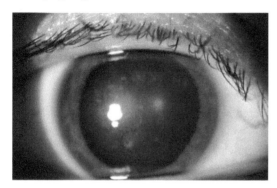

A. Epithelial basement membrane dystrophy (EBMD)

B. Granular corneal dystrophy type 1 (GCD1)

C. Reis–Bucklers corneal dystrophy (RBCD)

D. Thiel–Behnke corneal dystrophy (TBCD)

39. A 25-year-old photographer presents with bilateral decreased visual acuity. Electron microscopy reveals "curly fibers." What is his correct diagnosis?

A. Thiel–Behnke corneal dystrophy (TBCD)

B. Granular corneal dystrophy type 1 (GCD1)

C. Macular corneal dystrophy (MCD)

D. Reis–Bucklers corneal dystrophy (RBCD)

40. A patient presents for a second opinion. He visited his local ophthalmologist due to progressive blurry vision and was found to have bilateral corneal opacifications. He has had recurrent bilateral pain upon awakening since childhood. Slit lamp examination reveals a honeycomb pattern and curly fibers on electron microscopy. All of the following may be appropriate management options, except:

A. Superficial keratectomy

B. Phototherapeutic keratectomy (PTK)

C. Lamellar keratectomy

D. Descemet's membrane endothelial keratoplasty (DMEK)

41. A 15-year-old female has the following corneal findings (see the figure provided). Which of the following stains will help you make a diagnosis?

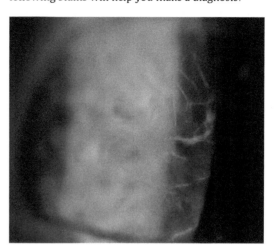

A. Masson trichrome stain

B. Congo red stain

C. Alcian blue

D. Oil red O

42. A 20-year-old male with history of myopic LASIK presents with progressive corneal opacities (see the figure provided). Histology reveals hyaline granular material accumulation that stains with Masson trichrome. What is the most likely diagnosis?

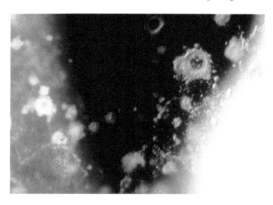

A. Granular corneal dystrophy type 1 (GCD1)

B. Reis–Bucklers corneal dystrophy (RBCD)

C. Macular corneal dystrophy (MCD)

D. Granular corneal dystrophy type 2 (GCD2)

43. A 25-year-old with history of bilateral epidemic keratoconjunctivitis, 10 years ago, is referred to the cornea clinic due to bilateral superficial stromal opacities (see the figure provided) that did not resolve with topical steroids. Which of the following is the most likely genetic inheritance?

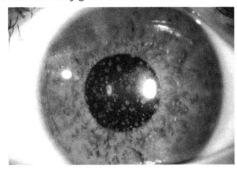

A. Autosomal dominant
B. X-linked dominant
C. Autosomal recessive
D. Sporadic

44. A 35-year-old male presents to your practice for evaluation of progressive blurry vision in both eyes for the past 8 years. This is his first time visiting an eye doctor. Slit lamp examination reveals diffuse haze with no clear intervening spaces. You suspect a pathology with the following histology (see the figures provided):

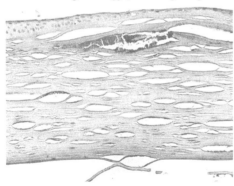

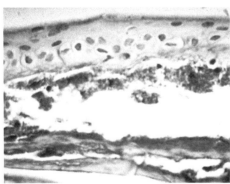

A. Cholesterol
B. Amyloid deposits
C. Glycosaminoglycan deposits
D. Hyaline deposits

45. A 23-year-old male presents with progressive blurry vision and glare associated with central corneal opacification since early childhood. The patient states vision in dim light is better than bright light. Which of the following blood test you should order?

A. Hemoglobin A1C
B. Liver function test
C. Fasting lipid profile
D. Serum electrolytes

46. All of the following are possible management options for a patient with the following corneal finding on specular microscopy (see the figure provided), except?

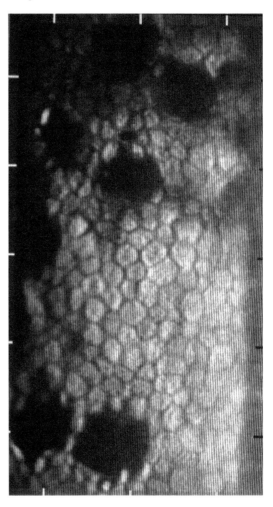

A. Sodium chloride drops
B. Descemet's membrane endothelial keratoplasty
C. Penetrating keratoplasty
D. Deep anterior lamellar keratoplasty

47. How might you advise this 16-year-old female with the following corneal topography (see the figure provided)?

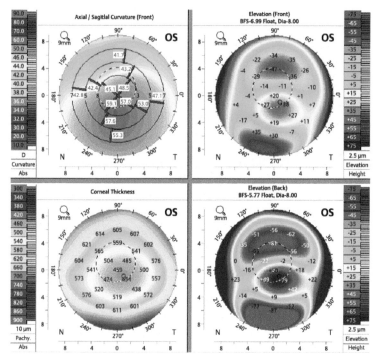

A. Limit your contact lens wear

B. Start antibiotic drops

C. Obtain autoimmune blood work-up

D. Stop rubbing your eyes

48. A 10-year-old male with a history of an ascending aorta aneurysm repair presents with generalized corneal thinning on topography. What is the most likely diagnosis?

A. Keratoconus

B. Keratoglobus

C. Pellucid margin degeneration

D. Ectasia post refractive surgery

49. A 2-year-old patient diagnosed with an autosomal recessive syndrome presents with bilateral corneal clouding. What is the most likely diagnosis?

A. Hurler syndrome

B. Hunter syndrome

C. Fabry disease

D. Tay–Sachs disease

50. A 5-year-old with renal failure, peripheral neuropathy, and psychomotor retardation is found to have the findings as shown in the given figure. What is the most likely diagnosis?

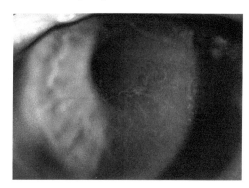

A. Hunter syndrome

B. Tay–Sachs disease

C. Scheie syndrome

D. Fabry disease

51. A 15-year-old with history of dwarfism and progressive renal dysfunction presents with the corneal crystals. The patient has noticed improvement of visual acuity after initiating which one of the following?

A. Moxifloxacin drops

B. Prednisolone acetate drops

C. Cysteamine eye drops

D. Ketotifen drops

11

52. A patient diagnosed with tyrosinemia during newborn screening will have which of the following corneal findings?

A. Interstitial keratitis

B. Corneal clouding

C. Pseudodendrites

D. Corneal verticillata

53. An 8-year-old male presents to clinic accompanied by his parents. They have noticed bilateral black deposits in both eyes along medial rectus. The mother comments that he has noticed his urine has had a very dark color. All of the following is true, except?

A. Ocular manifestations are usually symmetric.

B. Pigmentation is usually localized to the endothelium.

C. Scleral pigmentation occurs in over 80% of cases.

D. It has an autosomal recessive inheritance.

54. A 38-year-old male with a history of left peripheral facial palsy and corneal transplant presents to the emergency room due to left eye foreign body and photophobia for the past 3 days. Clinical findings reveal left lagophthalmos, bilateral dermatochalasis, and corneal opacities (see the figure provided). Which of the following histological stains is most likely to be positive?

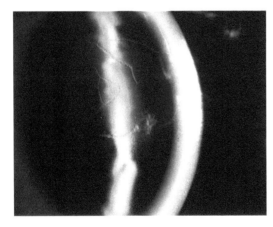

A. Alcian blue

B. Masson trichrome

C. Oil red O

D. Crystal violet dye

55. A 45-year-old male presents to the emergency room due to progressive yellow discoloration on the skin and conjunctiva along with involuntary tremor. Which of the following would be the most likely ocular finding?

A. Fleischer ring

B. Sunflower cataract

C. Polychromatic cataract

D. Coats white ring

56. A 15-year-old male with hyperextensibility of his joints presents with worsening visual acuity and high irregular astigmatism. Corneal topography reveals an asymmetric bowtie pattern. Which of the following patterns is most likely to be present?

A. Protrusion below the area of maximal thinning

B. Protrusion above the area of thinning

C. Steepening 90 degrees away from the area of thinning

D. Thinning nasal and temporally

57. A 25-year-old male with Marfan syndrome present with sudden monocular double vision. In which of the following quadrants you would classically expect the findings to be present?

A. Inferotemporal

B. Superonasal

C. Superotemporal

D. Inferonasal

58. A 5-year-old is referred from his pediatrician due to a failed vision screening. At arrival you note preauricular skin tags and this corneal finding (see the figure provided). Which of the following may also be present?

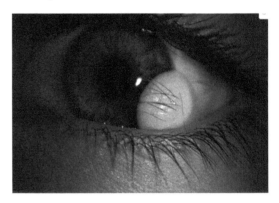

A. Iris coloboma

B. Optic nerve staphyloma

C. Eyelid coloboma

D. Conjunctival nevi

59. All of the following are associated with enlarged corneal nerves except:

A. Multiple endocrine neoplasia type 2B

B. Refsum syndrome

C. Hansen's disease

D. Meretoja syndrome

60. A 20-year-old male with xeroderma pigmentosum presents with multiple small nodules coalescing between 3 and 9 o'clock positions. He has experienced photophobia and irritation for the past 5 years. All of the following are appropriate therapies, except:

A. Ethylenediaminetetraacetic acid (EDTA) chelation

B. Superficial keratectomy

C. Lamellar keratoplasty

D. Penetrating keratoplasty

61. A corneal scraping from a 23-year-old male who presented to the emergency room was obtained. The patient presented with right eye pain, photophobia, and tearing. On initial examination, visual acuity was 20/70 in the affected eye with a central 3 × 3 mm epithelial infiltrate with feathery edges. Cultures revealed a microorganism that can invade an intact epithelium. Which of the following is the most likely pathogen?

A. *Fusarium species*

B. Candida albicans

C. Acanthamoeba

D. Pseudomonas aeruginosa

62. A 24-year-old male photography student presents for a second opinion. He returned from overseas recently, where he was treated with tobramycin and vancomycin fortified antibiotics every hour with no improvement. The patient has a history of contact lens wear. On examination, the patient has a visual acuity of 20/80 and the following corneal finding on slit lamp examination (see the figure provided). After careful examination, you notice prominent corneal nerves. Which of the following culture methods should you use?

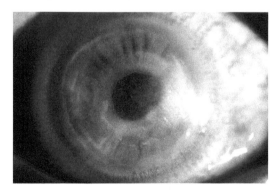

A. Non-nutrient agar with *Escherichia coli (E. Coli)* overlay

B. Sabouraud dextrose agar

C. Blood agar

D. Gomori methenamine silver (GMS)

63. A 5-year-old presents with a history of bilateral corneal dendritic lesions. Which of the following conditions is most like to be present?

A. Diabetes mellitus

B. Atopic dermatitis

C. Human immunodeficiency virus (HIV)

D. Seborrheic dermatitis

64. A 45-year-old male presents with photophobia and left eye pain for past 3 days. On exam, he is noted to have ptosis, ciliary flush, stromal edema, and inferior keratic precipitates. At the time of examination, visual acuity was 20/25 OU. Intraocular pressure was 26 in the affected eye and 1+ cell was found in the anterior chamber. The rest of the exam was within normal limits. Which of the following is proven to shorten the duration of his keratitis?

A. Oral acyclovir

B. Oral valacyclovir

C. Topical corticosteroids

D. Topical trifluridine

65. A 7-year-old male presents with painful swelling of the left lateral upper eyelid and a follicular conjunctivitis. The mother reports a maculopapular rash after a dose of amoxicillin. Which of the following is the most likely diagnosis?

A. Herpes simplex virus

B. Epstein–Barr virus (EBV)

C. Herpes zoster virus

D. Adenovirus

66. A 42-year-old male presents for a third opinion. The patient has experienced four episodes of right eye follicular conjunctivitis. He has been treated with topical corticosteroid eye drops, however the episodes recur shortly after tapering the drops. Which of the following would be the best treatment for this patient?

A. Valacyclovir

B. Doxycycline

C. Systemic steroids

D. Topical antibiotics

67. A 65-year-old female visits your clinic for a third opinion. The patient had been experiencing left eye redness, tearing, and photophobia for 3 weeks. She was diagnosed with iritis after YAG capsulotomy at an outside hospital and managed with topical steroids with recurrent bouts after tapering attempts. At examination, visual acuity is 20/40 in the affected eye, intraocular pressure is 21, and keratic precipitates are observed. There is no retained lens material on gonioscopy. Which of the following pathogens are you most concerned for?

A. Gram-positive cocci in clusters

B. Gram-positive cocci in pairs

C. Gram-positive rods

D. Gram-negative diplococci

68. A 35-year-old male presents to your clinic to establish care. The patient was diagnosed with a corneal ulcer 1 week ago. He states corneal cultures were obtained at the time of initial diagnosis. The microbiology lab reports a septate filamentous fungus. Which of the following is the most likely pathogen?

A. *Mucor*

B. *Rhizopus*

C. *Fusarium*

D. Candida

69. A 45-year-old male is referred to your office with concern for possible corneal ulcer of the left eye. He presented 1 week prior to the emergency room with tearing, irritation, and redness. Moxifloxacin was initiated. However, his symptoms worsened. On examination, visual acuity is 20/20 in the right eye, 20/40 in the left eye, the lashes have collaretes OU and there is bulbar injection. The cornea has a perilimbal opacity superotemporally with overlying epithelial defect (see the figure provided). What is the most likely diagnosis?

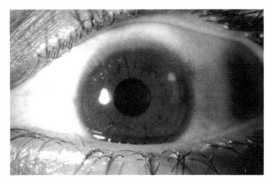

A. Mooren's ulcer

B. Peripheral ulcerative keratitis

C. Staphylococcal marginal keratitis

D. Exposure keratopathy

70. A 25-year-old male is referred from urgent care with right eye redness and hyperpurulent discharge for the past 3 days. The patient denies any significant ocular history. On examination, there is periauricular lymphadenopathy, 3+ bulbar injection, and 3 × 3 mm peripheral corneal ulcer associated with corneal edema. Which of the following is the most appropriate management?

A. Topical vancomycin and tobramycin

B. Doxycycline 100 mg every 12 hours

C. Ceftriaxone 1 g IV every 12 hours for 3 days plus topical vancomycin and tobramycin

D. Moxifloxacin drops, every hour

71. A 4-day-old male born at 38 weeks of gestation presents with acute left eye purulent discharge for the past 24 hours. What is the most likely diagnosis?

A. Chlamydia trachomatis

B. Neisseria gonorrhoeae

C. Herpes simplex virus

D. Pseudomonas aeruginosa

72. A 47-year-old Egyptian male presents with a history of foreign body sensation, redness, and tearing for more than 1 year. The patient was diagnosed with dry eyes and managed with topical cyclosporine without improvement of symptoms. Slit lamp examination reveals bilateral conjunctival follicular reaction, eyelid margin erythema, and a superior pannus of the cornea with interdigitated round pigmented scars. Which of the following is the most appropriate management?

A. Azithromycin

B. Ceftriaxone

C. Acyclovir

D. Vancomycin

73. A 55-year-old female with a past ocular history of bilateral penetrating keratoplasty 10 years ago due to advanced keratoconus presents with a history of mild discomfort in the right eye, redness, and photophobia. On examination, her visual acuity is 20/50 in the right eye and 20/30 in the left eye. Slit lamp examination reveals chemosis and conjunctival injection and an anterior stromal needle-like white infiltrate. Histological slides exhibit interlamellar aggregates of gram-positive cocci. Which of the following is the most likely pathogen?

A. Streptococcus pneumoniae

B. Staphylococcus aureus

C. Streptococcus viridans

D. Staphylococcus epidermidis

74. A 23-year-old male presents with eye redness and tearing 6 weeks after a myopic LASIK procedure. On exam, he has a stromal infiltrate along the flap. Scrapings are obtained from the stromal bed after lifting the flap and placed the specimen on Lowenstein–Jensen medium. All the following are appropriate therapies except:

A. Clarithromycin

B. Amikacin

C. Linezolid

D. Vancomycin

75. An 88-year-old female with a history of Crohn's disease presents due to progressive visual loss over the past 10 years. Her past ocular history includes an uneventful bilateral cataract surgery. On examination, her initial visual acuity is 20/40 OU, with intraocular pressure of 12 mm Hg on the right and 10 mm Hg on the left. Ishihara color plates are within normal limits. Slit lamp exam reveals the finding in the photograph below (see the figure provided). Automated perimetry shows central constriction bilaterally. Electroretinography reveals reduced scotopic and photopic responses. Which of the following pathogens have been associated with this condition?

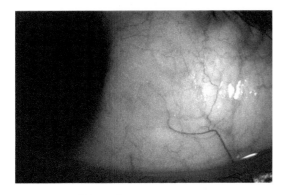

A. Gram-positive rods

B. Gram-negative cocci

C. Gram-positive cocci

D. Gram-positive filaments

76. A 25-year-old male patient with history of uneventful LASIK surgery 2 months ago presents with right eye pain, photophobia, and blurry vision for the past 2 weeks. On examination, his visual acuity is 20/50 on the right and 20/20 on the left. Slit lamp examination revealed a corneal epithelial defect 2 × 2 mm at 3 to 5 o'clock, originating from the flap and intrastromal infiltration. Corneal scraping revealed gram-positive aerobic filaments. Which of the following growth media was most likely to be used?

A. Blood agar

B. MacConkey agar

C. Lowenstein–Jensen medium

D. Thayer Martin agar

77. A 45-year-old female with no significant past medical history presents with chronic left eye redness for the past 2 years. She has visited multiple eye care providers and has been prescribed low-potency steroids without resolution of her symptoms. She presents to your office another opinion. On examination, her visual acuity is 20/20 on the right and 20/30 on the left. Slit lamp examination reveals right eye palpebral injection with two raised hyperemic granulomas in the inferior tarsal conjunctiva. Head and neck exam is noted for submandibular and preauricular lymph nodes. Which of the following is not part of the differential?

A. Tuberculosis

B. Sarcoidosis

C. Tularemia

D. Trachoma

78. A 46-year-old female contact lens wearer presents with 3 days of left eye photophobia and redness. She has no past medical or ocular history. On examination, visual acuity is 20/20 on the right and hand motion on the left. Slit lamp examination reveals the findings as shown in the given figure. Fundus exam was difficult to assess due to haze. Which of the following is the most likely pathogen?

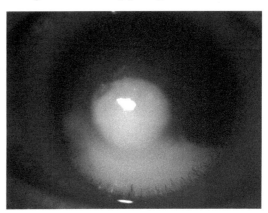

A. Acanthamoeba

B. Staphylococcus aureus

C. Streptococcus viridans

D. Pseudomonas aeruginosa

79. A 49-year-old female contact lens wearer presents with redness and photophobia for 2 weeks. Initial examination reveals a central corneal ulcer with a dense underlying infiltrate, purulent discharge, and 1 mm hypopyon. She was started on fortified antibiotics, including tobramycin and vancomycin every hour. One week later, the corneal infiltrate and thinning have worsened and the hypopyon size has increased. Which of the following is the next step in management?

A. Stop all drops and add prednisolone acetate.

B. Stop all drops and perform penetrating keratoplasty.

C. Obtain confocal microscopy.

D. Change antibiotics to fluoroquinolones every hour.

80. A 51-year-old male presents with a history of left eye injection and severe pain for the past 7 days. The patient states symptoms started after trauma with a tree branch during gardening. On examination, visual acuity is 20/20 on the right and light perception on the left. Slit lamp examination reveals severe bulbar injection and a 4 × 4 mm central infiltrate in the left eye. Gomori methenamine silver staining is positive. Which of the following is the best next step in management?

A. Tobramycin

B. Vancomycin

C. Moxifloxacin

D. Natamycin

81. A 43-year-old male was diagnosed with herpes simplex virus (HSV) keratitis. The patient has been on topical trifluridine for 3 days and develops periorbital redness and foreign body sensation. On examination, he is noted to have periorbital skin thickening, conjunctival papillary reaction, and corneal punctate epithelial erosions. Which of the following is the most likely hypersensitivity reaction?

A. Hypersensitivity type I

B. Hypersensitivity type II

C. Hypersensitivity type III

D. Hypersensitivity type IV

82. A 10-year-old male with seasonal allergies presents with foreign body sensation and itching. The patient reports recurrences every year during the spring. On examination, his lids and cornea show the following findings (see the figures provided). All of the following are appropriate management options except:

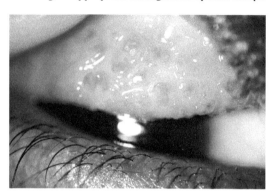

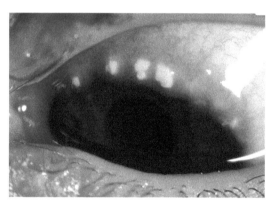

A. Prednisolone acetate

B. Azithromycin

C. Cyclosporine

D. Tacrolimus

83. A 14-year-old male presents with worsening perioral bullous lesions and target like lesions on his limbs for the past 4 days associated with fever and malaise. He recently finished a course of antibiotics for an upper respiratory tract infection. On examination, the patient is noted to have bilateral bulbar conjunctival injection and inferior punctate epithelial erosions. Which of following management options provides significant long-term benefit?

A. Aggressive lubrication

B. Topical steroids

C. Oral steroids

D. Amniotic membrane graft

84. A 42-year-old with history of epilepsy is admitted to the intensive care unit due to status epilepticus. The patient is managed with a variety of antiepileptic drugs, including phenytoin, valproic acid, and carbamazepine. During the second day of admission, he starts having fever spikes and bilateral eyelid erythema progressing rapidly to bilateral eyelid swelling and erythema with epidermal scaling. After examining the patient, you are mostly concerned for a disease associated with which of the following characteristic?

A. Rapidly progressive skin exfoliation and target-like lesions

B. Honey-colored crusted lesions with an erythematous base

C. Exudative pharyngitis and bright red exanthem

D. Raised target lesions on the extremities

85. A 65-year-old male presents to your clinic with a chief complaint of chronic red eye and epiphora. The patient has no past medical or ocular history. On examination, bilateral findings include: visual acuity of 20/40 OU, eyelid margin erythema, misdirected lashes, upper eyelid tarsal fibrosis, inferior coalescent punctate epithelial erosions, and a fornix depth of 4 mm. All of the following are associated with your most likely diagnosis, except:

A. IgA localized to the epidermis.

B. Cyclophosphamide is the mainstay of therapy.

C. Lubrication can be helpful in milder cases.

D. Fornix reconstruction surgery can be beneficial after immunosuppression.

86. A 47-year-old male with a history of bone marrow transplant for acute myelogenous leukemia presents with a history of 1 year of foreign body sensation and photosensitivity. He reports using artificial tear drops and ointment on the regular basis without much improvement. On examination, visual acuity is 20/20 OU; while the lids and lashes are within normal limits, the cornea reveals inferior punctate erosions with mucoid strands. Which of the following is not indicated in the next step of management?

A. Aggressive ocular lubrication and punctal plugs

B. Autologous serum tears

C. Prosthetic replacement of the ocular surface ecosystem (PROSE) lens

D. Keratoprosthesis

87. A 31-year-old with a recent history of diarrhea and vomiting presents to the emergency room with fever, lymphadenopathy, and oligoarticular arthritis. Which of the following would be the most common ocular manifestation in this patient?

A. Episcleritis

B. Conjunctivitis

C. Iridocyclitis

D. Keratitis

88. A 15-year-old presents with a recurrent episode of photophobia, tearing, and foreign body sensation in both eyes. This is the third episode in less than 2 years. Upon examination, visual acuity is 20/30 OU, the lids and lashes are within normal limits, the conjunctiva is white, and the cornea has multiple elevated punctate lesions centrally (see the figure provided). Fluorescein reveals negative staining of these lesions. Which is the most likely associated finding?

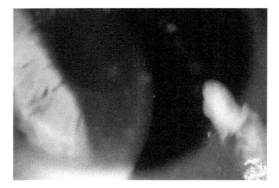

A. Interpalpebral fluorescein staining

B. Dramatic response to low-dose steroids

C. Stromal opacities with intervening haze

D. Inferior corneal fluorescein staining

89. A 45-year-old female with a history of vertigo and hearing loss presents with severe periorbital pain and redness. The patient states that her ocular symptoms began 1 week ago. She has severe photophobia and conjunctival injection. Examination reveals a visual acuity of 20/60 OU. The cornea appears hazy and there is 1+ anterior chamber cell. Posterior exam is grossly within normal limits. Infectious and immune blood panel are unremarkable. Which of the following is the most likely diagnosis?

A. Susac syndrome

B. Cogan's syndrome

C. Vogt–Koyanagi–harada syndrome

D. Sarcoidosis

90. A 65-year-old male with no significant past medical history presents with left eye severe pain, photophobia, and tearing. The patient mentions that he has been experiencing hand pain, swelling, stiffness, and mild joint deformities. The patient states that he has had worsening foreign body sensation in the affected eye for the past year. Slit lamp examination reveals the following (see the figure provided). Which of the following is the next step in diagnosis?

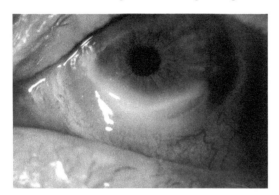

A. Anterior segment fluorescein angiography
B. Corneal topography
C. Corneal biopsy
D. Autoimmune panel

91. A 74-year-old female with no significant past medical history presents to your office. She had been followed by an outside ophthalmologist for peripheral ulcerative lesions of the right for the past 5 years. She complains of left eye pain, photophobia, and redness. On examination, the right eye appears phthisical and she has hand motion vision. The visual acuity in the left eye is 20/40. Slit lamp exam reveals an oval ulcer with sharp borders in the nasal cornea near the limbus and mild conjunctival injection. Corneal scrapings and autoimmune work-up are negative. The diagnosis of Mooren's ulcer is entertained. Which of the following has been linked to this pathology?

A. Rheumatoid arthritis
B. Hepatitis C virus
C. Syphilis
D. Tuberculosis

92. A 10-year-old male presents for evaluation of a recurrent slow-growing mass in the left eye for the past year despite surgical excision (see the figure provided) The patient has no significant past medical or ocular history. Slit lamp exam reveals a pedunculated and fleshy growth along the plica semilunaris. Biopsy of the mass reveals multiple branching fronds branching from a central vascularized core. All of the following are management options, except:

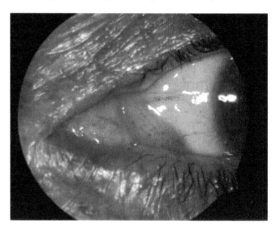

A. Topical interferon
B. Oral cimetidine
C. Dinitrochlorobenzene
D. Infliximab

93. A 60-year-old female with a history of diabetes mellitus and hypertension presents for her first annual diabetic exam. The patient has no eye related complaints. Slit lamp exam reveals a gelatinous conjunctival mass extending to the nasal limbus and cornea, with multiple feeder vessels. The rest of the anterior and posterior exam are within normal limits. Which of the following statements is correct regarding the most likely diagnosis?

A. Immunosuppression is not an associated risk factor.
B. Ninety-five percent occur at the fornix.
C. Neoplastic cells frequently penetrate Bowman's layer.
D. Hyperreflective thickened epithelium with a transition zone can be seen on anterior segment optical coherence tomography (OCT).

94. A 26-year-old female presents with the following finding (see the figure provided). What is her lifetime risk of uveal melanoma?

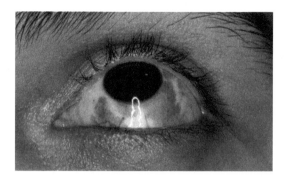

A. 1 in 10,000
B. 1 in 1,000
C. 1 in 400
D. 1 in 100

95. All of the following are factors associated with a poor conjunctival melanoma prognosis, except:

A. Melanomas arising from primary acquired melanosis (PAM)
B. Nonlimbal tumor
C. Pagetoid spread
D. Thickness > 1.8 mm

96. A 37-year-old male presents with a history of 5 days of a fleshy, friable, and pedunculated mass. He had a recent chalazion excision. Biopsy was obtained and revealed exaggerated granulation tissue with proliferating capillaries in a radiating pattern. Which of the following is the most likely diagnosis?

A. Necrobiotic xanthogranuloma
B. Juvenile xanthogranuloma
C. Fibrous histiocytoma
D. Pyogenic granuloma

97. A 56-year-old male with HIV presents to the emergency room complaining of blood in his eye. The patient is not compliant with highly active anti-retroviral therapy (HAART) therapy and had been experiencing a slow progressive painless inferior conjunctival red growth for the past 8 months. Clinical examination reveals a red and slightly elevated lesion with numerous fine vessels and petechial hemorrhages. Which of the following is the most likely diagnosis?

A. Kaposi's sarcoma
B. Subconjunctival hemorrhage
C. Episcleritis
D. Viral conjunctivitis

98. A 47-year-old female with no significant ocular history presents with redness, tearing, and foreign body sensation in both eyes for 8 months. She was diagnosed with chronic follicular conjunctivitis at an outside hospital and managed with chronic low-dose steroid drops. Slit lamp examination reveals the following (see the figure provided) and biopsy showed distinct marginal centers and mature lymphocytes. The rest of the examination was within normal limits. What is the best next step in management?

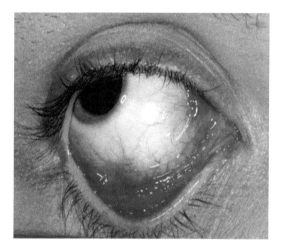

A. Continue low-potency topical steroids and add erythromycin ointment at bedtime
B. Conjunctival biopsy
C. Start higher-potency topical steroids
D. Viral swab

99. A 47-year-old female presents at the emergency room 3 hours after an unknown agent was thrown at her face. Upon arrival, she was noted to have facial burns and left eye injection. Initial pH was 10.0. The emergency room staff started irrigation with normal saline until pH of 7.0 was achieved. On exam, the left eye had a visual acuity of count fingers, madarosis, conjunctival sloughing, moderate to severe corneal haze with extensive limbal ischemia, and a difficulty view of the posterior pole. Right eye examination was within normal limits. B-scan revealed that the retina was attached in the left eye. What next step would best maximize her visual prognosis?

A. Place a contact lens
B. Perform a tarsorrhaphy
C. Place amniotic membrane
D. Hourly artificial tears

100. Six months after a severe alkali burn to the right eye, a patient is noted to have worsening conjunctival scarring, keratinization, and corneal haze. Which of the following is the next step in management?

A. Penetrating keratoplasty

B. Keratoprosthesis

C. Lamellar keratoplasty

D. Limbal epithelial transplantation

101. A 25-year-old male presents to the emergency room after a work-related accident with hydrofluoric acid. The patient states that a moderate amount of acid splashed in both of his eyes. On initial examination, visual acuity is 20/40 in both eyes, there are no facial burns or madarosis, there is mild to moderate conjunctival injection, mild to moderate corneal haze, and superonasal area of focal limbal ischemia is noted. After adequate management was instituted, he is noted to have an elevation of intraocular pressure of > 30 mm Hg in the right eye. Which of the following is the most appropriate next step in management?

A. Brimonidine 0.15%

B. Timolol 0.5%

C. Acetazolamide 500 mg bid

D. Dorzolamide 2%

102. A 28-year-old presents with sudden bilateral eye pain, tearing, foreign body sensation, photophobia, and blurred vision 6 hours after skiing. On slit lamp examination, conjunctival injection and interpalpebral corneal punctate epithelial erosions are noted. Which of the following wavelengths penetrates the entire thickness of the cornea?

A. UV-A

B. UV-B

C. UV-C

D. UV-D

103. A 25-year-old Asian male with no significant past medical or ocular history presents to the emergency room after left eye trauma during a baseball game. At his initial presentation, his visual acuity in the affected eye is 20/50, and there is periorbital ecchymosis, chemosis, and 2 mm layering hyphema. The rest of his exam is within normal limits. Which of the following is an indication for surgical intervention?

A. Intraocular pressure (IOP) average > 60 mm Hg for 2 days

B. IOP average > 25 mm Hg for 4 days

C. Total hyphema that persists for 1 day

D. Any hyphema failing to resolve completely within 8 days

104. A 5-year-old African American male presents to the emergency room with a hyphema after being hit in the eye while playing basketball. He is initiated on medium-potency topical steroids and cycloplegia with adequate improvement of symptoms and size of hyphema. Which of the following laboratory tests should be ordered prior to discharge?

A. 50:50 mixing study

B. Hemoglobin electrophoresis

C. Ultrasound biomicroscopy

D. Viral cultures

105. A 34-year-old male with keratoconus and previous penetrating keratoplasty in the right eye returns for a follow-up. Latest topography reveals a K1 49.93 @ 15, K2 at 44.60 @ 100. He has no sutures remaining and has a spherical equivalent of -9.00 in the operated eye and -4.00 in his left eye. The patient is extremely bothered by anisometropia. Which of the following is the next best step in management?

A. Relaxing incision at the steep meridian

B. Laser in situ keratomileusis

C. Photorefractive keratectomy

D. Contact lens trial

106. A 65-year-old female presents status post penetrating keratoplasty in the left eye with progressive blurry vision for the past year. Examination reveals a visual acuity of 20/25 in the right eye and 20/50 in the left eye. Slit lamp reveals a clear graft (see the figure provided) with no signs of rejection and a 1–2+ nuclear sclerosis. The rest of her exam is within normal limits. What is the next best step of management?

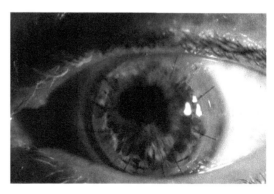

A. Cataract surgery is indicated at this moment.

B. Remove half of the sutures before cataract surgery.

C. Cataract surgery should be performed after suture removal is completed.

D. Penetrating keratoplasty is an absolute contraindication for cataract surgery.

107. Which of the following is the most likely disadvantage of Descemet stripping automated endothelial keratoplasty (DSAEK) over penetrating keratoplasty?

A. Light scattering

B. Small incision

C. Preservation of the anterior corneal curvature

D. More postoperative astigmatism

108. A 45-year-old patient presents for Descemet stripping automated endothelial keratoplasty (DSAEK) postoperative day one follow-up. Anterior segment optical coherence tomography reveals the following (see the figure provided). What is the best next step in management?

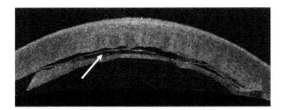

A. Observation

B. Rebubbling in the office

C. Prednisolone acetate

D. Take the patient to the operating room for a repeat DSAEK

109. A 45-year-old female presents to your clinic due to bilateral foreign body sensation for the past 3 months. Slit lamp examination revealed punctate epithelial erosions limited to the superior cornea. All of the following are associated with the following staining pattern, except?

A. Vernal keratoconjunctivitis

B. Superior limbic keratoconjunctivitis

C. Floppy eyelid syndrome

D. Eye drop toxicity

110. A 15-year-old male with past medical history of asthma presents with right eye pain, redness, and photophobia for the past 3 weeks. Past ocular history is also significant for bilateral allergic conjunctivitis. On examination, visual acuity is 20/60 on the right and 20/20 on the left, there is superior limbal injection and pannus. Corneal examination reveals the following (see the figure provided). Which of the following would you expect to find?

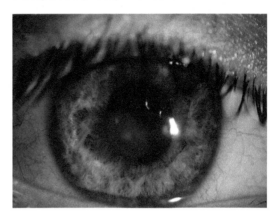

A. Arlt's line

B. Giant papillae

C. Pseudomembranes

D. Herbert's pits

111. A 25-year-old presents with 4 days of left eye redness and mucopurulent discharge associated with tender preauricular lymph node. On examination, visual acuity is 20/20 on the right and 20/40 on the left. A follicular reaction is noted in the inferior tarsal conjunctiva, and there are superficial punctate erosions in the inferior cornea. Giemsa stain reveals basophilic intracytoplasmic bodies. Which of the following culture media is indicated?

A. McCoy cell culture

B. Sabouraud agar

C. Non-nutrient agar with *Escherichia Coli*

D. Lowenstein–Jensen medium

112. A 40-year-old female presents with a history of chronic conjunctival injection, chemosis, and tearing. She has a history of mild to moderate asthma since childhood. On examination, she is noted to have bilateral eyelid erythema, scaliness of the lid skin, and lid thickening. Slit lamp examination reveals bilateral inferior tarsal papillary reaction and punctate epithelial erosions over the inferior third of the cornea. All of the following are associated with this condition except:

A. Anterior subcapsular cataracts

B. Higher risk of retinal detachment

C. Dennie–Morgan folds

D. Exposed Bowman's membrane

113. A 56-year-old female with no past medical history presents with right eye redness for the past 3 years. She has no other past ocular history. On examination, visual acuity is 20/150 OD and 20/20 OS. Slit lamp examination reveals an intense diffuse papillary conjunctivitis of both eyes, severe forniceal shortening of the right eye, and a large epithelial corneal defect with peripheral neovascularization. Immunofluorescence reveals antibodies binding at the basement membrane. Which of the following statements is false?

A. Dapsone is the first line of treatment with mild-moderate disease.

B. Stem cell failure is characterized by keratinization.

C. Reconstructive surgery is indicated in this patient.

D. Subconjunctival mitomycin can be used a temporizing treatment.

114. A 15-year-old presents with mucosal blistering and lip crusting for the past 10 days. He was admitted to the burn unit and found to have bilateral eye redness. On examination, visual acuity was 20/20 in both eyes, there is mild lid margin crusting and a papillary tarsal reaction, and few punctate epithelial erosions. There is conjunctival staining with fluorescein. All of the following are appropriate next steps except:

A. Prokera ring

B. Amniotic membrane graft fixed with sutures

C. Amniotic membrane graft fixed with glue

D. Frequent topical lubricants without amniotic membrane

115. A 55-year-old female with thyroid eye disease presents with foreign body sensation, burning, and photophobia. Slit lamp examination reveals upper lid papillary hypertrophy, superior redundant conjunctiva, superior punctate corneal epithelial erosions, and mild superior pannus. The rest of her exam is within normal limits. Which of the following statements is incorrect?

A. The patient has superior bulbar conjunctiva that stains with fluorescein but not with rose Bengal.

B. Acetylcysteine can be used to break down the filaments.

C. Retinoic acid can be used to retard keratinization.

D. This patient should have thyroid labs tested.

116. A 5-year-old presents with a gradually enlarging red conjunctival masses bilaterally. On review of systems, she is noted to have similar lesions in vagina and oral mucosa. As per the patient's parents one of the of the lesions was removed with forceps 1 week ago. After removal a white thickened avascular mass was noticed. All of the following statements are correct except:

A. Amorphous subepithelial deposits of eosinophilic material can be seen in histopathology.

B. Complete excisional biopsy is necessary.

C. Antifibrinolytic drugs are part of the management.

D. Amniotic membrane graft can be placed after lesion removal.

117. A 2-day-old female born with hydrops fetalis was found to have a rapid plasma reagin (RPR) 1:32. Which of the following statements regarding interstitial keratitis secondary to syphilis is correct?

A. Interstitial keratitis is usually present at birth.

B. Interstitial keratitis is associated with enlarged corneal nerves.

C. Interstitial keratitis is bilateral in 20% of cases.

D. Sectoral superior stromal inflammation is often seen in early disease.

118. A 45-year-old male with chronic blepharitis presents with left eye redness and tearing for the past 3 weeks. He has no past medical history. On examination, visual acuity is 20/20 in both eyes. Slit lamp examination reveals several peripheral corneal opacities. All of the following statements are correct, except:

A. These findings are secondary to a hypersensitivity reaction to staphylococcal exotoxin.

B. Stromal marginal infiltrates with no clearing space from the limbus.

C. There is usually no anterior chamber reaction.

D. Treatment consist of low- to medium-potency topical steroids.

119. A 40-year-old male presents complaining of a growth onto the cornea stemming from the nasal conjunctiva, associated with progressive visual decline for the past 2 years. He has no past medical history. On examination, corrected visual acuity is 20/80 on the right and 20/20 on the left. Slit lamp examination reveals a fibrovascular growth associated with moderate corneal thinning in the superonasal aspect of the cornea. Before planning for surgery, Scheimpflug imaging was obtained and revealed steepening of the cornea surface approximately 90 degrees away from the lesion. Which of the following statements is likely to be associated with this condition?

A. On histopathology, basophilic degeneration of elastotic fibers can be seen.
B. Tissue excision with bare sclera provides the maximum success rate.
C. Lamellar or penetrating keratoplasty for severe cases may be necessary.
D. There is anterior and posterior elevation on corneal topography.

120. A 36-year-old female contact lens wearer presents with bilateral chronic foreign body sensation and eye redness. She has been wearing contact lenses for 15 years. She has been using artificial tears without improvement. Examination is remarkable for bilateral multiple mucoid strands attached to corneal epithelium. All the following statements are correct in regard to this condition except:

A. This condition may be present in patients with thyroid eye disease.
B. Mucoid strands stain well with fluorescein and to a lesser extend with rose Bengal.
C. Acetylcysteine is part of the management.
D. Mechanical removal gives short-term relief.

121. Which of the following statements is correct regarding penetrating keratoplasty?

A. Large diameter grafts cause higher astigmatism.
B. Donor button is usually about 1 mm larger than the trephination site.
C. Small-diameter grafts are associated with lower tendency to cause peripheral anterior synechiae.
D. Host tissue cornea excision precedes preparation of donor cornea.

122. A 3-year-old diagnosed with an X-linked lysosomal storage disease presents for annual eye exam. The systemic manifestations of the disease are characterized by acroparesthesias, angiokeratomas, cardiomyopathy, and renal disease. All of the following are eye-related manifestations, except:

A. Vortex keratopathy
B. Wedge-shaped posterior cataract
C. Conjunctival aneurysm
D. Pseudodendrites

123. A 65-year-old with a progressive decline in visual acuity presents for evaluation. He is found to have visually significant cataracts in both eyes with 0.75 D of corneal astigmatism. Which of the following is correct regarding limbal relaxing incisions?

A. Incisions are placed in the steep meridian.
B. Incisions are approximately 200 μm in depth.
C. Hyperopic shift occurs with coupling ratios less than 1.
D. Cylinder correction depends on the depth of the incision.

124. Which of the following statements is correct regarding post radial keratotomy outcomes?

A. Intraocular lens (IOL) calculation should be done using a regression formula.
B. Corneal curvature becomes flat in the center and steeper in the periphery.
C. PERK study revealed a myopic shift in 43% of eyes between 6 months and 10 years postoperatively.
D. Greater hyperopic shifts occur with larger optical zones.

125. An 8-year-old male with no significant past medical history presents with 5 days of left eye redness, tearing, clear discharge, and blurry vision. On examination, visual acuity is 20/20. There is a follicular palpebral reaction and 2+ conjunctival injection. The rest of the anterior and posterior exams are within normal limits. Histology smear reveals multinucleated giant cells. Which of the following is the most likely diagnosis?

A. Adenovirus conjunctivitis
B. Herpes simplex virus (HSV) conjunctivitis
C. Toxic conjunctivitis
D. Inclusion conjunctivitis

126. A 34-year-old contact lens wearer presents to the eye clinic with a history of 6 days of right eye tearing, redness, pain, and discharge. The patient decided to use Polytrim drops prescribed previously for conjunctivitis, without much improvement. On examination, he is noted to have a central dendrite-like lesion. Confocal microscopy reveals the following (see the figure provided). Which of the following would treat the motile and dormant state?

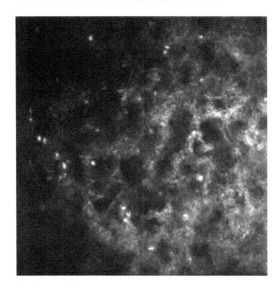

A. Hexamidine
B. Polyhexamethylene biguanide
C. Neomycin
D. Voriconazole

127. A 45-year-old male with HIV/AIDS presents with a history of 1 week of blurry vision, irritation, photophobia, and bilateral conjunctival injection. Slit lamp exam demonstrates multifocal fine punctate fluorescein staining lesions along with follicular conjunctival reaction. Brown and Hopps staining reveal small gram-positive spores. Which of the following is the most appropriate next step in management?

A. Polyhexamethylene biguanide
B. Voriconazole
C. Fumagillin
D. Vancomycin

128. Which of the following indications for PK has the highest rate of nonimmune mediated corneal graft failure?

A. Pseudophakic bullous keratopathy (PBK)
B. Fuchs endothelial dystrophy
C. Keratoconus
D. Corneal perforation

129. You examine a patient with the findings below (see the figure provided). Which of the following is the best step in management?

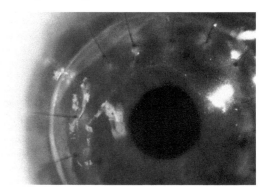

A. Prednisolone acetate drops
B. Moxifloxacin drops
C. Corneal scraping
D. Confocal microscopy

130. A 38-year-old female presents following a penetrating keratoplasty in the left eye due to progressive keratoconus. The patient complains of blurry vision in the operated eye for the past month. On examination, there are multiple subepithelial infiltrates. Which of the following slit lamp illumination technique would better identify these lesions?

A. Diffuse illumination
B. Direct illumination
C. Tangential illumination
D. Indirect illumination

131. Your patient presents for a postoperative month 1 follow-up with the findings below (see the figure provided). Which of the following is the most likely diagnosis?

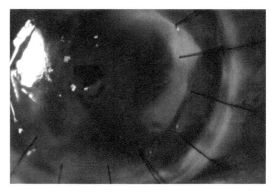

A. Epithelial rejection
B. Subepithelial rejection
C. Stromal rejection
D. Endothelial rejection

132. Femtosecond laser works through which type of energy?

A. Infrared light

B. Ultraviolet light

C. Natural light

D. Microwave

133. You performed LASIK 2 days ago in a 28-year-old female. The procedure was uneventful. She returns to your office complaining of slightly hazy vision. On exam, you note a fine granular appearing infiltrate within the flap interface. The eye is otherwise quiet. What would be the best first step?

A. Start broad-spectrum antibiotics

B. Lift up her flap and culture

C. Start topical corticosteroids

D. Start antifungals

134. What is the mechanism of laser action for the excimer laser?

A. Photoablation

B. Photodisruption

C. Photocoagulation

D. All of the above

135. Which of the following factors is associated with haze following photorefractive keratectomy (PRK) treatment?

A. Patients who tend to develop keloids

B. High myopic treatment (greater than 6 D)

C. Postoperative medical noncompliance

D. All of the above

136. A 70-year-old man presents complaining about fluctuations in his vision. He notes that the vision seems different in the morning than at the end of the day. It also seems to vary depending on his location. He is an avid skier and he finds it harder to see when he goes to the mountains. He had refractive surgery in the 1980s and states that a procedure was done "before LASIK to treat my near sightedness." Overall, his vision is blurry. What do you expect that his prescription will be?

A. Myopic

B. Hyperopic

C. Plano

D. Irregular astigmatism with a topography that looks like keratoconus

137. Which of the following is not a contraindication for refractive surgery for myopia?

A. History of a bacterial corneal ulcer

B. Pregnancy

C. Human immunodeficiency virus (HIV)

D. Accutane use

138. A 40-year-old man presents to you for a second opinion. He had LASIK surgery performed 5 years ago for myopia and has been doing well. On routine follow-up, he was found to have a peripheral corneal opacity (see the figure provided). He asks you what the next steps would be for the management of this finding. Of these, what would you recommend?

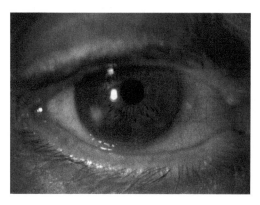

A. Observation

B. Start empiric antibiotics

C. Lift the LASIK flap and culture

D. Lift the LASIK flap and gently irrigate/scrape the stromal bed.

139. Which patient would be at highest risk for a button hole during LASIK flap creation?

A. A patient with a history of cataract surgery

B. A patient with moderate cylinder

C. A patient with very flat corneas

D. A patient with very steep corneas

140. A 23-year-old female with a history of herpetic simplex keratitis as well as recurrent corneal erosions presents for an evaluation of phototherapeutic keratectomy (PTK) for the treatment of her erosions. How might you council her?

A. The recurrent erosions can recur after PTK.

B. PTK may reactivate herpes simplex virus (HSV).

C. You may have a change in refraction.

D. All of the above.

141. A 25-year-old patient is interested in refractive surgery. He asks you to briefly explain the difference between LASIK, LASEK, and PRK. You explain:

A. LASIK involves creation of a stromal flap.

B. LASEK involves the creation of a stromal flap.

C. PRK involves the preservation of a sheet of epithelium.

D. None of the above.

142. You have a university-based practice. A 45-year-old woman presents with the following clinical picture (see the figure provided). She also complains of arthralgia, epistaxis, sinusitis, and shortness of breath. Who might you initially consult to help co-manage this patient?

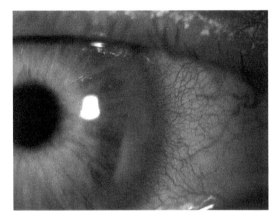

A. Rheumatology
B. Pulmonology
C. Nephrology
D. Cardiology

143. A 25-year-old female presents 2 weeks after conjunctivitis with the following findings (see the figure provided). She had a previous cold, conjunctival injection, and discharge, all of which resolved. She now complains of blurry vision and photophobia. You suspect that she had a previous virus and offer topical corticosteroids. She insists on getting antibiotics and tells you that a previous viral swab was negative. How do you respond?

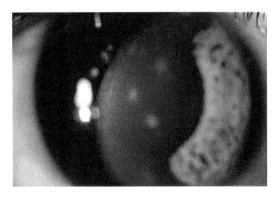

A. Agree to a short course of antibiotics.
B. Repeat viral swab.
C. Explain that the test may not have been sensitive enough to pick up the underlying virus or that the responsible virus was not tested. Because clinical presentation suggests postviral inflammation, you encourage steroid use.
D. Have her return in 1 week to monitor progress.

144. You are planning to perform a Descemet's membrane endothelial keratoplasty (DMEK) on a 68-year-old female with Fuchs dystrophy. Your corneal tissue arrives at the beginning of the day, and upon review of the tissue information you learn that you were actually provided with ultrathin Descemet stripping automated endothelial keratoplasty (DSAEK) tissue. The tissue remains unopened and in the proper storage settings. What should be your next step?

A. Proceed with the surgery as scheduled; ultrathin DSAEK and DMEK have comparable outcomes and the patient will not know the difference.
B. Cancel the surgery.
C. Call the eye bank and see if there is available DMEK tissue and if the DSAEK tissue can be exchanged.
D. Offer the option of ultrathin DSAEK to the patient.

145. A 25-year-old contact lens wearer presents asking you for a lens that he does not need to worry about. He would like to be able to swim, shower, and sleep in his lenses, and change them minimally. How would you advise this patient?

A. Contact lenses are safe to swim in, but they must be removed every night.
B. Contact lenses are foreign material that you are putting in your eye. They must be regularly cleaned or changed. Swimming and sleeping in lenses increases the risk of infection.
C. Extended wear lenses are safer than daily lenses.
D. It is probably safe to occasionally sleep in your lenses.

146. A 34-year-old man presents with foreign body sensation, blurry vision, and the following corneal finding (see the figure provided). He wants this to clear immediately and wants to make sure he never experiences an episode like this again. Per the Herpetic Eye Disease Study (HEDS) study, what should you advise:

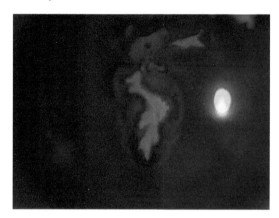

A. Starting a topical steroid will clear this faster.

B. Topical antiviral prophylaxis will reduce chances of recurrence.

C. Oral antiviral prophylaxis will reduce chances of recurrence.

D. The HEDS study did not show reduced rates of recurrence with antiviral prophylaxis.

147. A 25-year-old contact lens wearer presents with irritation and the following corneal finding (see the figure provided). According to the Steroid for Corneal Ulcer Trial (SCUT), adding topical corticosteroids to his treatment will result in which one of these?

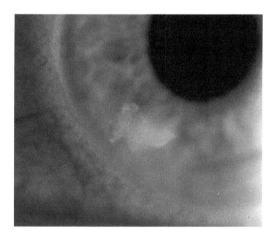

A. A faster time to reepithelialization

B. Worse visual outcome at 3 months

C. No difference in visual outcome at 3 months

D. A slower time to reepithelialization

148. An 84-year-old man with corneal edema in the setting of Fuchs dystrophy presents for consideration of Descemet's membrane endothelial keratoplasty (DMEK). He wants to optimize his chances of graft survival. According to the collaborative corneal transplant treatment study (CCTS), which factor(s) may be associated with increased risk of rejection?

A. Patients who are not human leukocyte antigen (HLA) matched

B. ABO blood type incompatibility

C. Patients over the age of 65 years

D. All of the above

149. A 54-year-old man presents with irritation and the following corneal lesion (see the figure provided). You predict that his corneal topography will show:

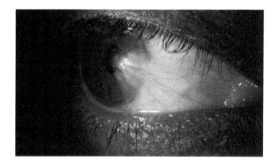

A. With-the-rule astigmatism

B. Against-the-rule astigmatism

C. Steep corneas

D. Flat corneas

150. A 68-year-old renal transplant recipient presents with the following corneal finding in the setting of a forehead rash (see the figure provided). All of the following are true about his condition except:

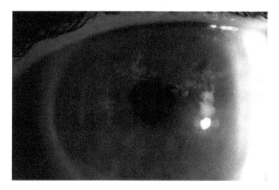

A. They stain well with fluorescein and rose Bengal.

B. The cornea may show decreased sensation.

C. These findings can recur in the future.

D. The patient should have a dilated fundus exam.

1.2 Answers and Explanations

Easy	Medium	Hard

1. Correct: Sebaceous gland carcinoma (B)

Sebaceous gland carcinoma classically arises from the meibomian glands of the tarsal plate and upper eyelids. It is less commonly associated with Zeiss glands. If a patient presents with a history of multiple chalazia on the same eyelid as the patient in the question (**A**), special attention should be given to eyelash misdirection, madarosis, thickening, and ulceration, as this could represent masquerading sebaceous glands carcinoma. Sebaceous gland carcinoma tends to masquerade as benign lesions or as other malignant tumors such as basal cell and squamous cell carcinoma (**C and D**).

2. Correct: Schirmer I test (B)

Schirmer I test is done without topical anesthetics and measures both basic and reflex tearing. Less than 5.5 mm of wetting after 5 minutes is diagnostic for dry eye. Basic secretion test (**A**) is performed after instillation of topical anesthetic and blotting of residual fluid from the inferior fornix. Less than 3 mm of wetting after 5 minutes with anesthetic is suggestive of dry eye. Schirmer II (**C**) measures reflex tearing. It is performed after applying anesthetics and irritating the nasal mucosa. Less than 15 mm of wetting after 2 minutes is consistent with a defect in reflex secretion. Schirmer IV (**D**) does not exist.

3. Correct: Lactoferrin (A)

Quantitative tear film test includes lactoferrin (**A**), immunoglobulin E, and matrix metalloproteinase. Lactoferrin is an iron-binding protein secreted by acinar cells of the lacrimal gland. Lactoferrin levels are directly correlated to aqueous production. Schirmer testing is a measurement of tear production. Meibography (**D**) is an imaging test demonstrating meibomian gland structure. Immunoglobulin E, not G (**B**) is part of quantitative testing of tear film. Elevated values (> 40 ng/mL) might indicate evaporative dry eyes, but this is not specific for dry eyes, as high values might be associated with allergies and infections. Schirmer testing (**C**) is used to measure tear production.

4. Correct: Meibomian gland dysfunction (D)

Meibomian gland dysfunction (MGD) is a condition of gland obstruction, and it is the most common cause of evaporative dry eye. Meibomian glands may appear capped with oil, dilated, or obstructed. Secretions are usually turbid and thicker than normal; tear meniscus may appear foamy. The dry eye workshop 2017 classified dry eye into "tear deficient" or "evaporative" in etiology. The tear deficient class is subclassified into Sjogren's syndrome dry eye and non-Sjogren's dry eye syndrome. Evaporative dry eye is due to excessive water loss from the exposed ocular surface in the presence of normal lacrimal secretory function. Sjogren's syndrome (**A**) is an autoimmune exocrinopathy of the lacrimal and salivary glands causing acinar and ductular cell death, and hyposecretion of tears and saliva. Age-related dry eye presents with periductal fibrosis and acinar atrophy (**B**). Trachoma is a combination of tarsal and conjunctival scarring, trichiasis, and cicatrizing meibomian gland obstruction caused by the bacterium *chlamydia trachomatis* (**C**).

5. Correct: Rosacea (A)

Rosacea is associated with neutrophil recruitment, angiogenesis, and cytokine release. It is associated with an excessive sebum secretion, meibomian gland dysfunction, and chronic blepharitis progressing to chronic conjunctivitis. If left untreated, it can cause stromal keratitis or keratitis, sterile corneal ulceration, or episcleritis. Repeated episodes of ocular surface inflammation can cause corneal neovascularization and scarring. The management includes oral antibiotics (tetracyclines or macrolides) and topical therapy to the face (e.g., metronidazole or azelaic acid). Warm compresses and lid scrubs can be helpful for meibomian gland function. Topical steroids can be initiated for patients with ulcerative keratitis and neovascularization, once infectious causes are ruled out. Staphylococcal blepharitis (**B**) is characterized by erythema and edema of the eyelid margin, eyelash loss and/or misdirection, and hard scales/collarettes. Keratoconjunctivitis sicca (**C**) is associated with Sjogren's syndrome, not rosacea. There is no evidence of chalazion in the given figure (**D**).

6. Correct: Failure to close the eye completely on the affected side (C)

This patient most likely has peripheral facial palsy (e.g., Bell's palsy) complicated by exposure keratopathy due to lagophthalmos. Exposure keratopathy can develop as a result of any condition that causes a poor blink or limited eyelid closure. Lagophthalmos is commonly associated with seventh nerve palsy. On exam, the patient may have punctate epithelial erosions involving the inferior cornea, or, in severe cases, the entire corneal surface. The management includes ocular surface lubrication as a first-line treatment. A lubricating ointment can be used at night. For more advanced cases, eyelid taping during sleep, bandage contact lenses, or tarsorrhaphy can be employed. Corneal sensitivity is associated with fifth cranial nerve (**A**), which is not affected in facial paralysis. Ptosis surgery can be associated with lagophthalmos but should not present with weakness of the forehead (**B**). Uncontrolled high blood pressure can cause a central facial paralysis (**D**).

7. Correct: Human immunodeficiency virus (D)

The most common cause of neurotrophic keratopathy is secondary to herpetic keratitis (**A**). The keratopathy associated with neutrophilia is typically seen in the central or paracentral cornea and tends to be located inferiorly or inferonasally because of the protective effect of the Bell's phenomenon. The lesions frequently have elevated gray white edges of heaped up epithelium ("rolled edges") with underlying stromal inflammation. If neurotrophic keratopathy is left untreated, it can advance to cause corneal ulceration, scarring, and neovascularization. Other causes of neurotrophic keratitis are cerebrovascular accidents, diabetes mellitus, familial dysautonomia or Riley–Day syndrome (**B**), leprosy or Hansen's disease (**C**), and topical medication toxicity. Management includes aggressive lubrication, bandage or specialty contact lenses, tetracyclines to prevent keratolysis, and in advanced cases corneal cross-linking or amniotic membrane graft. HIV is not associated with neurotrophic keratopathy (**D**).

8. Correct: Floppy eyelid syndrome (A)

Floppy eyelid syndrome is characterized by chronic ocular surface changes due to a lax eyelid that everts with minimal force. Eversion can often take place during sleep, as the eyelid rubs against the pillow. It is associated with obesity and sleep apnea. Clinical exam reveals corneal epitheliopathy associated with large palpebral papillae. It is a known biomechanical predisposing factor to the development of keratoconus due to chronic inflammation and irritation. Patients can be treated with lubrication, especially an ointment at night, and tape, patch or shields at night. If it persists, a horizontal eyelid tightening procedure can be considered. Superior limbic keratoconjunctivitis (**B**) is associated with thyroid eye disease. Dermatochalasis (**C**) refers to the presence of redundant eyelid skin due to aging. Rosacea is a chronic inflammatory skin condition. Ocular rosacea includes bilateral chronic blepharitis and meibomian gland dysfunction (**D**). Options B, C, and D are not associated with laxity of the eyelids.

9. Correct: Superior limbic keratoconjunctivitis (D)

Superior limbic keratoconjunctivitis is a chronic bilateral and often asymmetric inflammatory condition involving the superior tarsal and mainly the superior bulbar conjunctiva. It is often associated with autoimmune thyroid disease, graft versus host disease, and postoperative complication of blepharoplasty. Ocular findings may include a fine papillary reaction on the superior tarsal conjunctiva, injection and thickening of the superior bulbar conjunctiva hypertrophy of the superior limbus, and/or superior filamentary keratitis. Floppy eyelid syndrome (**A**) is usually associated with sleep apnea and includes findings of papillary reaction and eyelid laxity. Exposure keratopathy (**B**) can often be seen after blepharoplasty, especially if it results in poor closure of the lid, but the findings are usually in the inferior cornea, where the eye is most likely to be exposed. A foreign body under the superior eyelid (**C**) would be visible on slit lamp examination.

10. Correct: Laser-assisted in situ keratomileusis (LASIK) (D)

Recurrent corneal erosions are characterized by the sudden onset of eye pain, usually during the night or upon first awakening. Many patients seem to experience ocular discomfort out of proportion to exam findings. During the attack, the epithelium often looks heaped up and edematous, though most of the patients have an intact epithelium or minimal epithelial irregularity at the time of examination. The contralateral eye should be carefully examined to detect dystrophic erosions. Recurrent erosion syndrome is associated with epithelial basement membrane dystrophy in 50% of patients, and map lines and cysts can occasionally be seen on careful examination. Management includes aggressive lubrication (**A**) or hypertonic saline solution (**B**) at night. The lubrication helps the lid glide off the epithelium upon opening without causing an erosion. The hypertonic saline ointment helps stick the epithelium to the underlying basement membrane by minimizing the natural swelling of the cornea overnight. In many patients, the use of contact bandage lenses provides temporary relief of symptoms. If erosions persist despite conservative measures, surgical options can be offered including epithelial debridement, anterior stromal puncture, or PTK (**C**). Refractive therapies (LASIK/PRK) are not indicated in the management of recurrent corneal erosions (**D**).

11. Correct: Topical anesthetic abuse (A)

Topical anesthetic abuse is characterized by inhibition of epithelial cell migration, loss of microvilli, reduction of desmosomes, and swelling of mitochondria and lysosomes. It mimics infectious causes and can follow a similar clinical course. In severe cases, patients present with hypopyon, dense stromal infiltrates, and a large ring opacity. Suspicion should be raised in patients not improving despite adequate medical management and those involved in a health care setting as the patient in question, especially after abrasions or keratitis. Given the patient is a health care worker associated with no improvement, anesthetic abuse should be high in your differential. Fungal keratitis is usually associated with a history of trauma to the cornea with plant or vegetable material (**C**), and *Acanthamoeba* (**B**) is almost always in the setting of contact lens wear. Fungal keratitis and acanthamoeba keratitis should be always considered in the diagnosis of corneal ulcers, especially those with no improvement with antibiotic therapy. In the early stages of anesthetic abuse, patients may present with a neurotrophic-like appearance but herpetic lesions (**D**) do not progress to ring opacity.

12. Correct: Stem cell deficiency (B)

The patient in question has a history of a recent bone marrow transplantation making the diagnosis of graft versus host disease-associated stem cell deficiency likely. Limbal stem cell deficiency is characterized by a loss of stem cells at the limbus. Impression cytology can be used to evaluate for stem cell deficiency. It may show goblet cells on the cornea (which are normally not present). Epithelial cells are critical for wound healing and repopulation of corneal epithelium. Patients with limbal stem cell deficiency may exhibit a "whorl like" epitheliopathy, persistent epithelial defects, and corneal conjunctivalization and neovascularization. Keratoconjunctivitis sicca may be associated with loss of the palisades of Vogt, but the patient in question had a recent bone marrow transplant and does not have Sjogren's syndrome (**C**). Toxic keratoconjunctivitis and rosacea should not lead to a destruction of the palisades of Vogt. (**A, D**)

13. Correct: Cornea plana (C)

Sclerocornea is a nonprogressive, noninflammatory scleralization of the cornea. It might be limited to the periphery or involve the entire cornea. Sclerocornea is usually sporadic and in 80% of cases it is associated with cornea plana (**C**). Cornea plana is a rare condition in which the radius of curvature is less than 43 D and keratometry readings are between 30 and 35. Patients usually present with hyperopia > 10 D. Microcornea (**A**) is defined as a < 10 mm corneal diameter. It can be associated with sclerocornea, but cornea plana has a stronger association. Patients with microcornea are predisposed to angle closure glaucoma. Megalocornea (**B**) is defined as bilateral corneal diameters > 13 mm, is typically seen in males, and has no association with sclerocornea. Patients are usually myopes, have with-the-rule astigmatism, and often present a challenge to cataract surgeons due to lens instability and subluxation, iridodonesis, and poor zonular integrity. Megalocornea should be distinguished from buphthalmos seen in congenital glaucoma, which also causes an increase in corneal diameter. Posterior embryotoxon (**D**) is a thickened and anteriorly displaced Schwalbe's line; it has no association with sclerocornea.

14. Correct: Axenfeld–Rieger syndrome (ARS) (C)

Axenfeld–Rieger syndrome corresponds to a spectrum of disorders characterized by an anteriorly displaced Shwalbe's line or posterior embryotoxon. ARS examination reveals iris strands, iris hypoplasia, corectopia, and glaucoma. ARS is associated with craniofacial, dental, skeletal, and umbilical abnormalities. None of the other options present with posterior embryotoxon.

15. Correct: Peters anomaly (B)

Peters anomaly is characterized by the presence of central or paracentral corneal opacity due to the absence of corneal endothelium and Descemet's membrane beneath the area of opacity. Eighty percent of cases are bilateral. There are two types. Type I is characterized by iridocorneal adhesions and a central opacity that is usually avascular. Type II is characterized by corneolenticular adhesions, corneal opacity, and/or cataract. Glaucoma is present in 50% of cases. Other eye abnormalities include microcornea, aniridia, retinal detachment, and persistent fetal vasculature. Peter plus syndrome refers to Peters anomaly associated with systemic abnormalities, as in the patient in this question. A useful mnemonic for the differential of corneal opacities is STUMPED (sclerocornea, tears in Descemet's membrane, ulcers, metabolic, congenital hereditary endothelial dystrophy [CHED], dermoid). Pediatric corneal ulcers (**A**) are rare and most often caused by herpetic and bacterial infection, and would present with conjunctival injection, fluorescein uptake, and underlying infiltrate. Birth trauma can cause corneal clouding when there are breaks in Descemet's membrane secondary to the use of forceps (**C**). There is no mention of birth trauma in this question stem. Dermoid presents as a well circumscribed, elevated fleshy to pale yellow color limbal mass (**D**). A limbal dermoid is a choristoma, a benign tumor consisting of normal tissue derived from germ cell layers foreign to that body site. Limbal dermoids may contain fat, cartilage, and hair.

16. Correct: IV penicillin (A)

Congenital syphilis is acquired in utero and caused by infection with *Treponema pallidum*. Interstitial keratitis typically presents between 6 and 12 years of age in patients with untreated syphilis. Keratitis presents as rapidly progressive corneal edema and abnormal vascularization in the deep stroma. The cornea assumes a pink salmon color due to the neovascularization. There are many possible etiologies associated with interstitial keratitis, including but not limited to Epstein–Barr virus, herpes simplex virus, Lyme disease, and tuberculosis. The patient in question has hearing deficits and dental abnormalities, hence congenital syphilis is high on the differential. Definitive treatment is with penicillin. Ceftazidime (**B**), acyclovir (**C**), and voriconazole (**D**) are not part of the treatment for congenital syphilis.

17. Correct: Forceps trauma (A)

Vertical striae after birth are characteristic of forceps-induced trauma (**A**). Horizontal striae or Haab's striae are due to corneal stretching secondary to increased intraocular pressure in the setting of congenital glaucoma (**B**). Cortical cataracts would not have corneal findings (**C**). Corneal ulcer presents with corneal thinning, often in the setting of an infiltrate or infection. There should not be associated striae (**D**).

18. Correct: Stocker's line (A)

The most likely underlying diagnosis in the question is pterygium. Pterygium is wing-shaped growth of conjunctiva and fibrovascular tissue on the superficial cornea, and it can have iron deposition in the cornea, known as a Stocker's line. It is strongly correlated with UV light exposure. All answer questions are related to iron deposition in the cornea. Hudson–Stahli is line associated with normal aging and is present between the middle and lower third of the cornea (**B**). Fleischer's ring is seen at the base of the cone in keratoconus (**C**). Ferry's line is a corneal epithelial iron line at the edge of filtering blebs (**D**).

19. Correct: Photorefractive keratectomy (D)

Spheroidal degeneration is characterized by translucent, golden-brown, spheroidal deposits in the subepithelium, Bowman's layer, or superficial stroma. The deposits are bilateral and initially located in the nasal and temporal cornea. Histopathologic studies reveal extracellular, proteinaceous, hyaline deposits with elastotic degeneration. The deposit composition is not lipid, despite the oil droplet appearance. Ocular lubrication is recommended (**A**) to smooth the cornea and decrease symptoms. Superficial keratectomy (**B**) and phototherapeutic keratectomy (**C**) are indicated when central cornea is involved. Photorefractive keratectomy (**D**) is a refractive procedure which is not indicated in the management of spheroidal degeneration.

20. Correct: Phototherapeutic keratectomy (PTK) (B)

Band keratopathy is a degeneration of the superficial cornea that involves the calcification and destruction of Bowman's membrane. Band keratopathy usually first appears in the 3 and 9 o'clock positions and can progress across the interpalpebral zone of the cornea, affecting the visual axis. It is associated with chronic ocular inflammatory diseases, hypercalcemic and hyperphosphatemic states (such as renal failure), and silicone oil in the eye. The calcium can be removed from Bowman's layer by chelation with EDTA. Artificial tears and bandage contact lenses (**C, D**) are appropriate options to manage symptoms. PTK (**B**) should not be used as primary treatment because calcium ablates at a different rate than stroma and could produce a severely irregular surface.

21. Correct: Carotid doppler (C)

Arcus senilis is an involution change caused by the deposition of lipids in the peripheral cornea. Lipids accumulate at the level of Bowman's layer and Descemet's membrane. Unilateral arcus senilis is associated with contralateral carotid disease, which should prompt you to obtain carotid doppler (**C**). The remaining options are not part of the work-up for unilateral arcus senilis (**A, B, D**).

22. Correct: Terrien's marginal degeneration (D)

Terrien's marginal degeneration is a noninflammatory, slowly progressive, painless thinning of the peripheral cornea. It is usually bilateral. The cause is unknown. Patients initially present with superonasal thinning that spreads circumferentially. Mooren's ulcer (**B**) presents with painful peripheral thinning of unknown etiology. It will often start temporally or nasally and spread circumferentially. There may be an association with hepatitis C. PUK (**A**) is peripheral, often unilateral, painful ulceration of the cornea due to elevated collagenase. It is often associated with rheumatologic disease (rheumatoid arthritis, Sjogren's syndrome, and polyarteritis nodosa). Staphylococcal marginal degeneration (**C**) is characterized by a subepithelial infiltrate near the limbus, separated from the limbus by a small clear zone. It is caused by a hypersensitivity reaction to staphylococcus and usually heals well with topical steroids.

23. Correct: Corneal topography (A)

The question stem describes Terrien's marginal degeneration, which is a corneal stromal degeneration. It is slowly progressive, painless thinning of the peripheral cornea. It is usually bilateral. The cause is unknown. Patients initially present with superonasal thinning that spreads circumferentially. Corneal topography reveals flattening of the peripheral thinned cornea, with steepening of the corneal surface 90 degrees away from the midpoint. This produces against-the-rule astigmatism. The other options will not contribute to identification of this condition (**B, C, D**). Corneal scraping could potentially cause perforation.

24. Correct: Salzmann's nodular degeneration (C)

Salzmann's nodular degeneration is a noninflammatory corneal degeneration that can be seen in the setting of chronic inflammation such as phlyctenulosis, trachoma, interstitial keratitis or a history of multiple surgeries. The nodules are gray-white and elevated, as shown in the provided figure. Histologic examination reveals replacement of Bowman's layer with hyaline and fibrillar material. Treatment includes ocular lubrication for mild cases. Superficial keratectomy can be used if irritation persists despite lubrication. Phlyctenulosis and corneal ulcer present with inflammatory changes (**A, D**). Band keratopathy presents with calcific deposits, usually at 3 and 9 o'clock positions (**B**).

25. Correct: Superficial keratectomy (C)

The question stem describes a well demarcated and anteriorly located lesion. The OCT shows hyper-reflective material in the anterior cornea, anterior to the stroma and clearly demarcated. This is likely Salzmann's nodular degeneration, which are benign nodules composed of irregularly arranged collagen fibers. The nodules can be removed by superficial keratectomy, although patients should be counseled that these can recur 20% of the time. Lamellar and penetrating keratoplasty should be used with deep stromal involvement (**A and B**). Corneal biopsy with cryotherapy and adjuvant chemotherapy is indicated in cases of malignancy (**D**).

26. Correct: Specular microscopy (B)

The female patient described in this question has corectopia and unilateral angle closure glaucoma and therefore has the likely diagnosis of iridocorneal endothelial syndrome. Specular microscopy would reveal the characteristic light-dark reversal, along with endothelial cell pleomorphism, and polymegathism. Corneal topography, anterior segment OCT, and ultrasound biomicroscopy can be used to acquire additional information about the cornea and the eye, but would not give a definitive diagnosis (**A, C, and D**).

27. Correct: Amiodarone (B)

Amiodarone, an antiarrhythmic agent, is the most common cause of cornea verticillata. On exam, cornea verticillata presents as a clockwise whorl-like pattern of golden-brown or gray deposits in the inferior interpalpebral portion of the cornea. Other inciting agents include chloroquine, hydroxychloroquine, indomethacin, tamoxifen, and phenothiazines. Metoprolol, diltiazem, and apixaban are systemic drugs for the management of atrial fibrillation and are not associated with corneal verticillata (**A, C, and D**).

28. Correct: Fabry disease (A)

The question refers to corneal verticillata. In addition to systemic medications such as amiodarone, chloroquine, hydroxychloroquine, indomethacin, tamoxifen, and phenothiazines, corneal verticillata is associated with Fabry disease. Fabry disease is an X-linked genetic disease due to a deficiency of the enzyme alpha galactosidase causing a glycolipid known as globotriaosylceramide to accumulate within blood vessels and multiple organs including kidneys, heart, peripheral nervous system, and skin. Hunter, Scheie, and Hurler syndromes (**B, C, and D**) present with corneal clouding.

29. Correct: 9.5–10.5 mm (A)

The corneal diameter measures 9.5–10.5 mm horizontally, it is approximately 500 to 600 µm thick, and it gradually increases in thickness toward the periphery. (**B**) and (**D**) correspond to megalocornea. (**C**) corresponds to microcornea.

30. Correct: Collagen type I (A)

The corneal stroma consists mostly of type I collagen, with smaller amounts of III, V, and VI collagens also present. Corneal collagen cross-linking is now an FDA-approved treatment to halt the progression of keratoconus. It works through the combination of riboflavin (vitamin B2) and UV light to promote new collagen bonds, thus "strengthening" the cornea to prevent further ectatic disease.

31. Correct: Specular microscopy (A)

Specular microscopy provides an objective measurement of corneal endothelial cells, including density, coefficient of variation, and percentage of hexagonal cells. All of the other options are not objective tests for endothelial cells (**B, C, and D**). The question stem describes a patient with pseudophakic bullous keratopathy, for which specular microscopy would show decreased endothelial cell count.

32. Correct: Confocal microscopy (B)

Confocal microscopy allows for in vivo imaging of the cornea through a slit scanning microscope. The scan takes serial images across many layers of the cornea, comparable to in vitro histochemical analysis. The patient in question is at high risk for acanthamoeba keratitis, given his contact lens use history and recent swimming. Confocal microscopy can identify the protozoan. The other options will not aid in the diagnosis of this infection. Specular microscopy is used to assess endothelial cell count, coefficient of variation, and percentage of hexagonal cells (**A**). Anterior optical coherence tomography (**C**) produces two-dimensional, high-resolution, and high-definition cross-sectional images of the anterior segment allowing delineation of the layers of the cornea, anterior chamber, and iris. It is not used for the microbiologic diagnosis of corneal ulcers. Ultrasound biomicroscopy (**D**) provides high-resolution ultrasonic images of the anterior segment, including the cornea, iris, lens, angle and ciliary body. It can be used for patients with anterior segment opacities and is especially helpful for ciliary body pathologies (cysts and tumors), angle abnormalities (angle recession, pupillary block, plateau iris, malignant glaucoma, and cyclodialysis), and interocular lens (IOL) positioning.

33. Correct: Neural crest (B)

This patient most likely has the diagnosis of Peters anomaly, which is due to the absence of Descemet's membrane and endothelium. Descemet's membrane and endothelium are derived from the neural crest. The corneal epithelium is derived from the surface ectoderm (**A**). Bowman's membrane and stroma are derived from mesoderm (**C**). There are no eye structures that are derived from the endoderm (**D**).

34. Correct: Epithelial basement membrane dystrophy (EBMD) (C)

Recurrent epithelial erosions can present with any of the options in this question. However, slit lamp examination using retroillumination reveals fingerprint/dot lesions which are characteristic of EBMD. Fluorescein staining aids in the diagnosis by making the lesions more evident (see the figure provided). EBMD occurs in 6 to 18% of the population, more commonly in women, with increasing frequency in patients older than 50 years. Clinical findings and their correlating histopathology are as follows: Fingerprints: thin and relucent hairlike lines. Maps: geographic and irregular sheets of thickened epithelium with circumscribed borders. Dots: irregular, oval, or comma-shaped intraepithelial opacities. Blebs: irregular and subepithelial accumulation of fibrogranular material. Symptoms are typically related to recurrent epithelial erosions and/or blurred vision. Due to the irregularity of the basement membrane and epithelium, patients with EBMD may have irregular astigmatism. Recurrent epithelial erosions occur in 10% of patients, who often present with characteristic pain upon awakening. As with EBMD, Meesmann epithelial dystrophy affects epithelium and subepithelium. It presents with bubble-like blebs (**D**). Options a and b are dystrophies of the epithelium-stroma. Reis-Bucklers corneal dystrophy (RBCD) presents as confluent, irregular, and coarse geographic opacities (**A**). Thiel-Behnke corneal dystrophy (TBCD) presents with symmetric subepithelial reticular opacities in a honeycomb pattern (**B**).

35. Correct: Lisch epithelial corneal dystrophy (LECD) (C)

LECD is an X-linked dominant corneal dystrophy. Clinical findings include whorled, flame-shaped, or feather-like corneal opacities that radiate from the limbus to the central cornea. Histopathology reveals diffuse cytoplasmic vacuolization. Recurrent corneal erosions present in most corneal dystrophies (**A, B, and D**), but not in LECD.

36. Correct: Meesmann epithelial corneal dystrophy (MECD) (B)

MECD is an autosomal dominant dystrophy with a mutation in the gene keratin 3 (KRT3), characterized by electron-dense intraepithelial cysts consisting of Periodic acid-Schiff (PAS)-positive degenerated epithelial cell products surrounded by tangles of cytoplasmic filaments, known as peculiar substance. MECD appears very early in life. The cornea will have multiple, tiny epithelial vesicles that are diffusely distributed. The presence of peculiar substance in pathologic studies is not characteristic of the remaining options (**A, C, and D**).

37. Correct: Lisch epithelial corneal dystrophy (LECD) (C)

LECD has an X-linked dominant inheritance. Using retroillumination or direct light, a characteristic band shaped with feathery lesion in a whorl-like pattern is found. Pathology reveals diffuse cytoplasmic vacuolization and scattered staining with Ki-67 evidence of increased mitotic activity. MECD (**A**) presents with bubble-like blebs with indirect illumination. EBMD presents with fingerprints, maps, and/or dots using sclerotic scatter or retroillumination (**B**). Thiel-Behnke corneal dystrophy (TBCD) presents with subepithelial reticular opacities (honeycomb pattern) with a broad oblique slit of light (**D**).

38. Correct: Reis-Bucklers corneal dystrophy (RBCD) (C)

In RBCD, Bowman's layer is disrupted or absent and replaced by a sheet of connective-like tissue with granular deposits that stain red with Masson trichrome stain. RBCD presents in the first few years of life with confluent, irregular, and coarse geographic opacities at the level of Bowman's layer and superficial stroma. These opacities vary in density and are mostly central. Granular corneal dystrophy type 1 (GCD1) can present early in life and stains bright red with Masson trichrome as well; however, the cornea has characteristic crumb-like opacities with clear intervening spaces (**B**). Epithelial basement membrane dystrophy (EBMD) and Thiel-Behnke corneal dystrophy (TBCD) do not stain with Masson trichrome (**A, D**). EBMD does not occur early in life. TBCD can occur in the first or second decade of life as solitary lesions that progress overtime to a honeycomb pattern.

39. Correct: Thiel-Behnke corneal dystrophy (TBCD) (A)

Clinically, Reis-Bucklers corneal dystrophy (RBCD) and TBCD could be hard to distinguish. Curly fibers seen on electron microscopy at the level of Bowman's membrane are pathognomonic for TBCD. TBCD is often confused with RBCD, as both involve Bowman's layer, hence electron microscopy is needed to distinguish these two dystrophies. Granular corneal dystrophy type 1 (GCD1) (**B**) has electron-dense material made up of rod-shaped bodies on seen on electron microscopy. Macular corneal dystrophy (MCD) (**C**) electron microscopy reveals extracellular clumps or fibrogranular material.

40. Correct: Descemet's membrane endothelial keratoplasty (DMEK) (D)

Thiel–Behnke corneal dystrophy is a corneal dystrophy at the level of Bowman's membrane. Over time, reticular opacities develop in a honeycomb pattern, sparing the peripheral cornea. Corneal dystrophies at the level of Bowman's membrane can be managed with superficial keratectomy (**A**), PTK (**B**), and lamellar keratectomy (**C**). DMEK is indicated for endothelial dystrophies.

41. Correct: Congo red stain (B)

Lattice corneal dystrophy is characterized by refractile branching lines in the corneal stroma (see the figure provided). On pathology, lattice dystrophy has arborizing amyloid deposits in the anterior stroma, positive staining with Congo red stain and crystal violet dye. Lattice lines develop as the condition progresses. They start centrally and superficially and spread centrifugally. The peripheral cornea typically remains clear. Masson trichrome stain is used for Reis–Bucklers corneal dystrophy, and granular corneal dystrophy 1 and 2 (**A**). Alcian blue stains macular corneal dystrophy (**C**). Oil red O stains Schnyder corneal dystrophy (**D**).

42. Correct: Granular corneal dystrophy type 1 (GCD1) (A)

GCD1 stains bright red with Masson trichrome stain. The opacities are composed of granular hyaline material. Onset occurs early in life with crumb-like opacities in the superficial cornea; the opacities are separated by clear spaces (see the figure provided). GCD is the most common dystrophy and is autosomal dominant. Laser refractive surgery should be avoided in patients with granular dystrophy because of the risk of postoperative haze. RBCD and GCD2 stain with Masson trichrome. RBCD presents with confluent, irregular, and coarse geographic opacities (**B**). GCD2 presents with stellate-shaped, snowflake-like opacities (**D**). Macular corneal dystrophy stains with Alcian blue (**C**).

43. Correct: Autosomal recessive (C)

In this patient, the history of epidemic keratoconjunctivitis does not explain his clinical course. He suffers from macular corneal dystrophy, an autosomal recessive dystrophy with superficial, irregular, whitish, fleck-like opacities that evolve into focal,

gray-white, superficial stromal opacities with intervening haze. The opacities present in the first decade of life and can be seen limbus to limbus with no intervening clear spaces and diffuse haze. Gelatinous drop-like corneal dystrophy and congenital hereditary endothelial dystrophy (CHED) are also autosomal recessive. Gelatinous drop-like corneal dystrophy presents with subepithelial amyloid nodules similar to those in band keratopathy (The patient in the given figure is noted to have deep stromal haze; in comparison, gelatinous drop-like corneal dystrophy is characterized by subepithelial lesions that can protrude forward in a mulberry configuration. CHED examination reveals a milky appearance on diffuse illumination with diffuse stromal thickening and presents in early childhood. Lisch epithelial corneal dystrophy is X-dominant and presents as a feathery, whorled pattern (**B**). Epithelial basement membrane dystrophy is sporadic and has the characteristic fingerprint, map, and dot pattern. Fuchs endothelial corneal dystrophy can be sporadic or autosomal dominant in inheritance. Fuchs is an endothelial dystrophy presenting with guttae and stromal edema. All the other dystrophies not mentioned in this stem are autosomal dominant, including Meesman, Reis–Bucklers, Thiel–Behnke, Lattice type 1 and 2, Schnyder, and posterior polymorphous corneal dystrophy.

44. Correct: Glycosaminoglycan deposits (C)

Macular corneal dystrophy stains with Alcian blue or colloidal iron; it is characterized by glycosaminoglycan deposits and presents in young patients between 10 and 30 years of age. Examination reveals diffuse haze with no clear intervening spaces as seen in this patient. Cholesterol (**A**) stains with oil red O and it is characteristic for Schnyder dystrophy. Amyloid deposits (**B**) in lattice dystrophy stain with Congo red and examination reveals branching refractile lines. Hyaline deposits (**D**) in granular dystrophy stain with Masson trichrome and examination demonstrates a breadcrumb appearance in type 1 and stellate fleck opacities in type 2.

45. Correct: Fasting lipid profile (C)

Schnyder corneal dystrophy is a rare autosomal dominant stromal dystrophy that can be present as early as in the first year of life. However, diagnosis is usually made by the second or third decade of life. It disproportionately reduces photopic vision compared to retained normal scotopic vision. The exact pathogenesis is unknown but is thought to be secondary to a defect in lipid metabolism. A fasting lipid profile (**C**) should be done to detect possible hyperlipoproteinemia or hyperlipidemia. Abnormalities of glucose metabolism (**A**), liver function (**B**), and serum electrolytes (**D**) have not been linked.

46. Correct: Deep anterior lamellar keratoplasty (D)

Fuchs endothelial corneal dystrophy is caused by dysfunctional or reduced endothelial cells, which can lead to corneal edema and scarring over time. On exam, corneal guttae are usually first evident centrally and may become confluent over time, taking on a beaten metal appearance. Later stages are characterized by endothelial decompensation and stromal edema causing bullous keratopathy. Specular microscopy reveals areas of endothelial loss—guttata (see the figure provided). Fuchs dystrophy usually presents in the fourth decade of life or later. Sodium chloride drops can be helpful in managing stromal edema (**B**). Both Descemet's membrane endothelial keratoplasty (**B**) and penetrating keratoplasty (**C**) can be used in severe cases. Deep anterior lamellar keratopathy is not indicated for endothelial dystrophies as the corneal endothelium will not be replaced.

47. Correct: Stop rubbing your eyes (D)

This patient has keratoconus. It is a common disorder of central or paracentral corneal thinning and protrusion at the maximal point of thinning. The onset is most commonly during puberty, and progression continues through young adulthood. Nearly all cases are bilateral, but asymmetry is common. Topography reveals irregular astigmatism and inferior steepening with an asymmetric bow tie pattern, as shown in the given figure. Eye rubbing has been associated with progression of keratoconus and patients with keratoconus should be advised to refrain from rubbing their eyes. While contact lenses may be helpful to correct the refractive error, they do not prevent keratoconus from progressing or permanently correct the ectasia that has already occurred (**A**). Keratoconus is not associated with any infectious process (**B**). Keratoconus is not an autoimmune condition (**C**).

48. Correct: Keratoglobus (B)

Keratoglobus is globular corneal deformation typically present at birth associated with generalized thinning. It is strongly associated with blue sclera syndrome, Ehlers–Danlos syndrome type VI. Pathology reveals a fragmented or absent Bowman's layer, thinned stroma, and a thin Descemet's membrane. The corneal curvature may be as steep as 50 to 60 D. The prognosis for penetrating keratoplasty is much poorer than in other corneal ectasias. Keratoconus (**A**) has been associated with collagen disorders and presents with central or paracentral steepening, and inferior steepening. Pellucid margin degeneration presents in adults and topography reveals flattening of the peripheral thinned cornea with steeping 90 degrees away (**C**). The patient would have needed a history of a refractive procedure in order to develop postrefractive ectasia (**D**).

49. Correct: Hurler syndrome (A)

Hurler syndrome is a systemic mucopolysaccharidosis, an inherited lysosomal disease characterized by corneal clouding due to accumulation of incompletely degraded glycosaminoglycans within the keratocytes, corneal epithelium, and endothelium. Hunter syndrome and Fabry disease are X-linked (**B**, **C**). Hunter syndrome does not present with corneal clouding at birth. Fabry disease is associated with corneal verticillata. Tay–Sachs disease is autosomal recessive and ocular manifestations are mostly retinal (**D**).

50. Correct: Fabry disease (D)

Fabry disease is part of the sphingolipidoses spectrum. It is caused by a deficiency of alpha-galactosidase, leading to accumulation of ceramide trihexoside in the renal and cardiovascular system. The cornea exhibits a whorl-like pattern or cornea verticillata in the basal layers of the epithelium. Scheie syndrome (**C**) presents with slow progressive corneal opacification and Hunter syndrome may present with mild corneal opacity later in life. Tay–Sachs disease primarily involves the retina (**B**).

51. Correct: Cysteamine eye drops (C)

Cystinosis is a rare autosomal recessive metabolic disorder characterized by the accumulation of cystine by-products within lysosomes. It is caused by a defect in the cysteine transporter cystinosin. There are three types: Infantile or nephropathic cystinosis, characterized by growth failure and renal Fanconi syndrome. Juvenile cystinosis, in which kidney dysfunction occurs during adolescence. Nonnephropathic or ocular cystinosis, crystal deposition begins in the anterior periphery of the cornea and extends inward and posteriorly. Topical cysteamine (**C**) has been proven to decrease corneal crystals if used every 1 to 2 hours during the day. Moxifloxacin (**A**), prednisolone (**B**), and ketotifen (**D**) are not part of the treatment for ocular cystinosis unless an associated pathology occurs.

52. Correct: Pseudodendrites (C)

Tyrosinemia type II is an autosomal recessive disorder resulting from tyrosine aminotransferase deficiency. Corneal exam reveals pseudodendrites. The treatment consists of dietary tyrosine restriction. Tyrosinemia type I is not associated with corneal pathology. Interstitial keratitis (**A**) can be associated with *Mycobacterium tuberculosis*, Lyme, and syphilis, among others. Mucopolysaccharidoses, including Hurler and Scheie, can present with corneal clouding (**B**) in the newborn period. Corneal verticillata is associated with Fabry disease and medications, including amiodarone, chloroquine, hydroxychloroquine, indomethacin, and phenothiazine (**D**).

53. Correct: Pigmentation is usually localized to the endothelium (C)

Alkaptonuria is a rare autosomal recessive disorder (**D**) caused by a deficiency of the enzyme homogentisic acid oxidase, causing accumulation of homogentisic acid. The frequency of this disease is highest among patients from the Dominican Republic and Slovakia. Patients present with ochronosis or blue-black pigmentation due to alkapton accumulation; it is usually symmetric (**A**) and deposition occurs more commonly in the sclera (**C**). When it affects the cornea, depositions are localized usually at the level of epithelium and Bowman's layer.

54. Correct: Crystal violet dye (D)

The given figure reveals lattice lines present after corneal transplant, composed of amyloid, therefore it will stain with Congo red and crystal violet dye. Familial amyloidosis or Meretoja syndrome presents in the third to fourth decade of life. Clinical findings include "mask-like" facies, dermatochalasis, lagophthalmos, pendulous ears, cranial and peripheral nerve palsies, and dry skin with amyloid deposition. Corneal lattice lines are present, usually peripheral. Lattice can recur in corneal grafts. **A, B, and C** will not stain amyloid.

55. Correct: Sunflower cataract (B)

Wilson's disease is an autosomal recessive disorder linked to mutation ATP7b on chromosome 13 causing copper deposition in the liver, kidneys, brain, and Descemet's membrane, known as a Kayser–Fleischer ring (not Fleischer ring, which is an iron line seen in keratoconus, a). A sunflower cataract may be present. The cataract has a greenish central opacity of the anterior capsule with spoke-like radial cortical opacities. Patients present with liver cirrhosis, kidney failure, and parkinsonian-like symptoms. Polychromatic or christmas tree cataract presents in patients with myotonic dystrophy (**C**). Coats white ring is a circular or oval gray-white dot seen as remnant of metallic foreign body (**D**).

56. Correct: Protrusion below the area of thinning (A)

Ehlers–Danlos syndrome type VI (the oculo-scoliotic type), is an autosomal recessive disorder associated with joint and skin hyperextensibility, keratoconus, and keratoglobus. Keratoconus is characterized by irregular astigmatism, progressive inferior corneal thinning, and protrusion below or at the area of maximal thinning. Pellucid marginal degeneration presents with protrusion above the area of thinning (**B**) usually in the inferior cornea. Terrien's marginal degeneration reveals flattening of the peripheral thinned cornea with steeping 90 degrees away (**C**). Peripheral ulcerative keratitis can present with thinning in any quadrant of the cornea (**D**).

57. Correct: Superotemporal (C)

Marfan syndrome presents with ectopia lentis. Patients present with spontaneous or posttraumatic subluxation of their lens classically toward the superotemporal quadrant, though other directions (**A, B, and D**) are not uncommon. Homocystinuria is associated with inferonasal lens subluxation in 80% of the cases (**D**).

58. Correct: Eyelid coloboma (C)

Goldenhar–Gorlin syndrome (GGS) is a congenital condition characterized by incomplete development of the ear, nose, soft palate, lip, and mandible. Common clinical finding includes limbal dermoid, preauricular tags, strabismus, and eyelid colobomas. Corneal dermoid can cause corneal astigmatism as well as occlusion of the pupil, if large enough, both of which can cause amblyopia. GGS is not associated with optic nerve staphyloma, iris coloboma, or conjunctival nevi (**B, C, and D**).

59. Correct: Meretoja syndrome (D)

Meretoja syndrome presents with corneal lattice lines, which comprise amyloid, not enlarged corneal nerves. Multiple endocrine neoplasia type 2B, Refsum syndrome, Hansen's disease, and Riley–Day syndrome are associated with enlarged corneal nerves (**A, B, and C**).

60. Correct: Ethylenediaminetetraacetic acid (EDTA) chelation (A)

Xeroderma pigmentosum has been associated with gelatinous drop-like corneal dystrophy (GDLD) and keratoconus. GDLD is characterized by subepithelial stromal amyloid deposits. Onset occurs in the first to second decade of life. Findings are similar to those of band keratopathy, however EDTA is not part of the management as this is not related to calcium accumulation (**A**). GDLD management include medical management (lubrication) and surgical procedures including superficial keratectomy, lamellar keratoplasty, and penetrating keratoplasty (**B, C, and D**).

61. Correct: *Fusarium species* (A)

Few organisms can invade intact epithelium; these organisms include Neisseria gonorrhoeae, Neisseria meningitidis, Corynebacterium diphtheriae, Shigella, Haemophilus influenzae biotype III, Listeria monocytogenes, and Fusarium species. Fusarium is a filamentous fungus that may present with feathery or indistinct edges of the infiltrate; occasionally satellite infiltrates are found. Fungal keratitis presents with fewer symptoms compared to bacterial etiologies. Natamycin 5% is recommended. Systemic antifungals should be considered with intracameral fungal extension. Other options (**B, C, and D**) need an epithelial defect to invade corneal tissue. Candida keratitis (**B**) presents a superficial white plaque and responds better to amphotericin B (0.15–0.30%) suspension. Acanthamoeba keratitis (**C**) is associated to contact lens wear, presenting with severe ocular pain out of proportion to the initial presentation and a protracted clinical course. Acanthamoeba medical management includes diamidines (hexamidine), biguanides (polyhexamethylene biguanide, chlorhexidine), aminoglycosides (neomycin), and imidazoles (voriconazole miconazole, itraconazole, and ketoconazole). Pseudomonas keratitis (**D**) has a rapid onset of symptoms, presenting with a purulent stromal inflammation, severe anterior chamber reaction, and hypopyon.

62. Correct: Non-nutrient agar with *Escherichia coli (E. Coli)* overlay (A)

Prominent corneal nerves or radial perineuritis are nearly pathognomonic of amebic keratitis. The patient in question has been managed with broad-spectrum antibiotics without improvement, therefore, *Acanthamoeba* infection should be high on your differential especially given the history of contact lens wear. Non-nutrient agar with *E. coli* or *Enterobacter aerogenes* is the preferred culture media for *Acanthamoeba*. Sabouraud dextrose agar is a good media for fungus (**B**). Blood agar is a good media for most bacteria (**C**). GMS is a stain that can be used to identify fungi (**D**).

63. Correct: Atopic dermatitis (B)

Herpes simplex virus (HSV) keratitis is typically unilateral, but patients with atopy may present with bilateral HSV. Bilateral HSV is more common in primary than recurrent ocular infection. There is no proven relationships HSV and diabetes mellitus, HIV, and seborrheic dermatitis (**A, C, and D**).

64. Correct: Topical corticosteroids (C)

The combination of uveitis, elevated intraocular pressure, and corneal edema in this patient suggests a likely herpetic etiology. The Herpetic Eye Disease Study (HEDS) showed that topical corticosteroids given with a prophylactic antiviral significantly decreased stromal inflammation and shortened the duration of keratitis. Adding oral acyclovir (**A**) showed no benefit in the management of stromal keratitis when added to trifluridine and steroids. Valacyclovir was not used in HEDS (**B**). Topical trifluridine (**D**) alone was inferior when compared to topical steroid plus trifluridine in reducing keratitis duration, with no impact on uveitis duration.

65. Correct: Epstein-Barr virus (EBV) (B)

EBV is the most common cause of acute dacryoadenitis. It can also present with acute follicular conjunctivitis, Parinaud oculoglandular syndrome, and bulbar conjunctival nodules. EBV, also called human herpesvirus 5, is best known as the cause of infectious mononucleosis. Infection occurs by the oral transfer of saliva. The development of a maculopapular rash following amoxicillin intake is frequent in patient with infectious mononucleosis, ranging from 27 to 69%. The exact mechanism is not clear but is thought to be secondary to viral sensitization to the drug. Herpes simplex virus (**A**), herpes zoster virus (**C**), and adenovirus (**D**) are not typically associated with an amoxicillin-induced rash unless the patient has a true allergy to the antibiotic.

66. Correct: Doxycycline (B)

This patient may have Chlamydia trachomatis, which should be suspected in patients with recurrent follicular conjunctivitis despite adequate treatment. The differential diagnosis also includes toxic conjunctivitis from topical medications and molluscum contagiosum. Oral doxycycline can be used for 7 to 14 days. Some patients also respond well to azithromycin 1 g × 1 dose. Valacyclovir is used when herpes simplex virus is suspected (**A**). Systemic steroids and topical antibiotics are not indicated (**C, D**).

67. Correct: Gram-positive rods (C)

Propionibacterium species is the most common causative pathogen of chronic postoperative bacterial endophthalmitis. *Propionibacterium acnes* is an anaerobic gram-positive rod, commonly found on the eyelid skin or on the conjunctiva. *P. acnes* can present as a plaque on the posterior capsule and cause an indolent uveitis. The diagnosis is confirmed by obtaining aerobic, anaerobic, and fungal cultures of the aqueous, capsular plaques, and vitreous. *Staphylococcus epidermidis* (**A**) and *Corynebacterium* species (**B**) may also cause a similar chronic infection but are less common than *P. acnes* infection. *Neisseria gonorrhoeae* (**D**) causes a hyperacute conjunctivitis.

68. Correct: *Fusarium* (C)

Fungi are classically divided into 2 groups: yeast and mold. Molds can be septated, as in the case of *Fusarium* (**C**) or nonseptated, as in the case of *Mucor*, *Rhizopus*, and *Absidia* (**A, B**). Candida and cryptococcus are yeasts (**D**).

69. Correct: Staphylococcal marginal keratitis (C)

Staphylococcal marginal keratitis presents as peripheral infiltrates in the superficial cornea, often where the lids cross the cornea. Ulceration is in the marginal zone and separated from the limbus by a clear corneal zone as seen in the provided figure. Staphylococcal marginal keratitis is a hypersensitivity (inflammatory not infectious) reaction and responds very well to topical steroids. Mooren's ulcer is an autoimmune peripheral stromal ulceration with progressive stromal thinning; there is no separation between the ulceration and the limbus (**A**). Peripheral ulcerative keratitis is associated with systemic disease (rheumatoid arthritis, polyarteritis nodosa, systemic lupus erythematous), and presents with ulceration and stromal infiltration at the limbus with no separation between ulcer and limbus (**B**). Terrien's marginal degeneration is an idiopathic thinning of the peripheral corneal, painless and without inflammation, usually occurring superonasally bilaterally (**D**).

70. Correct: Ceftriaxone 1 g IV every 12 hours for 3 days plus topical vancomycin and tobramycin (C)

Hyperacute gonococcal conjunctivitis presents with explosive and rapid onset of purulent conjunctivitis including injection, chemosis, and severe eyelid edema. Corneal involvement may consist of diffuse epithelial haze, marginal infiltrates, and ulcerative keratitis that can progress to perforation. Patients with gonococcal conjunctivitis with corneal ulceration should be treated with ceftriaxone 1 g IV every 12 hours for 3 days along with fortified antibiotics if necessary. Patients are often treated with concomitant oral azithromycin, because coinfection with chlamydia is very common. Topical vancomycin with tobramycin or moxifloxacin are used to treat bacterial corneal ulcers not related to gonorrhea (**A, D**). Doxycycline (**B**) can be used for the treatment of gonorrhea; however, resistance has become more prevalent, therefore, ceftriaxone has become first line of treatment.

71. Correct: Neisseria gonorrhea (B)

Neonatal gonococcal conjunctivitis presents as a hyperacute purulent conjunctivitis between 3 to 5 days of life. In severe cases, it can present as keratitis with a high risk of perforation, endophthalmitis, or systemic infection. *Chlamydia trachomatis* and *Pseudomonas aeruginosa* present between 5 and 14 days of life (**A, D**). Herpes simplex virus presents after 2 weeks of life (**C**).

72. Correct: Azithromycin (A)

Trachoma is caused by *Chlamydia trachomatis* serotypes A–C. Initial symptoms include foreign body sensation, redness, tearing, and mucopurulent discharge. Patients present with large tarsal follicles, linear scarring of the superior tarsus (Arlt line), and Herbert's pits, which are necrotic follicles that progress to corneal limbal depressions. The description of the round scars in the question stem refers to Herbert's pits. Trachoma requires at least two of the following criteria: follicles on the upper tarsal conjunctival, limbal follicles, tarsal conjunctival scarring, and/or vascular pannus. Management consist of macrolides or tetracyclines. Ceftriaxone, acyclovir, and vancomycin (**B, C, and D**) are not appropriate treatments for trachoma.

73. Correct: Streptococcus viridans (C)

Infectious crystalline keratopathy (ICK) is a rare infection of the cornea that results in gray-white branching stromal opacities. ICK is associated with chronic use of topical steroids. The most common pathogen is *S. viridans*. Obtaining adequate samples through a corneal scraping can be difficult because the bacteria harbors below an intact epithelium, sometimes at the level of deep stroma. Diagnostic keratectomy provides a higher yield. Histology slides reveal aggregates of gram-positive cocci within the anterior stroma. Treatment in patients with previous penetrating keratoplasty consists of steroid taper, aggressive antibiotic regimens, and in refractory cases graft excision with repeat penetrating keratoplasty. **A, B, and D** have not been associated with ICK.

74. Correct: Vancomycin (D)

Lowenstein–Jensen is a growth media used for mycobacteria. Atypical mycobacteria are important pathogens following laser in situ keratomileusis, characterized by a protracted course requiring a prolonged treatment with antifungal therapy. Vancomycin inhibits bacterial cell wall synthesis but does not have antimycobacterial activity. Clarithromycin, amikacin, and linezolid (**A, B, and C**) are appropriate treatment modalities for mycobacteria. Fluoroquinolones can also be used.

75. Correct: Gram-positive rods (A)

Bitot's spots are patches of dry looking conjunctiva with overlying frothy material composed of colonies of *Corynebacterium*, a gram-positive rod. It is associated with vitamin A deficiency, xerophthalmia, which also manifests with nyctalopia, conjunctival and corneal xerosis, and keratomalacia. The remaining answers are not associated with bitot's spots.

76. Correct: Lowenstein–Jensen medium (C)

This medium is used to isolate *Mycobacteria*, a weak gram positive, aerobic, nonmotile, acid fast rod. Atypical *Mycobacteria*, including *Mycobacterium fortuitum* and *M. chelonae*, are associated with post-LASIK keratitis in up to 30% of reported cases. LASIK keratitis is characterized by a delayed and protracted onset of nonsuppurative infiltrates. Bloor agar (**A**) isolates *Haemophilus influenzae*, *Streptococcus pneumoniae*, and *Neisseria*. MacConkey agar (**B**) isolates Enterobacteriaceae. Thayer Martin agar (**D**) isolates *Neisseria gonorrhoeae*.

77. Correct: Trachoma (D)

Granulomatous conjunctivitis in association with preauricular lymphadenopathy is known as Parinaud oculoglandular syndrome. Granulomatous conjunctivitis has been associated with bacteria such as *M. tuberculosis* (**A**), and *Francisella tularensis* (**C**). Conjunctival biopsy typically reveals infectious granulomas with central necrosis. Sarcoidosis is a noninfectious cause of chronic granulomatous conjunctivitis (**B**). Trachoma (**D**), caused by *Chlamydia trachomatis*, presents with chronic follicular conjunctivitis, Herbert's pits, and tarsal conjunctival scarring.

78. Correct: Pseudomonas aeruginosa (D)

Bacterial keratitis in contact lens wearers is a common sight-threatening condition, presenting with a sudden onset of pain and often decreased vision. The corneal infiltrate can lead to tissue necrosis and perforation if left untreated. The most common cause of bacterial keratitis in contact lens wearers is *P. aeruginosa*. *Acanthamoeba* (**A**) is a protozoan found in freshwater and soil associated with ~ 90% of contact lens wearers, however *P. aeruginosa* is more frequently encountered as the cause of infection. *Streptococcus viridans* (**C**) has been associated with infectious crystalline keratopathy. *Staphylococcus aureus* (**B**) has been linked to bacterial keratitis, however the clinical presentation of the patient is most likely due to pseudomonas.

79. Correct: Obtain confocal microscopy (C)

Corneal ulcers not improving on empiric fortified antibiotics should raise the suspicion for other etiologies, including fungal keratitis and *Acanthamoeba*. On confocal microscopy, fungal keratitis can be seen as branching filaments or individual septa. The cysts of *Acanthamoeba* can often also be identified on confocal microscopy. Steroids should not be used in the absence of appropriate antibiotic therapy (**A**). Penetrating keratoplasty is indicated if the disease progresses despite adequate therapy or in the setting of perforation (**B**). Changing to fluoroquinolones would not provide as broad a coverage as the fortified antibiotics (**D**), and this patient is already showing worsening on appropriate antibiotic therapy.

80. Correct: Natamycin (D)

Fungal cell walls stain with Gomori methenamine silver. Fungal keratitis often begins with fewer inflammatory signs and symptoms than bacterial keratitis, but over time intense suppuration develops with rapidly progressive hypopyon and anterior chamber reaction. Fungus grows well on sabouraud dextrose agar. Natamycin (**D**) is recommended for the treatment of fungal keratitis; other options include amphotericin (which is very good against yeast) and voriconazole. Tobramycin (**A**) and vancomycin (**B**) are indicated in the management of bacterial keratitis. Moxifloxacin (**C**) is a fourth-generation fluoroquinolone with some activity against atypical mycobacterial coverage, but voriconazole is the best option.

81. Correct: Hypersensitivity type IV (D)

Contact dermatoblepharitis can be due to type I (immediate) or type IV hypersensitivity (delayed). Type IV hypersensitivity or cell-mediated response usually begins 24 to 72 hours following instillation of a topical agent resulting in a chronic allergic reaction seen in the question stem. This can sometimes lead to hyperpigmentation and scarring if the agent is not discontinued. Trifluridine is a topical antiviral for the treatment of epithelial keratitis caused by HSV. It is one of the many agents associated with contact dermatoblepharitis. Allergic conjunctivitis is a type of type I or immediate hypersensitivity and occurs within minutes after exposure to an allergen (**A**). Type I is mediated by immunoglobulin E and mast cell release. Mucous membrane pemphigoid is a type II or cytotoxic hypersensitivity, in which autoantibodies are found in the basement membrane zone (**B**). Type III hypersensitivity reactions are the result of immune complex deposition (antigen–antibody complex), with examples including reactions like scleritis and subepithelial infiltrates (**C**).

82. Correct: Azithromycin (B)

Vernal keratoconjunctivitis (VKC) is an atopic condition of the anterior segment. It usually affects young males in a seasonal manner (peaking around spring time). VKC can be due to hypersensitivity type I or type IV reactions. Patients present with itching, photophobia, blurred vision, and mucoid discharge. Some of the characteristic manifestations of VKC include giant papillae resembling cobblestones (see figure i), Horner-Trantas dots, aggregates of eosinophils, and epithelial cells at the limbus (see figure ii), pannus or shield ulcer (a noninfectious epithelial ulcer with underlying stromal opacification in the superior cornea). Therapy includes topical antihistamines, steroids, cyclosporine, or tacrolimus (**A, C, and D**). Azithromycin (**B**) is used to treat trachoma.

83. Correct: Amniotic membrane graft (D)

Steven Johnson syndrome (SJS) is a hypersensitivity reaction to infectious agents or drugs. SJS pathogenesis consists of keratinocyte cell apoptosis via the perforin–granzyme pathway. Bullous lesions appear in mucous membranes of the eyes, mouth, and genitalia. All the options mentioned are part of the management of SJS patients; however, during the acute phase if there is conjunctival involvement and corneal involvement, amniotic membrane graft has been proven to provide a significant long-term benefit. If left untreated, significant long-term conjunctival and corneal scarring may develop.

84. Correct: Rapidly progressive skin exfoliation and target-like lesions (A)

Steven Johnson syndrome (SJS) is the result of a hypersensitivity reaction to medication or infection. Several drugs have been identified, including antiepileptics such as phenytoin, valproic acid, phenobarbital, and carbamazepine. Patients initially present with prodromal symptoms of fever, malaise, cough, arthralgias, anorexia, and/or headaches. Conjunctivitis might occur 1 to 3 days before skin lesions appear. Intense erythema progressing to epidermolysis, mucous membrane erosion, and severe pain might occur. SJS is a rapidly progressive condition with skin exfoliation and target-like lesions leading to severe dehydration, hypovolemic shock and death, if left untreated. Impetigo is an acute, contagious infection of the superficial epidermis. It presents as honey-colored crusted lesions due to *Streptococcus pyogenes* or *Staphylococcus aureus* (**B**). Scarlet fever, also caused by *S. pyogenes*, is characterized by exudative pharyngitis, fever, and an exanthem (**C**). Erythema multiforme is an acute and self-limited skin type IV hypersensitivity reaction to medication and infections; it presents as localized raised eruptions (**D**) of the skin with minimal or no mucosal involvement.

85. Correct: IgA localized to the epidermis (A)

Mucous membrane pemphigoid (MMP), also known as ocular cicatricial pemphigoid, is a hypersensitivity type II reaction, in which autoantibodies (IgA, IgG, IgM, or complement 3) are directed against the basement membrane, not the epidermis as in pemphigus vulgaris (**A**). The disease is characterized by subepithelial fibrosis, loss of goblet cells, and shortening of the fornices. Later stages present with symblepharon, restricted extraocular movements due to adhesions, punctal stenosis, ectropion, trichiasis, corneal neovascularization, and/or corneal perforation. MMP is a systemic disease. Mild cases can be managed with topical therapy, including lubrication, steroids, cyclosporine, and tacrolimus, but these therapies will only provide symptomatic relief (**C**). Cyclophosphamide (**B**) remains the mainstay of therapy when sight is threatened. Surgical reconstructive procedures (**D**) should wait until immunosuppression is initiated and the patient's inflammatory process is controlled.

86. Correct: Keratoprosthesis (D)

Ocular graft versus host disease is a complication of allogeneic bone marrow transplantation. Graft cells attack the transplanted patient's tissues, including skin, gut, lungs, liver, gastrointestinal tract, and eyes. Management includes aggressive lubrication, punctal occlusion, mucolytic agents, bandage contact lenses, topical cyclosporine, or tacrolimus (**A, B**). PROSE scleral lens is an option for the management of complex corneal disease. It is a custom-made lens for the patient which serves as a fluid reservoir, improving corneal stability and healing (**C**). Keratoprosthesis, or replacement of the cornea with an artificial cornea, would not be indicated as a next step in management for this patient (**D**).

87. Correct: Conjunctivitis (B)

Reactive arthritis is a disorder characterized by ocular, urethral, and joint inflammation. It (previously called Reiter's syndrome) occurs after dysentery due to gram-negative bacteria or nongonococcal urethritis. Ocular manifestations include scleritis, conjunctivitis, keratitis and iridocyclitis (**A, C, and D**), but the most common ocular finding is bilateral papillary conjunctivitis with mucopurulent discharge.

88. Correct: Dramatic response to low-dose steroids (B)

Thygeson's superficial punctate keratitis is characterized by multiple intraepithelial opacities extending to the anterior stroma. These lesions are usually bilateral, found in the central cornea, and multiple in number (20–40 elevated lesions) with negative staining. Patients present with tearing, photophobia, burning, and foreign body sensation during episodes. It has been linked to immune and viral etiologies. Lesions respond dramatically to low-dose steroids with recurrences after tapering attempts (**B**). Recurrent corneal erosions present as sudden episodes of eye pain, usually at night or upon awakening. Most of the times patients have minimal findings on exam or very faint fluorescein staining, as the irregular epithelium heals very quickly. Management consists of aggressive lubrication, patching, hypertonic agents, or short-term use of steroids. Surgical interventions include stromal micropuncture or phototherapeutic keratectomy (PTK). Exposure keratopathy is characterized by coalescing punctate epithelial erosions, and are often interpalpebral in location due to ineffective lid closure (**A**). Punctate epithelial erosions stain positively with fluorescein and tend to be inferiorly based (**D**). Macular corneal dystrophy consists of superficial, irregular, whitish stromal opacities with intervening haze (**C**). Lesions usually progress to involve all layers of the cornea and extend to the corneal periphery.

89. Correct: Cogan's syndrome (B)

Cogan's syndrome is a rare autoimmune disease characterized by progressive ocular and audiovestibular symptoms. It is usually associated with a nontreponemal interstitial keratitis, though multiple cases of scleritis and uveitis had been reported. Cogan's syndrome is a diagnosis of exclusion. Patients presenting with hearing loss and ocular posterior findings should be managed with systemic steroids. Susac syndrome is characterized by hearing loss, branch retinal artery occlusions, and encephalopathy (**A**). Vogt-Koyanagi–Harada syndrome is a bilateral granulomatous panuveitis associated with alopecia, poliosis, and dysacusia (**C**). Sarcoidosis is characterized by a granulomatous uveitis and scleritis (**D**). Patients with sarcoidosis may have bilateral hilar lymphadenopathies and elevated angiotensin-converting enzyme (ACE) or lysozyme levels. Sarcoid can infiltrate cranial nerve VIII and cause hearing loss.

90.   Correct: Autoimmune panel (D)

The differential diagnosis for peripheral corneal ulceration includes: peripheral ulcerative keratitis, Mooren's ulcer, Terrien's marginal degeneration, senile furrow degeneration, pellucid marginal degeneration, and herpetic disease. The patient in the question presents with joint inflammation and deformities raising concerns for rheumatoid arthritis. Rheumatoid arthritis is strongly associated with peripheral ulcerative keratitis (PUK; 32–42%). PUK presents as a crescent-shaped juxtalimbal corneal lesion with overlying epithelial defect leading to descemetocele and corneal perforation. Anterior segment fluorescein angiography (**A**) is used for the diagnosis and differentiation of anterior segment tumors. Corneal topography (**B**) is not indicated in the acute phase of PUK. Corneal biopsy (**C**) can be useful in elucidating infectious etiologies.

91.   Correct: Hepatitis C virus (B)

Mooren's ulcer is a painful peripheral ulceration of unknown etiology that has been associated with hepatitis C. The ulcer starts in the periphery and spreads circumferentially and centrally over months. The bed of the ulcer becomes vascularized, ultimately progressing to stromal thinning and perforation. The diagnosis requires the absence of any ocular infection or systemic rheumatologic disease. The medical treatment typically includes topical and systemic immunosuppression. Surgical approaches include limbal conjunctival excision and lamellar keratoplasty. Rheumatoid arthritis, rosacea, syphilis, and tuberculosis have been associated with peripheral ulcerative keratitis (**A, C, and D**).

92.   Correct: Infliximab (D)

Infliximab is a chimeric monoclonal antibody against tumor necrosis alpha used to treat autoimmune diseases. Conjunctival papillomas are composed of multiple branching fronds emanating from a pedunculated base with a central vascularized core, and are most frequently associated with HPV 6 and 11. In cases of recurrence, adjunct therapies to surgical excision include: cryotherapy, dinitrochlorobenzene, interferon, mitomycin-C, or cimetidine (**A, B, and C**).

93.   Correct: Hyperreflective thickened epithelium with a transition zone can be seen on anterior segment OCT (D)

The patient's exam is concerning for conjunctival intraepithelial neoplasia (CIN). CIN is considered a premalignant condition which stays superficial to Bowman's layer (**C**). There are three types: papilliform, gelatinous, and leukoplakic. CIN has been associated with ultraviolet light exposure, immunosuppression (**A**), and human papillomavirus. Patients are usually unaware of the lesion initially. Approximately 95% occur at the limbus (**B**). Corneal involvement is the result of the spread of abnormal epithelium from the adjacent limbus. OCT (**D**) can reveal a hyperreflective, thickened epithelium with an abrupt transition from normal to abnormal tissue. CIN can be managed with topical chemotherapy or surgical excision with a "no touch" technique.

94.   Correct: 1 in 400 (C)

Ocular melanocytosis is a focal proliferation of subepithelial melanocytes. It presents as episcleral slate gray pigmentation, usually immobile and unilateral. The lifetime risk of uveal melanoma is about 1 in 400. All the other options are incorrect.

95.   Correct: Melanoma arising from primary acquired melanosis (A)

Melanoma may arise from PAM (70%), nevi (5%), or de novo (25%). Lesions are usually found in the bulbar conjunctiva or at the limbus. Poor prognostic indicators include: nonlimbal locations, invasion into deeper tissues, thickness > 1.8 mm, involvement of the eyelid margin, pagetoid spread, lymphatic invasion, and mixed cell type (**B, C, and D**). Treatment should be initiated promptly given the risk of metastasis.

96.   Correct: Pyogenic granuloma (D)

Pyogenic granuloma is a reactive hemangioma characterized by granulation tissue and proliferation of immature capillary channels. Pyogenic granulomas are red, pedunculated growths with a smooth surface. Management consists of surgical excision or topical/intralesional steroids. Juvenile xanthogranuloma (**B**) is a histiocytic disorder. Fibrous histiocytoma (**C**) is composed of fibroblasts and histiocytes with lipid vacuoles. Necrobiotic xanthogranuloma (**A**) is a rare histiocytic disease characterized by foamy histiocytes and giant cells.

97.   Correct: Kaposi's sarcoma (A)

Kaposi's sarcoma is a malignant neoplasm of vascular endothelium associated with herpes virus 8. It is commonly associated with AIDS, organ transplantation, or any other immunosuppressive state. It may present as

41

a reddish subconjunctival lesion. Therapeutic options include surgical debulking, radiotherapy, and/or chemotherapy. Episcleritis is usually acute and transient (**C**). Subconjunctival hemorrhage and viral conjunctivitis usually resolve in a few weeks (**B**).

98. Correct: Conjunctival biopsy (B)

Benign lymphoid hyperplasia and conjunctival lymphoma are commonly misdiagnosed as chronic follicular conjunctivitis. It presents as salmon-colored subepithelial tumor with a pebbly appearance. Given the fact that the patient had been treated chronically with steroids without improvement, the next step in management is to obtain a conjunctival biopsy. Benign lymphoid hyperplasia can be clinically indistinguishable from conjunctival lymphoma. Continuing the same management (**A**) will not supply the underlying diagnosis. Increasing the potency could be an appropriate change in therapy, but a diagnosis should be obtained first (**C**). Obtaining a viral swab is not indicated (**D**).

99. Correct: Place amniotic membrane (C)

Alkali burns are more severe than acid exposure, with a higher chance of corneal melting and perforation. Alkali are lipophilic and continue to cause necrosis until the agent is removed by irrigation. Acids coagulate protein, hence producing a natural barrier to penetration. Visual prognosis depends on the extent of ocular surface injury. The patient in question is likely a grade III on the severity score—severe corneal haze and extensive limbal ischemia. The most important step in the management of chemical injuries is irrigation. Early amniotic membrane transplant has been shown to lead to better final visual acuity in patients with moderate to severe burns than medicine alone. While frequent artificial tears (**D**) may also be helpful, particularly in less severe burns, the patient in this question stem has limbal ischemia and is at high risk for corneal scarring. A bandage contact lens (**A**) can be helpful in healing epithelial defects but should be used with caution in patients with chemical injury as it may trap residual chemical and lead to further ischemia. A tarsorrhaphy (**B**) in this acute phase is not beneficial.

100. Correct: Limbal epithelial transplantation (D)

For a patient with alkali burn with extensive damage, limbal cell transplantation is the best option, especially given the patient in question with unilateral damage. The stem cells can be harvested from her healthy eye. Grafts (**A, B, and C**) are most likely to fail given the loss of goblet and limbal cells. Most patients are better candidates for keratoplasty or keratoprosthesis after limbal cell repopulation.

101. Correct: Acetazolamide 500 mg bid (C)

Chemical burns should always be managed initially with copious irritation until normalization of the pH. The second stage of management should be aimed at decreasing inflammation, controlling intraocular pressure, and promoting healing. In the early stages, an increase in intraocular pressure might occur, which should be controlled with oral lowering agents (**C**) as all possible surface irritants should be avoided (**A, B, and D**).

102. Correct: UV-A (A)

Ultraviolet radiation (UVR) can be divided in UV-A, B, and C. UV-C is absorbed by ozone in the atmosphere, thus terrestrial light is composed of UV-A (96%) and UV-B (4%). The patient in question has snow blindness or photokeratitis due to UVR exposure. Shorter wavelengths such as UV-B are primarily absorbed by the corneal epithelium (**B**) and longer wavelengths such as UV-A (**A**) can penetrate the entire thickness of the cornea and reach the lens (and is used in the treatment of keratoconus). Management of photokeratitis includes patching, aggressive lubrication, and cycloplegia.

103. Correct: IOP average > 60 mm Hg for 2 days (A)

Traumatic hyphema results from injury to the vessels of the peripheral iris, iris sphincter, or anterior ciliary body. Prognosis is generally good even in cases with total hyphema. Surgical intervention is indicated to prevent optic atrophy, corneal blood staining, or peripheral anterior synechia. To prevent optic atrophy, surgical intervention is indicated for IOP averages of > 60 mm Hg for 2 days (**A**) or > 35 mm Hg for 7 days. To prevent corneal blood staining, surgery is indicated with an IOP average > 25 mm Hg for 5 days, not 4 days (**B**). To prevent peripheral anterior synechiae (PAS), a total hyphema that persists for 5 days, not 1 day (**C**) or any hyphema that fails to resolve < 50% within 8 days (**D**), should be surgically cleared. Note that indications for surgical intervention for traumatic hyphema in sickle cell patients are stricter, including IOP > 25 mm Hg for 24 hours or IOP with transient elevations to > 30 mm Hg for 2 to 4 days, despite medical intervention.

104. Correct: Hemoglobin electrophoresis (B)

Traumatic hyphema in African American patient should prompt a sickle cell work-up. Sickle cell patients are prone to more complications, including corneal blood staining and elevated intraocular pressure (IOP) due to restricted outflow in the trabecular meshwork. Indications for surgical intervention for traumatic hyphema in sickle cell patients include IOP > 25 mm Hg for 24 hours or IOP with transient elevations to > 30 mm Hg for 2 to 4 days, despite medical intervention. Clotting abnormalities, interocular lens abnormalities, and herpes infection are causes of spontaneous hyphema (**A, B, and D**).

105. Correct: Contact lens trial (D)

Contact lenses can be used to correct anisometropia after sutures have been removed. After removal of all sutures, relaxing incisions (**A**) can help with residual astigmatism, but would not eliminate anisometropia. Refractive surgery (**B and C**), especially photorefractive keratectomy (**C**) can be used, but it would be helpful to understand if his symptoms are eliminated with a contact lens. A contact lens also offers a long-term alternative solution.

106. Correct: Cataract surgery should be performed after suture removal is completed (C)

In this patient with early cataracts, blurry vision may indeed be from a worsening cataract, but her final visual refraction and astigmatism has yet to be optimized with suture removal (**B**). Sutures should be removed to determine final corneal astigmatism and better inform IOL calculation, should cataract extraction still be indicated (**A**). Penetrating keratoplasty is not a contraindication for cataract surgery (**D**).

107. Correct: Light scattering (A)

Reduced postoperative visual acuity can be due to preexisting corneal pathologies and light scattering due to long-standing corneal edema and the graft–host interface. Small incision is an advantage of DSAEK over penetrating keratoplasty (**B**). DSAEK is associated with preservation of the anterior corneal curvature and thickening of the posterior corneal curvature (**C**). Penetrating keratoplasty is associated with higher astigmatism compare to DSAEK (**D**).

108. Correct: Rebubbling in the office (B)

The risk for DSAEK dislocation has been reported as high as 14.5% within the first 1 to 2 days. Immediate rebubbling has been advocated if there is significant detachment to restore the donor–host interface. Detached DSAEKs might spontaneously reattach (**A**); however, rebubbling provides better outcomes for graft success, especially if there is substantial detachment. Prednisolone acetate is used to manage corneal edema and prevent rejection (**C**). DSAEK replacement may be indicated if rebubbling fails or if there is a late detachment presentation with decreased best-corrected visual acuity (**D**).

109. Correct: Eye drop toxicity (D)

Eye drop toxicity presents with inferior or diffuse punctate epithelial erosions. All the other options are associated with superior punctate epithelial erosions. Vernal keratoconjunctivitis (**A**) is a recurrent, bilateral disorder presenting with upper tarsal conjunctival hyperemia and diffuse velvety papillary hypertrophy that evolves into cobblestones and giant papillae; it is associated with limbal disease (Horner-Trantas dots) and superior punctate epithelial erosions. Superior limbic keratoconjunctivitis (**B**) is associated with thyroid eye disease, possibly due to blink-related trauma, tear film insufficiency, and excess laxity of conjunctival tissue leading to a hyperemic band of superior bulbar conjunctiva and punctate epithelial erosions separated from the limbus by a zone of normal epithelium. Floppy eyelid syndrome (**C**) presents as extreme laxity of the eyelids; easy eversion of the eyelids, and lids that can be pulled away easily from the eye.

110. Correct: Giant papillae (B)

Vernal keratoconjunctivitis (VKC) is a recurrent and bilateral disorder. It primarily affects boys and the onset is usually in early childhood. VKC can present as upper tarsal conjunctival hyperemia and diffuse velvety papillary hypertrophy that evolves into cobblestones and giant papillae, limbal disease (Horner-Trantas dots), or keratopathy. Keratopathy most frequently is associated with palpebral disease and presents as superior punctate epithelial erosions, epithelial macroerosions, plaques, and shield ulcers. Mechanical irritation from giant papillae and eye rubbing may predispose to shield ulcers. Arlt's line (**A**) is associated with trachoma. Pseudomembranes (**C**) are a fibrin-rich exudate lacking blood or lymphatic vessels resulting from an inflammatory state, seen commonly with epidemic keratoconjunctivitis. Herbert's pits (**D**) are superior limbal shallow depressions in trachoma.

111. Correct: McCoy cell culture (A)

Adult chlamydial conjunctivitis is an oculogenital infection caused by serotypes D–K. *Chlamydia trachomatis* cannot replicate extracellularly, and therefore depends on a host. McCoy cells are applied to a culture of microorganisms dependent on a eukaryotic host. Polymerase chain reaction, when available, can also be used to detect chlamydia. Clinical presentation is characterized by a watery or mucopurulent discharge, tender preauricular lymphadenopathy, and follicular reaction. Corneal findings include superficial punctate keratitis, perilimbal subepithelial corneal infiltrates, and a superficial pannus. Giemsa staining reveals basophilic intracytoplasmic bodies. Sabouraud agar (**B**) is used for Fungi. Non-nutrient agar with *E. coli* (**C**) is used for *Acanthamoeba*. Lowenstein–Jensen (**D**) is used for *Mycobacteria* and *Nocardia*.

112.   Correct: Exposed Bowman's membrane (D)

The question stem here describes atopic keratoconjunctivitis (AKC). AKC typically develops in adulthood following a history of atopy. The patient in question presents with atopic findings of the eyelids (erythema, scaliness, thickening, and inferior tarsal findings). AKC has been associated with anterior and posterior subcapsular cataracts (**A**), higher risk of retinal detachment than the rest of the population (**B**), and Dennie–Morgan folds (**D**) caused by persistent rubbing. Vernal keratoconjunctivitis (VKC) is more common in young boys and findings usually involve superior tarsus and upper third of the cornea. Shield ulcers (**D**) are areas of exposed Bowman's membrane that are sometimes coated with mucus and calcium in patients with VKC.

113.   Correct: Reconstructive surgery is indicated in this patient (C)

Mucous membrane pemphigoid is a type II hypersensitivity response characterized by antibodies binding the basement membrane. Conjunctival features include: chronic papillary conjunctivitis, an initial subtle fibrosis leading to symblepharon, plica flattening, and keratinization of the caruncle if left untreated. Patients initially complain of dry eye related symptoms due to the loss of goblet cells or foreign body sensation due to aberrant lashes. Corneal examination reveals epithelial defects and peripheral vascularization; these progress to keratinization and conjunctivalization of the cornea due to stem cell failure (**B**). Dapsone is usually first line of treatment (**A**) in mild to moderate cases. Systemic steroids are usually used for rapid disease control. Subconjunctival mitomycin (**D**) or steroid injection can be used as temporary options in patients who cannot tolerate systemic treatment. The patient in the question stem presents with active disease, therefore, reconstructive surgery is not indicated. Surgery may be required in some patients, but only after treatment and stabilization of the underlying condition.

114.   Correct: Frequent topical lubricants without amniotic membrane (D)

Steven Johnson syndrome patients benefit from early surgical management with amniotic membrane to prevent conjunctival and corneal keratinization. Early amniotic membrane graft has been shown to be anti-inflammatory, promote epithelial cell migration, inhibit epithelial cell apoptosis, and suppress scar formation and neovascularization. Early use, within 2 to 3 weeks of the beginning of symptoms, has the highest yield in preventing complications. Amniotic membrane can be fixated with sutures or glue (**B, C**). Prokera ring is a polycarbonate ring with amniotic membrane across the lumen (**A**). The patient in question has signs of early epitheliopathy and conjunctival reaction which can result in devastating surface complications, so topical lubrication is not enough.

115.   Correct: Superior bulbar conjunctiva that stain with fluorescein but not with rose Bengal (A)

Superior limbic keratoconjunctivitis (SLK) presents with papillary hypertrophy of the superior tarsal plate, and stains with rose Bengal and fluorescein. Corneal findings present in the superior third including punctate corneal epithelial erosions, superior filamentary keratitis and pannus. Acetylcysteine can be used to break down filaments (**B**) and retinoic acid can be used to prevent keratinization (**C**). Approximately 3% of patients with thyroid eye disease have SLK (**D**).

116.   Correct: Antifibrinolytic drugs are part of the management (C)

Ligneous conjunctivitis presents as bilateral membranous lesions on the tarsal conjunctiva associated with systemic involvement including periodontal tissue, respiratory tract, kidneys, and female genitalia. Histopathology reveals amorphous subepithelial deposits of eosinophilic material consisting of fibrin (**A**). It is important to discontinue any antifibrinolytic drug (**C**) given plasmin-mediated fibrinolysis deficiency has been associated with this disease. Very careful and complete surgical removal is indicated as the lesion can grow back if not completely removed (**B**). Excision should be followed by topical heparin and steroids until epithelialization. Amniotic membrane transplant can be used to promote healing and prevent scarring after removal of lesions (**D**).

117.   Correct: Sectoral superior stromal inflammation is often seen in early disease (D)

Interstitial keratitis is an immune-mediated stromal inflammation commonly related to congenital syphilis and less so to acquired syphilis. It begins as a sectoral superior stromal inflammation with granulomatous anterior uveitis, progressing to limbitis, stromal vascularization, and clouding (salmon patch appearance). It usually manifests between ages 5 and 25 years (**A**), not at birth. If a patient less than 2 years of age presents with concerns for interstitial keratitis, infectious causes should be entertained including *Mycobacterium tuberculosis*, *M. leprae*, *Borrelia burgdorferi*, Measles, Epstein–Barr virus, *Chlamydia trachomatis*, *Leishmania*, herpes simplex virus, and *Onchocerca volvulus*. Interstitial keratitis following congenital syphilis is bilateral in 80% (**C**) and is associated with ghost vessels (**B**), not enlarged corneal nerves. Ghost vessels are part of the chronic phase of interstitial keratitis. Other chronic changes include with stromal scarring, thinning, astigmatism, and band keratopathy.

118. Correct: Stromal marginal infiltrates with no clearing space from the limbus (B)

Marginal keratitis is thought to be a hypersensitivity reaction to *Staphylococcus* (**A**); patients usually have a history of chronic blepharitis. It is characterized by epitheliopathy that progresses to subepithelial marginal infiltrates with a clear space between the infiltrate and limbus (**B**). Despite the intense reaction in areas of involvement, the cornea is usually clear and there is mild to no anterior chamber reaction (**C**). Treatment consists of low-potency steroid drops to hasten recovery (**D**). Long-term treatment includes control of blepharitis.

119. Correct: Lamellar or penetrating keratoplasty for severe cases may be necessary (C)

Terrien's marginal degeneration is an idiopathic thinning of the peripheral cornea. It is usually bilateral but can be very asymmetric. It usually affects those older than 40 years. The thinning initially begins in the superonasal cornea and spreads circumferentially, separated from the limbus by a clear zone. Slit lamp findings include a fine vascular pannus, superior thinning, and lipid deposits. Corneal topography reveals flattening of the peripheral thinned corneal with steepening 90 degrees away from the midpoint of the thinned area, causing a high against-the-rule or oblique astigmatism, as noted with the patient on this question stem. It is important to distinguish pseudopterygium from pterygium; the latter has edges that can be elevated with forceps and causes with-the-rule astigmatism. A true pterygium arises from elastotic degeneration of the conjunctiva (**A**); a pseudopterygium arises from destruction of the marginal corneal epithelium. A true pterygium should not cause significant corneal thinning. Pterygia should not be excised with bare sclera (**B**). Studies have found lower recurrence rates with amniotic membrane or conjunctival autograft. Option d refers to topographic findings consistent with keratoconus.

120. Correct: Mucoid strands stain well with fluorescein and to a lesser extend with rose Bengal (B)

Filamentary keratopathy occurs due to a deposition of mucus in areas of loose epithelium. It has been associated with keratoconjunctivitis sicca, excessive contact lens wear (as in the patient in question stem), corneal epithelial instability (postsurgical and refractive patients), superior limbic keratoconjunctivitis, thyroid eye disease (**A**), bullous keratopathy, and neurotrophic keratopathy. Filaments stain well with rose Bengal and to a lesser extent with fluorescein. Treatment consists of managing the underlying causes, mechanical removal (**D**) to provide symptomatic relief, mucolytics (**C**), lubrication, sodium chloride drops, nonsteroidal anti-inflammatory drops, and bandage contact lenses.

121. Correct: Small-diameter grafts are associated with lower tendency to cause peripheral anterior synechiae (C)

A common graft size is 8 mm; smaller grafts—not larger—give high astigmatism (**A**). The donor button is usually about 0.25 to 0.50 mm larger in diameter than host tissue (**B**). Donor cornea should always be prepared before excision of host cornea (**D**).

122. Correct: Pseudodendrites (D)

Fabry disease is an X-linked lysosomal storage disease caused by deficiency of the enzyme alpha-galactosidase. Systemic manifestations include acroparesthesias, angiokeratomas, cardiomyopathies, and renal disease. Ocular manifestations include vortex keratopathy (**A**), wedge-shaped posterior cataracts (**B**), corkscrew vessels and conjunctival aneurysms (**C**). Pseudodendrites are associated with tyrosinemia, not with Fabry disease.

123. Correct: Incisions are placed in the steep meridian (A)

Limbal relaxing incisions (LRI) are partial thickness incisions made at the corneal periphery for the treatment of corneal astigmatism. LRIs are incisions set at approximately 600 μm depth or 50 μm less than the thinnest pachymetry measurement at the limbus (**B**). Incisions are placed just anterior to the limbus at the steep axis. Coupling refers to a compensatory steepening at the meridian 90 degrees away from the LRIs; coupling ratio is the relationship of the flat meridian divided by the steep meridian. When this ratio is greater than 1.0, a hyperopic shift occurs (**C**). Increasing the length, not the depth, of LRIs increases the magnitude of astigmatic correction (**D**). Arcuate keratotomy is another incisional surgical procedure made at the steep meridians of the midperiphery of the cornea (7 mm zone) with a greater depth compared to LRI's.

124. Correct: Corneal curvature becomes flat in the center and steeper in the periphery (B)

Radial keratotomy is now considered an obsolete procedure; however, many previously treated patients are now in need of cataract surgery, which can pose a challenge for cataract surgeons due to IOL calculations. Radial keratotomy consists of radial incisions made with a diamond knife in the corneal stroma leading to a change in corneal topography—flattening in the center and steepening in the periphery or an oblate cornea. It was one of the first refractive surgeries to treat −1.0 to −4.00 of myopia, but is complicated by spherical aberrations, diurnal fluctuation of vision due to hypoxic edema of the incisions during sleep leading to hyperopic shift upon awakening, and a progressive flattening effect leading to a hyperopic shift noted with smaller optical zones, not larger

(**D**). The PERK study found a hyperopic shift of 1.00 or greater in 43% of radial keratotomy patients (**C**). Cataract extraction can be challenging because cases are complicated by higher risk of corneal edema despite gentle phacoemulsification and difficult intraocular lens calculation due to a central flattening. Calculations should be performed with a third-generation formula (e.g., Hoffer Q, Holladay 2, or SRK/T) instead of a regression formula (e.g., SRK I or SRK II) (**A**). Newer formulas, including the ASCRS IOL calculator, account for previous radial keratotomy surgery.

125. Correct: HSV conjunctivitis (B)

Primary HSV infections without epithelial or stromal keratitis are commonly misdiagnosed as adenovirus conjunctivitis, given the similar clinical appearance. HSV conjunctivitis is usually unilateral and self-limited. HSV Tzanck smear reveals multinucleate giant cells. Other signs that can help distinguish primary ocular HSV from adenovirus are vesicles on the skin or eyelid margin and dendritic epithelial keratitis. Adenovirus conjunctivitis (**A**) presents with bilateral follicular conjunctivitis, sometimes with conjunctival membranes or pseudomembranes. Toxic conjunctivitis (**C**) occurs with chronic use of topical ocular medications. Chlamydial inclusion conjunctivitis causes a chronic follicular conjunctivitis (**D**).

126. Correct: Polyhexamethylene biguanide (B)

Amebic keratitis can affect the corneal epithelium, causing punctate epitheliopathy or pseudodendrites. Stromal infection manifests as an early gray-white superficial infiltrate progressing to a complete ring infiltrate. Inflamed corneal nerves or radial perineuritis are pathognomonic. The given figure shows a confocal microscopy of a patient with *Acanthamoeba* infection; cysts can be seen as bright white clusters, distributed throughout the scan. Biguanides have been shown to have activity against trophozoites and cysts. Biguanides include polyhexamethylene biguanide and chlorhexidine. Hexamidine (**A**), neomycin (**C**), and voriconazole (**D**) may be part of amebic keratitis management, but only have activity against.

127. Correct: Fumagillin (C)

Microsporidia is an intracellular protozoan that manifests as stromal keratitis in immunocompetent individuals, or as epitheliopathy in immunosuppressed patients. Stromal keratitis is caused by agents of the genus *Nosema* and keratoconjunctivitis is caused by the genera *Encephalitozoon* and Septata. Light microscopy using the Brown and Hopps stain reveals small gram-positive microsporidial spores. Fumagillin with or without fluoroquinolones are part of the management of microsporidiosis. Polyhexamethylene biguanide (**A**) and voriconazole (**B**) are part of the treatment for amebic keratitis. Voriconazole is also a therapeutic alternative for fungal keratitis. Vancomycin (**D**) is indicated for bacterial keratitis.

128. Correct: Pseudophakic bullous keratopathy (PBK) (A)

Late nonimmune mediated endothelial failure is characterized by corneal edema without acute inflammation or graft rejection, likely due to normal loss of endothelial cells in the donor. Nonimmune endothelial failure is most likely seen in patients treated for PBK compared to the number of patients treated for Fuchs corneal dystrophy (**B**), keratoconus (**C**), or corneal perforation (**D**).

129. Correct: Prednisolone acetate drops (A)

Corneal graft rejection is divided into epithelial, subepithelial, stromal, and endothelial. Epithelial graft rejection is characterized by a linear epithelial ridge that advances centripetally. Management includes early recognition and prompt initiation of steroid drops. Epithelial lines are not related to infectious pathogens (**B, C**). Confocal microscopy (**D**) is indicated in cases of epithelial ingrowth or infectious keratopathy (fungal, amebic).

130. Correct: Tangential illumination (C)

Corneal transplant rejection may present as subepithelial infiltrates resembling epidemic keratoconjunctivitis infiltrates. Subepithelial infiltrates are best seen on tangential illumination (medium wide beam of moderate height). In diffuse illumination, light is spread evenly over the entire observed surface (**A**). Direct illumination (**B**) uses a narrow focal slit beam at a 45- to 60-degree angle, and is useful in identifying the depth/layer of corneal pathology. Indirect illumination uses a short and narrow beam at the border of the pathology (**D**).

131. Correct: Endothelial rejection (D)

Corneal allograft rejection may occur years after penetrating keratoplasty. Endothelial rejection is the most common type of rejection. Patients present with pain, redness, or loss of vision. Slit lamp examination reveals an advancing rejection line or Khodadoust line, usually originating from a vascularized area. Associated findings include keratic precipitate deposition and corneal edema. Epithelial rejection presents with an epithelial line (**A**) that can be seen on indirect transillumination. Subepithelial rejection presents with subepithelial infiltrates similar to those of adenovirus conjunctivitis (**B**). Stromal rejection alone occurs most commonly with deep anterior lamellar keratoplasty (**C**).

132. Correct: Infrared light (A)

Both Nd-YAG laser (wavelength 1064 nm) and femtosecond laser (1053 nm) work through infrared light. Natural light is 510 nm and rhodopsin in the retina is most sensitive to this frequency (**C**). The excimer laser works through ultraviolet light (193 nm wavelength, b).

133. Correct: Start topical corticosteroids (C)

The question stem refers to diffuse lamellar keratitis (DLK), also known as sands of Sahara syndrome. DLK is an interface inflammation that usually presents immediately after LASIK surgery and typically causes few, if any, symptoms. The treatment is topical corticosteroids. In comparison, a post-LASIK infectious keratitis is generally painful and associated with photophobia and ciliary injection (**A, B, and C**). Mycobacterial and fungal infection usually presents several weeks after LASIK. Gram-positive bacteria can be seen shortly after the procedure but are usually discretely located at the flap margin.

134. Correct: Photoablation (A)

The excimer laser works through the disruption of covalent bonds. The laser pulses selectively ablate small areas of tissue without destroying adjacent tissue. Excimer laser is used to correct refractive errors (i.e., photorefractive keratectomy and excimer laser in situ keratomileusis). Photodisruption (**B**) uses laser energy to rupture or explode tissue. Examples of photodisruption include YAG capsulotomy and laser iridotomy. Photocoagulation (**C**) occurs when the tissue absorbs light energy delivered by the laser and converts it to heat. Panretinal photocoagulation (PRP) is an example of this.

135. Correct: All of the above (D)

Postoperative haze is a potential complication of PRK. Haze can be prevented with topical steroids, and patients who fail to take steroids after PRK are at increased risk of developing haze. Poor healing (keloid formation) and highly myopic treatments are also risk factors for the development of haze.

136. Correct: Hyperopic (B)

The question stem refers to radial keratotomy, which was a refractive procedure that preceded LASIK for the treatment of low myopia. A diamond knife was used to make radial incision in the cornea, thereby flattening it. Unfortunately, the procedure has several significant complications. Vision may fluctuate during the course of the day and at varying altitudes (as this patient has noted when he skies). In addition, patients often have a hyperopic shift over time. In the PERK study, 43% had greater than 1 D of hyperopic shift after 10 years. Myopic regression (**A**) can sometimes be seen after LASIK or photorefractive keratectomy (PRK) treatments or with the development of a cataract. It is unlikely that this patient is plano (**C**) given his visual complaints. Irregular astigmatism (**D**) is a potential complication of LASIK or PRK, especially in patients at risk for ectasia.

137. Correct: History of bacterial corneal ulcer (A)

Patients with a history of corneal ulcers can undergo refractive surgery, especially if there is minimal scar or the scar is not located centrally. Photorefractive keratectomy (PRK) may be a better option than LASIK as the scar may interfere with flap creation. All of the other choices—pregnancy, HIV, and Accutane use—are contraindications for refractive surgery treatments (**B, C, and D**). Other contraindications include history of herpes simplex or herpes zoster infection, unstable refraction, connective tissue disease, history of keloid formation, and active inflammatory disease of the eye.

138. Correct: Observation (A)

The photo here shows a picture of epithelial ingrowth. The ingrowth is peripheral and asymptomatic. Many cases of ingrowth, as in this patient, can be observed and may be self-limited. If the ingrowth progresses or causes astigmatism or visual disturbance, the flap can be lifted, and the stromal bed scraped (**D**). Alcohol can also be used on the stromal bed to limit further ingrowth. Infectious keratitis would be very unlikely 5 years after LASIK and in an asymptomatic individual (**B, C**).

139. Correct: A patient with very steep corneas (D)

Steep corneas are at higher risk for button hole formation, whereas flat corneas are at higher risk for free flap formation (**C**). Patients who have LASIK after cataract surgery or with moderate cylinder (**A, B**) are not necessarily at higher risk of free caps or button holes.

140. Correct: All of the above (D)

PTK uses the excimer laser to ablate superficial corneal pathology (limited to the anterior one-third of the cornea). In cases of recurrent corneal erosion, PTK can induce scarring or adhesion of the epithelium to the underlying Bowman's membrane to prevent recurrence. Since PTK is an ablative procedure, it can lead to a small hyperopic or astigmatic change in refraction. Unfortunately, erosions occasionally return after a single PTK treatment, in which case multiple treatments may be necessary. PTK, like most corneal surgeries, can reactivate latent HSV infections.

141. Correct: LASIK involves the creation of a stromal flap (A)

In LASEK (as opposed to PRK), a sheet of epithelium is preserved and placed over the ablated area at the conclusion of the procedure (**B**). In PRK, the overlying epithelium is removed, and the stromal bed is ablated (**C**).

142. Correct: Rheumatology (A)

This patient's clinical presentation is concerning for granulomatosis with polyangiitis (formerly Wegener's granulomatosis), which is a potentially fatal vasculitis that requires systemic immunosuppression and coordination with a rheumatologist. Granulomatosis with polyangiitis can affect the lungs and kidneys through damage to small- and medium-sized vessels. In advanced disease, it can also result in cardiac damage, so care may ultimately involve all answer choices (**B, C, and D**), but immediate attention should be given to immunosuppression, and therefore rheumatology is the best initial consultation option. Patients typically present with a history of recurrent nose bleeds and sinusitis. In granulomatosis with polyangiitis, eye findings present early in the disease, including peripheral corneal thinning as in peripheral ulcerative keratitis, orbital inflammation with proptosis, scleritis, uveitis, retinal vasculitis, acute ischemic optic neuropathy, retinal detachment, and choroidal detachment.

143. Correct: Explain that the test may not have been sensitive enough to pick up the underlying virus or that the responsible virus was not tested. Because clinical presentation suggests post-viral inflammation, you encourage steroid use (C)

The photograph (see the figure provided) depicts subepithelial infiltrates, which are often secondary to postviral inflammation. They are not infectious in nature but can cause blurry vision and photophobia. The proper treatment is steroids. The viral swab may not have picked up the particular viral culprit or may not have had the sensitivity to pick it up, but the virus is now cleared and so a second viral swab is of little utility (**B**). Since there is no bacterial infection, antibiotics are not indicated (**A**). Having her return in 1 week to monitor progress is reasonable, but steroids would be a better option and more likely to improve the patient's symptoms (**D**).

144. Correct: Cancel the surgery and alert the eye bank (B)

The **patient** expects and has prepared for a DMEK procedure and should not undergo a different procedure (**A**). Similarly, the patient has consented for this

procedure in advance of surgery, therefore proceeding with a different procedure without her permission would not be correct (**C**). She may feel pressured to accept a procedure that she had not desired because it is the day of surgery and she would like to proceed (**D**). It is appropriate to cancel the surgery (**B**) if there is no appropriate DMEK tissue available or the tissue cannot be exchanged, but it may be possible to get the correct tissue so that the patient can still proceed with surgery.

145. Correct: Contact lenses are foreign material that you are putting in your eye. They must be regularly cleaned or changed. (B)

Swimming and sleeping in lenses increase the risk of infection (**B**) Contact lens wear is the greatest risk factor for infectious keratitis and lenses must be properly cleaned, stored, and changed. Extended wear past the recommended usage date and swimming or showering in contact lenses increases the risk of infection, even if it is done occasionally (**A, C, and D**).

146. Correct: Oral antiviral prophylaxis will reduce chances of recurrence (C)

The HEDS study found that oral acyclovir reduces the risk of recurrent ocular disease during the treatment period (**D**). The HEDS study found that topical cortical steroids are useful for the treatment of stromal keratitis. Topical corticosteroids should not be used in herpetic keratitis as in our patient (see the figure provided), as there is live virus and this may prolong disease (**A**). Topical antiviral prophylaxis (**B**) was not used in the HEDS study.

147. Correct: No difference in visual outcome at 3 months (C)

The SCUT explored whether topical corticosteroids as adjunctive therapy for bacterial keratitis improve clinical outcomes at 3 months. The study found no difference in best uncorrected visual acuity at 3 months (**B**). Interestingly, however, patients who were count fingers or worse at baseline and patients with ulcers that were completely central did do better with topical corticosteroids. The time to reepithelialization did not differ significantly between the two groups (**A, D**).

148. Correct: ABO blood type incompatibility (B)

The CCTS showed that ABO blood type incompatibility is a possible risk factor for rejection. While most practitioners do not routinely consider blood type in their transplants because of the low risk of rejection, some may consider it in patients who are at high risk for rejection. HLA matching (**A**) is not cost-effective or advantageous. This study did not look at donor age (**C**), but the Cornea Donor Study (CDS) found that the

5-year cumulative probability of graft survival was the same in both the < 66-year-old donor group and the > 66-year-old donor group.

149. Correct: With-the-rule astigmatism (A)

A pterygium flattens where it inserts and causes steepening 90 degrees away. Since pterygia are almost always nasal or temporal, they classically lead to with-the-rule astigmatism. Pterygium excision can result in reduction of astigmatism postoperatively. With-the-rule astigmatism happens when the axis of the positive cylinder is oriented at 90 degrees, as is typically seen in children. Against-the-rule astigmatism (**B**) refers to the axis of the positive cylinder oriented at 180 degrees, as is typically seen in adults. Pterygia do not cause changes in sphere (**C, D**).

150. Correct: They stain well with fluorescein and rose Bengal (A)

The photograph and stem describe a pseudodendrite, seen in herpes zoster. Pseudodendrites are slightly raised with negative staining, and stain minimally with fluorescein and rose Bengal (unlike HSV). Zoster can result in neurotrophic cornea and can recur (**B, C**). Zoster can affect the posterior segment, particularly in immunosuppressed patients (like our patient here with a renal transplant), and a dilated fundus exam should be performed on initial evaluation (**D**).

Chapter 2

Glaucoma

Veena Rao

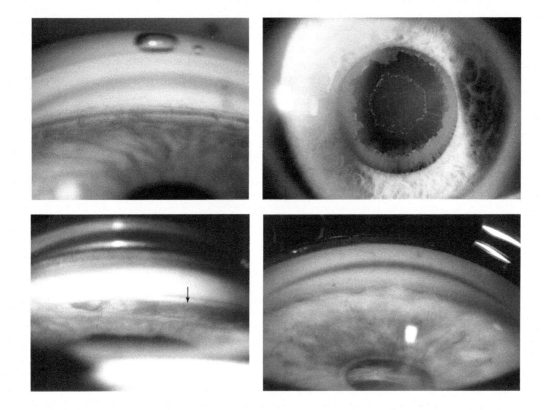

2.1 Questions

Easy | Medium | Hard

1. A patient is sent for evaluation for possible narrow-angle glaucoma. The view of the inferior angle with indirect gonioscopy appears as in the first figure. The second figure was acquired after which of the following?

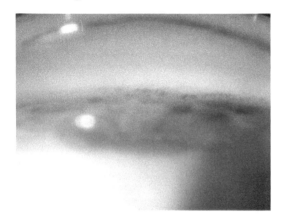

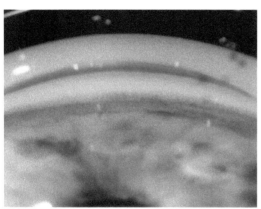

A. Asking the patient to look up or tilting the mirror up
B. Asking the patient to look up or tilting the mirror down
C. Asking the patient to look down or tilting the mirror up
D. Asking the patient to look down or tilting the mirror down

2. The image below was most likely taken from the autopsy of which of the following patients?

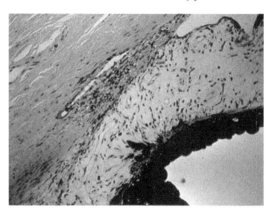

A. A patient who has an extensive family history of glaucoma
B. patient who was a poorly controlled diabetic who eventually went blind in this eye
C. A patient who has a history of episodic eye pain
D. A patient who was hit by a baseball in the eye at age 10 years

3. The secondary open-angle glaucoma shown here and caused by mutations in LOXL1 demonstrates characteristic histologic changes in each of the following tissues except which one?

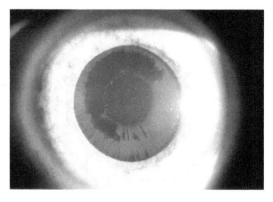

A. Lens epithelium
B. Iris stroma
C. Iris blood vessels
D. Conjunctival blood vessels

4. What is the most common complication of selective laser trabeculoplasty (SLT)?

A. Transient intraocular pressure increase
B. Iritis
C. Synechiae
D. Pain

5. A 55-year-old man underwent uncomplicated trabeculectomy in his left eye. On postoperative day 4, the intraocular pressure is 45 mm Hg. The anterior chamber is noted to be shallow and the bleb appears elevated. Which of the following is the next best intervention?

A. Start timolol eye drops in this eye.

B. Start acetazolamide pills.

C. Perform laser suture lysis.

D. Start atropine eye drops in this eye.

6. Which of the following options is most likely for the the patient whose gonioscopy is shown below?

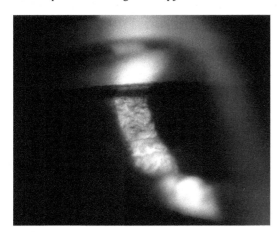

A. Experienced recent blunt trauma to the eye

B. Has an intraocular pressure of 8 mm Hg

C. Has a refraction of −4.00 diopters

D. Has a history of of juvenile idiopathic arthritis–associated uveitis treated with steroids

7. An 85-year-old man with a history of severe primary open-angle glaucoma in both eyes presents to the clinic with an intraocular pressure of 21 mm Hg in the right eye and 35 mm Hg in the left eye. His visual field shows severe constriction in both eyes due to advanced glaucoma. He reports difficulty in taking his eye drops regularly, due to his arthritis, and he lives alone. You discuss treatment options with him. Which of the following options should likely be avoided in this patient?

A. Glaucoma drainage device

B. Trabeculectomy with mitomycin C

C. Selective laser trabeculoplasty

D. Transscleral diode cyclophotocoagulation

8. Glaucoma is __× as prevalent in the black population versus the white population.

A. 2

B. 4

C. 8

D. 16

9. Which of the following components is less plentiful in aqueous humor versus plasma?

A. Hydrogen

B. Chloride

C. Bicarbonate

D. Ascorbic acid

10. A 79-year-old woman presents to your clinic with elevated intraocular pressure. She reports intolerance to several eye drops in the past. You review your treatment options and start her on a medication she has not tried previously, which works by decreasing uveoscleral outflow. Which drug class does this drop belong to?

A. Miotic drugs

B. Cycloplegic drugs

C. Beta blockers

D. Trauma

11. A 50-year-old male patient with a past medical history significant for hypothyroidism and alcohol abuse is undergoing strabismus surgery under general anesthesia. He begins to exhibit symptoms of malignant hyperthermia. Which of the following does not contribute to an increase in intraocular pressure?

A. Ketamine

B. Elevated body temperature

C. Alcohol

D. Hypothyroidism

12. What percentage of glaucoma patients may develop nerve fiber layer hemorrhages?

A. 10%

B. 33%

C. 50%

D. 60%

13. A 35-year-old man presents for a second opinion on a recent diagnosis of glaucoma. He has no known history of elevated intraocular pressure on his routine annual eye examinations. The patient presents with the below testing and a normal visual field. On dilated fundoscopy, the optic nerves appear symmetrical and tilted. Which of the following would be the next best step in his care?

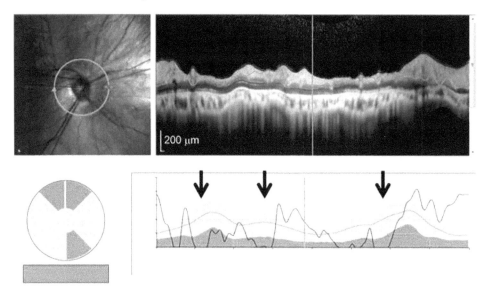

A. Plan laser trabeculoplasty to lower his intraocular pressure.

B. Obtain neuroimaging.

C. Careful observation with repeat visual field testing.

D. Initiation of latanoprost.

14. A patient with 20/25 vision in both eyes and intraocular pressure of 24 mm Hg presents with the following clinical appearance. Which treatment plan is least appropriate?

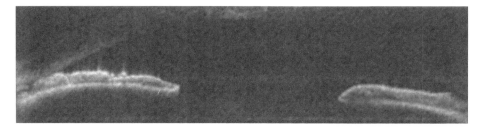

A. Laser peripheral iridotomy alone

B. Phacoemulsification with intraocular lens implantation

C. Initiation of timolol

D. A series of two laser procedures for each eye

15. A 69-year-old woman with a history of asthma, hypertension, and open-angle glaucoma treated with latanoprost has the following visual fields (in the figure below—top visual field from 1 year ago and bottom visual field from today). Her intraocular pressure readings in this eye over this time period have ranged between 8 and 9 mm Hg, and her optic disc shows a cup to disc ratio of 0.8 with inferior thinning. Which further evaluation is best indicated at this time?

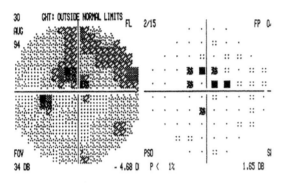

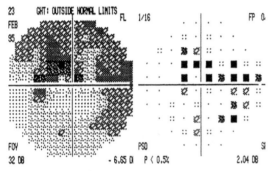

A. Referral to a neurologist for possible neuroimaging

B. Referral to her cardiologist to ensure adequate blood pressure control

C. Referral to her pulmonologist to see if timolol would be an appropriate agent for her glaucoma

D. Referral to a retina specialist for evaluation of possible occult macular degeneration

16. A patient undergoes valved glaucoma drainage device implanation. At postoperative week 8, the patient's intraocular pressure is noted to have increased to 28 mm Hg in the operative eye. This increase in eye pressure is most likely due to which of the following?

A. Steroid-related intraocular pressure rise

B. Prolonged intraocular inflammation leading to scarring of the trabecular meshwork

C. Encapsulation of the extraocular reservoir surrounding the implant

D. Progressive glaucoma

17. An 85-year-old man with uncontrolled eye pressure despite good compliance with his maximally tolerated eye drops refuses surgery to better control his glaucoma. You compromise on trying oral acetazolamide. In counseling the patient on acetazolamide use, you discuss potential side effects. Which of the following is not a potential adverse reaction?

A. Parasthesias

B. Aplastic anemia

C. Loss of libido

D. Fatty liver disease

18. A 63-year-old man with a history of brimonidine use for 8 years presents to your clinic with bilateral red, irritated, itchy eyes. You suspect an allergy to brimonidine. Which of the following is the incidence of blepharoconjunctivitis with chronic use of brimonidine tartrate?

A. 5%

B. 10%

C. 20%

D. 40%

19. A 72-year-old retired male physician is very cautious about interactions between his glaucoma drops and his systemic health. He has a history of high cholesterol, for which he takes an oral statin drug. He should be counseled about which of the following for the use of topical timolol?

A. Increases high-density lipoprotein (HDL) cholesterol levels.

B. Decreases HDL cholesterol levels.

C. Has no effect on serum cholesterol levels.

D. Decreases overall serum cholesterol levels.

20. A 9-month-old female infant with primary congential glaucoma requires surgery to control her eye pressure. The cornea has diffuse edema leading to a cloudy view of the iris and optic nerve on examination under anesthesia. Which of the following would be the best surgical approach in this setting?

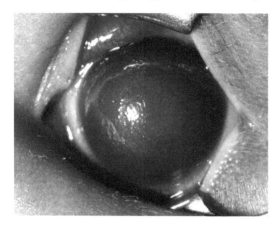

A. Goniotomy

B. Trabeculotomy ab externo

C. Glaucoma drainage device

D. Transscleral diode cyclophotocoagulation

21. Concerned parents of a newborn infant present to your clinic for an evaluation of their baby, who has an extensive family history of glaucoma. They are concerned he may have glaucoma because he is tearing, which the parents heard can be a sign of glaucoma in infants. You measure the intraocular pressure of the baby and reassure the parents that his eye pressure is normal. What is the most likely measurement obtained?

A. Less than 10 mm Hg

B. Low teens

C. Mid teens

D. Upper teens

22. A 35-year-old female patient with the clinical appearance below presents to your clinic. What is the most common cause of glaucoma in her condition?

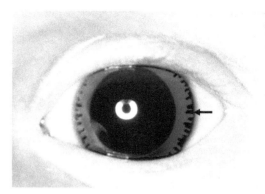

A. Rotation of the iris stump toward the angle, leading to synechial angle closure

B. Abnormal development of the trabecular meshwork

C. Abnormally high level of resistance in the trabecular meshwork

D. Overproduction of aqueous fluid

23. When performing trabeculectomy on a patient with this condition, what is the most concerning potential complication?

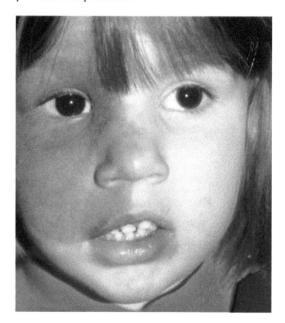

A. Choroidal hemorrhage

B. Hyphema

C. Neovascularization of the iris

D. Prolonged inflammation

24. A 64-year-old myopic man presents to your clinic. While traveling abroad several weeks ago, he recalls several days of flashing lights in his right eye, followed by slowly decreasing vision in that eye. On examination, his vision is counting fingers at his face with a dilated examination remarkable for a chronic-appearing retinal detachment with three peripheral retinal tears. What is the mechanism behind elevated intraocular pressure in this clinical scenario?

A. Decreased outflow due to perturbation of the retinal pigment epithelium

B. Increased pigment floating in the vitreous and anterior chamber, clogging the trabecular meshwork

C. Photoreceptor segments clogging the trabecular meshwork

D. Secondary angle closure from the retinal detachment rotating the iris anteriorly

25. A 29-year-old woman with congenital glaucoma typically controlled on latanoprost once daily in both eyes presents to your clinic for a routine check up. She tells you she is planning on becoming pregnant this year and asks which medication would be best for her if she does become pregnant?

A. Brimonidine

B. Timolol

C. Dorzolamide

D. Latanoprost

26. Among which group is the prevalence of primary angle closure highest?

A. Chinese

B. Inuit

C. Scandinavian

D. East African

27. Of the four scenarios presented below, in which case is the gene responsible located on chromosome 1?

A. An 85-year-old woman with scleral spur identified on gonioscopy 360 degrees and history of maximal intraocular pressure of 35 mm Hg OU

B. A 33-year-old woman with history of open-angle glaucoma and elevated intraocular pressures, now controlled by trabeculectomy in both eyes

C. A 65-year-old woman with history of elevated intraocular pressure and moth-eaten pupillary border

D. A 54-year-old man with posterior embryotoxon and history of elevated intraocular pressure

28. Which structure is responsible for aqueous humor production?

A. Capillaries within ciliary processes

B. Stroma of ciliary processes

C. Inner nonpigmented epithelial cells of ciliary processes

D. Outer pigmented epithelial cells of ciliary processes

29. What method measures the rate of aqueous humor formation?

A. Tonometry

B. Tonography

C. Fluorophotometry

D. Angiography

30. What is the area of greatest resistance in the trabecular outflow system?

A. Uveal meshwork

B. Corneoscleral meshwork

C. Scleral spur

D. Juxtacanalicular meshwork

31. What percentage of aqueous outflow is attributable to the uveoscleral pathway?

A. 2%

B. 15%

C. 25%

D. 35%

32. When using the Goldmann tonometry to measure intraocular pressure, corneal edema can cause a falsely ____ pressure reading, and an excess of fluorescein can cause a falsely ____ pressure reading.

A. Low; high

B. Low; low

C. High; high

D. High; low

33. A 55-year-old woman presents to your clinic for a glaucoma suspect evaluation. She has visual acuity of 20/20 OU, intraocular pressure 21 mm Hg OD and 20 mm Hg OS, central corneal thickness of 600 μm OU. She mentions her optometrist told her she has "thick corneas" and that was a reassuring sign against glaucoma. Which clinical trial is her optometrist referring to?

A. Blue Mountain Eye Study

B. Collaborative Initial Glaucoma Treatment Study

C. Ocular Hypertension Treatment Study

D. Early Manifest Glaucoma Trial

34. You present to a new eye clinic and observe each of the four technicians cleans the Goldmann applanation prism using a different technique. You note one technician did not perform an adequate job cleaning the prism. Which technique did he or she use?

A. Wiping the prism with an alcohol pad

B. Soaking the prism in 70% isopropyl alcohol

C. Soaking the prism in 1:10 sodium hypochlorite

D. Wiping the prism with 1:10 sodium hypochlorite

35. An optic nerve is measured as 1.5 mm in height on ophthalmoscopy with a 90 D lens. What is the actual height of the nerve?

A. 1.15 mm

B. 1.5 mm

C. 1.65 mm

D. 1.95 mm

36. You are examining a 49-year-old man for a glaucoma suspect evaluation. You find the right eye has a cup to disc ratio of 0.3 and the left eye has a cup to disc ratio of 0.65. You discuss the assymmetry with your patient, who asks you what is the chance that this is just normal asymmetry. You answer that asymmetry to this degree is present in __% of normal individuals.

A. 0%

B. 1%

C. 5%

D. 10%

37. The accuracy of visual field testing may decrease with pupil sizes smaller than which of the following option?

A. 2.0 mm

B. 2.5 mm

C. 1.5 mm

D. 3.0 mm

38. Frequency doubling technology (FDT) perimetry can be especially useful in patients with _____ glaucoma, possibly due to its emphasis on __ cells.

A. Late glaucoma, M cells

B. Early glaucoma, M cells

C. Late glaucoma, P cells

D. Early glaucoma, P cells

39. A 60-year-old woman presents for a new patient evaluation. This is her first eye examination in 10 years. Her best corrected visual acuity is 20/20 in the right eye and 20/80 in the left eye. The intraocular pressure is 15 mm Hg in the right eye and 38 in the left eye. There is no afferent pupillary defect. The optic nerve is notable for a cup to disc ratio of 0.2 in the right eye with a healthy rim and near total loss of the optic nerve rim tissue in the left eye. Which of the following glaucomas is most likely in this scenario?

A. Primary open angle

B. Pigmentary

C. Pseudoexfoliation

D. Iridocorneal endothelial syndrome

40. For a patient with pigmentary glaucoma compared to a patient with primary open-angle glaucoma, selective laser trabeculoplasty would be expected to have an effect lasting a _____ duration and require ____ energy settings:

A. Longer, higher

B. Longer, lower

C. Shorter, higher

D. Shorter, lower

41. A 90-year-old woman who is pseudophakic OD presents with a 4+ nuclear sclerotic cataract OS and intraocular pressure of 12 mm Hg OD and 48 mm Hg OS. She reports pain in the left eye and denies trauma. On slit lamp examination, you note microcystic corneal edema, 3+ anterior chamber cell, keratoprecipitates, and an open-angle OS. Which of the following cell types is uniquely seen in this subtype of glaucoma?

A. Basophils

B. Neutrophils

C. Eosinophils

D. Macrophages

42. A 49-year-old man presents with unilateral blurry vision, light sensitivity, and elevated intraocular pressure. You note anterior-chamber inflammation on his examination. Which of the following ocular inflammatory conditions is least likely in this scenario?

A. Herpes simplex uveitis

B. Toxoplasmosis uveitis

C. Fuchs' heterochromic iridocyclitis

D. HLA B27-associated uveitis

43. A 56-year-old man presents with decreased vision and a "red" right eye. He is found to have elevated episcleral venous pressure. Which comorbidity is most likely to be present?

A. Superior vena cava syndrome

B. Aortic regurgitation

C. Uncontrolled hypertension

D. Diastolic heart failure

44. What is normal episcleral venous pressure?

A. 4–6 mm Hg

B. 6–8 mm Hg

C. 8–10 mm Hg

D. 10–12 mm Hg

45. Four patients present to your emergency room on Sunday afternoon with eye trauma. Which patient is least likely to develop glaucoma?

A. Man hit in eye with baseball

B. Girl hit by tree branch leading to corneal abrasion

C. Woman with metal grinding injury

D. Man with bleach to eye

46. Which medication should be avoided in this patient?

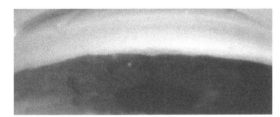

A. Rosuvastatin

B. Amiodarone

C. Oxybutynin

D. Fluticasone

47. Which of the following options is most likely the patient shown in the figure?

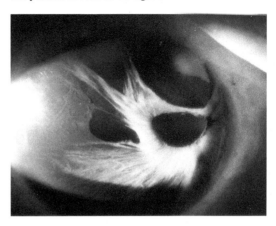

A. Has symmetrical clinical findings in both eyes

B. Is a woman

C. Is 70 years old

D. Has experienced ocular trauma

48. What is the most appropriate next step in treatment for a patient with intraocular pressure of 40 mm Hg on maximal tolerated medical therapy in an eye with with 20/100 vision following treatment for ocular melanoma?

A. Continue to observe on maximal medical therapy

B. Trabeculectomy with mitomycin C

C. Glaucoma drainage device

D. Transscleral diode cyclophotocoagulation

49. Which of the following conditions is not associated with glaucoma?

A. Sturge–Weber syndrome

B. Neurofibromatosis type 1

C. von Hippel–Lindau syndrome

D. Tuberous sclerosis

50. Two teenage parents bring their 6-month old male infant in for an examination, as they've noticed the baby makes strange "grimacing" facial movements. They also note that the baby's eyes tear up and he cries when being taken outside into the daylight. Which of the following is most often true for the condition the baby presents with here?

A. Occurs in males

B. Occurs within the first 3 years of life

C. Occurs in one eye

D. Has a better prognosis if diagnosed as a newborn infant

51. This finding is thought to develop due to which of the following reasons?

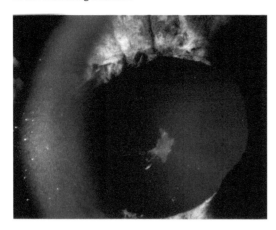

A. Chronic inflammation
B. Iris pigment deposition
C. Ischemia
D. Regressed neovascularization

52. A 58-year-old hyperopic woman presents to the emergency room with decreased vision, nausea, vomiting, and unilateral eye pain. Which of the following medical treatments are indicated for her most likely condition?

A. Brimonidine and pilocarpine 2%
B. Brimonidine and pilocarpine 4%
C. Apraclonidine and pilocarpine 2%
D. Apraclonidine and pilocarpine 4%

53. The patient shown below presents with unilateral eye pain and elevated eye pressure. The lens appears tilted on slit lamp examination and there are limited angle structures seen on gonioscopy. Which of the following is the least appropriate treatment?

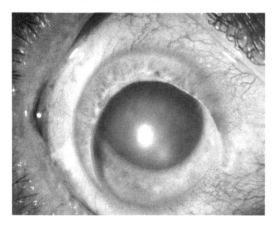

A. Laser iridotomy
B. Atropine
C. Pilocarpine
D. Acetazolamide

54. A 60-year-old woman complains of decreased visual acuity OD. Her vision is 20/60 OD. Her IOP is 36 mm Hg OD. Slit lamp examination is significant for a mid-dilated, fixed pupil associated with a mix of prominent and fine abnormal blood vessels in the anterior-chamber angle. Which answer would you least likely elicit upon taking further history?

A. Sudden onset of diffusely decreased vision
B. History of panretinal photocoagulation
C. Sudden onset of decreased vision in the upper half of the visual field
D. Episodes of dark vision that self-resolve

55. A 65-year-old woman with a history of central retinal vein occlusion presents several months after her initial diagnosis with eye pain and decreased vision in the affected eye. On gonioscopy, you note synechiae and abnormal blood vessels. The patient asks what percentage of patients like her develop this condition, and you answer as below:

A. 5%
B. 10%
C. 25%
D. 33%

56. A recently postoperative cataract surgery patient presents with a diffusely shallow anterior chamber and elevated intraocular pressure. Examination of the posterior segment appears within normal limits. Which of the following is the most appropriate treatment for the likely condition?

A. Nd:YAG laser treatment
B. Pilocarpine
C. Bandage contact lens
D. Suturing of the main cataract surgery wound

57. Which of the following is a diagnostic tool helpful in this condition?

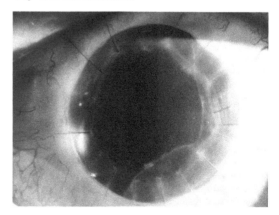

A. Ultrasound biomicroscopy
B. CT scan
C. Argon laser
D. Pachymetry

58. A small child is noted to have a white pupillary reflex. On further examination, a retrolental membrane is noted. Which of the following would be the most likely subtype of glaucoma to develop in this patient?

A. Inflammatory or uveitic

B. Chronic angle closure

C. Open angle

D. Steroid induced

59. A 26-year-old woman with a history of migraine and seasonal allergies presents to your clinic with bilateral eye pain and elevated eye pressure. She is currently using topiramate and fluticasone nasal spray for her medical conditions. What should not be used to treat the most likely etiology of her elevated intracranial pressure?

A. Acetazolamide

B. Immediate discontinuation of topiramate

C. Immediate laser peripheral iridotomy

D. Atropine

60. Which layer of the cornea is affected in this external photograph?

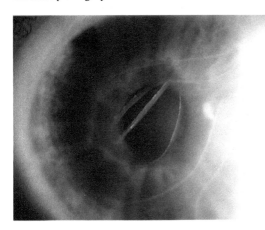

A. Epithelium

B. Bowman's layer

C. Descemet's membrane

D. Endothelium

61. What is the most common inheritance pattern of this condition?

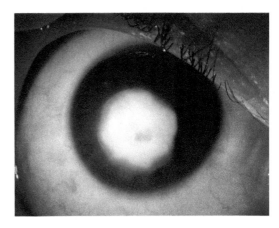

A. Autosomal recessive

B. Autosomal dominant

C. X-linked recessive

D. Sporadic

62. This infant would mostly benefit from a referral to which of the following specialists?

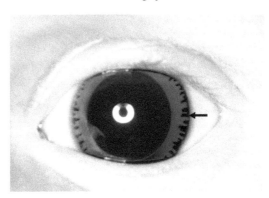

A. Cardiologist

B. Nephrologist

C. Gastroenterologist

D. Dermatologist

63. An infant is diagnosed with bilateral cataracts by her pediatrician. She subsequently undergoes cataract surgery in both eyes within the first few months of birth. Which factors may increase her risks of developing glaucoma?

A. Cataract surgery at the age of 2 years

B. Small corneal diameter

C. Uncomplicated cataract surgery

D. Density of cataract

64. What is the normal corneal diameter in a newborn infant?

A. 8 mm

B. 9 mm

C. 10 mm

D. 11 mm

65. At the normal rate of aqueous production, how long would it take for the eye to reaccumulate the volume removed in a 100-µL anterior-chamber paracentesis?

A. 30 minutes

B. 40 minutes

C. 50 minutes

D. 60 minutes

66. Diurnal variation in intraocular pressure greater than ___ mm Hg is suggestive of glaucoma.

A. 4

B. 8

C. 10

D. 12

67. Which factor is least likely to increase intraocular pressure?

A. Playing a trombone

B. Yoga

C. Chronic constipation

D. Pregnancy

68. A 32-year-old African American man presents with intraocular pressure of 25 mm Hg OU and cup to disc ratio of 0.7 OU. Which factor is least likely to promote progression of his glaucoma?

A. Younger age

B. Larger cup to disc ratio

C. Higher intraocular pressure

D. Race

69. A 32-year-old man presents with intraocular pressure of 34 mm Hg OD and 38 mm Hg OS. His cup to disc ratio is 0.9 OD and 0.95 OS. His visual field testing is revealing for superior and inferior arcuate scotomas OS worse than OD. Which gene is associated with his glaucoma diagnosis?

A. *GLC1A*

B. *GLC1B*

C. *GLC1C*

D. *GLC1E*

70. A patient presents for evaluation of progressive glaucoma. Her visual fields are shown below. Which of the following is the best course for the next step in management?

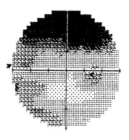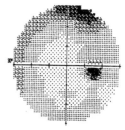

A. Start brimonidine in both eyes 2×/d

B. Observe closely

C. Obtain neuroimaging

D. External ocular examination

71. An 83-year-old woman with primary open-angle glaucoma controlled after trabeculectomy OU performed 10 years ago presents to your clinic with 1 day of right-sided eye pain and decreased vision. Your examination is notable for injection surrounding the trabeculectomy and 1-mm hypopyon. Which of the following is a risk factor for the development of this condition?

A. Wearing an eye shield at night

B. Moderate weight lifting

C. Swimming with watertight goggles

D. Thin, avascular bleb

72. A 45-year-old man who is undergoing trabeculectomy with mitomcyin C for his right eye due to progressive pigmentary glaucoma. What should be specifically considered during his postoperative period?

A. Wearing an eye shield at night indefinitely

B. Prolonged topical antibiotic course

C. Regular use of ocular lubrication

D. Delayed laser suture lysis

73. Which of the following is most likely the mechanism of action of selective laser trabeculoplasty?

A. Increased aqueous humor outflow due to small openings created in the trabecular meshwork

B. Increased aqueous humor outflow due to distortion of the junctions between cells in the trabecular meshwork

C. Increased aqueous humor outflow mediated by thermal changes to the trabecular meshwork

D. Increased aqueous humor outflow due to changes in matrix metalloproteinases in the trabecular meshwork

74. An 85-year-old man with elevated intraocular pressure that is not resposive to antihypertensive eye drops or acetazolamide. You discuss the risks and benefits of a trial of mannitol with the patient and his family. You should discuss all of the following potential side effects except which one?

A. Subdural hemorrhage

B. Subarachnoid hemorrhage

C. Congestive heart failure

D. Tinnitus

75. A postoperative month-1 trabeculectomy patient presents to clinic and you are asked to consent the patient for a 5-fluorouracil (5-FU) injection. What is a potential risk from the medication that should be discussed with the patient?

A. Progressive cataract formatoin

B. Retinal tear

C. Corneal endothelial disease

D. Blebitis

76. In planning for cataract extraction using phacoemulsification in a patient with an anatomic narrow angle and anterior-chamber depth of 1.9 mm, which of the following might be useful?

A. High-viscosity viscoelastic

B. Hydrodissection of the nucleus and phacoemulsification above the iris plane

C. Decreased bottle height

D. Creation of a larger main incision

77. An 88-year-old man referred to your clinic for advanced glaucoma notes good compliance with his three eye drops and eye visits. He has not noted any recent changes in vision. His best corrected visual acuity is 20/40 in the right eye and 20/200 in the left eye; intraocular pressure is 8 mm Hg in both eyes. The patient is pseudophakic in both eyes and has a cup to disc ratio of 0.95 in both eyes. Which of the following would you most recommend?

A. Discussion of treatment plan with a family member

B. Discussion of a low-vision evaluation

C. Discussion of insurance coverage of medication

D. Assistance with transportation costs to/from the clinic

78. Goldmann's applanation can yield falsely ___ intraocular pressure readings if excessive fluorescein was instilled and falsely ___ intraocular pressure readings in the setting of high myopia.

A. Low, low

B. Low, high

C. High, high

D. High, low

79. Which of the following lenses is not appropriate for performing the procedure seen here?

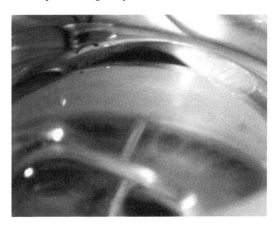

A. Koeppe's lens

B. Barkan's lens

C. Swan–Jacob lens

D. Posner's lens

80. The following patient would benefit from which of the following options?

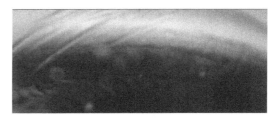

A. Cataract extraction

B. Laser peripheral iridotomy alone

C. Brimonidine

D. Panretinal photocoagulation

81. What systemic findings are associated with this condition?

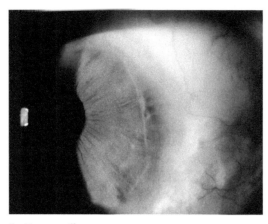

A. Hypospadias

B. Enlarged molars

C. Mottled skin pigmentation

D. Ataxia

82. The lamina cribrosa of the optic nerve is supplied by which of the following?

A. The circle of Zinn–Haller

B. Central retinal artery

C. Retinal capillaries

D. Cilioretinal artery

83. What is the usual visual field stimulus size on a standard automated visual field performed with a Humphrey perimeter?

A. ¼ mm²

B. 1 mm²

C. 4 mm²

D. 16 mm²

84. In which of the following patients malignant glaucoma is most likely to occur?

A. A patient with history of pigmentary glaucoma

B. A patient requiring an in-the-bag lens implant +28 diopters for emmetropia

C. A patient having axial length of 24 mm

D. A patient having history of requiring three medications to control intraocular pressure

85. How large is a Goldmann size III stimulus compared to a Goldmann size I stimulus?

A. Two times larger

B. Four times larger

C. Eight times larger

D. Sixteen times larger

86. A 50-year-old woman has an intraocular pressure of 26 mm Hg both eyes (OU) despite reliable use of dorzolamide–timolol OU twice a day and latanoprost OU before bed. She has an allergy to brimonidine. You discuss starting a trial of pilocarpine. The patient asks about potential side effects. All of the following should be discussed except which one?

A. Induced myopia

B. Retinal detachment

C. Band keratopathy

D. Iritis

87. A patient presents for a routine appointment with the following appearance. Which of the following is not a reasonable treatment course?

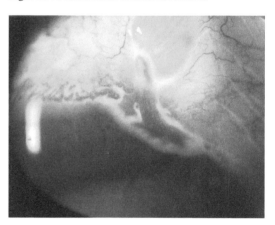

A. Observation

B. Autologous blood injection

C. Antibiotic ointment

D. Timolol

88. Which patient would likely benefit from the largest intraocular pressure lowering with selective laser trabeculoplasty?

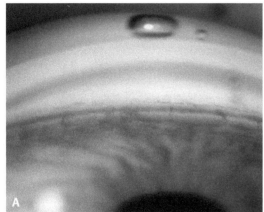

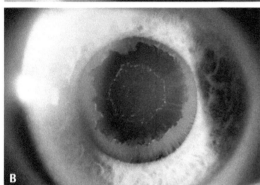

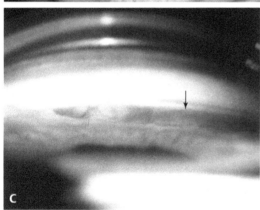

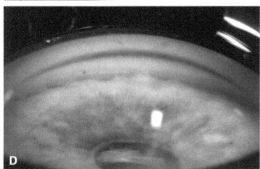

A. Image A

B. Image B

C. Image C

D. Image D

Consider the following story while answering the next two questions:

89. A 16-year-old African American patient with the examination shown is being treated in your emergency room for an intraocular pressure of 28 mm Hg. He is unsure of his past medical history but states he has been generally healthy.

Which medication should be used with caution in this situation?

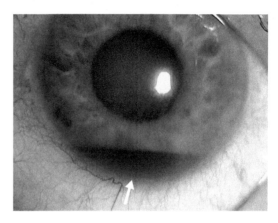

A. Latanoprost

B. Brimonidine

C. Timolol

D. Dorzolamide

90. The patient seen in the figure is tested and found to have normal blood work. He would not be recommended surgery in which of the following scenarios?

A. Corneal blood staining

B. Intraocular pressure of 35 mm Hg for 3 days

C. Intraocular pressure of 35 mm Hg for 36 hours and sickle cell trait

D. Intraocular pressure of 25 mm Hg for 36 hours and sickle cell anemia

91. What is the blood supply to the superficial nerve fiber layer of the optic nerve?

A. Central retinal artery

B. Short posterior ciliary arteries

C. Circle of Zinn–Haller

D. Contributions from both circle of Zinn–Haller and other short posterior ciliary arteries

92. A newborn of 1 month old is being treated for elevated intraocular pressure in the setting of congenital glaucoma. Which of the following medications should not be used?

A. Timolol

B. Brimonidine

C. Dorzolamide

D. Latanoprost

93. What is the most common pathogen in this condition?

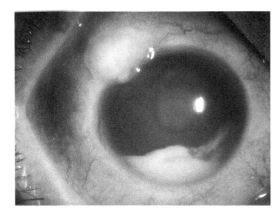

A. Streptococcus

B. Staphylococcus

C. Haemophilus influenzae

D. Fungi

94. The Ocular Hypertension Treatment Study identified which of the following as a protective factor against glaucoma development?

A. Central corneal thickness

B. Increased age

C. Increased cup to disc ratio

D. Higher baseline intraocular pressure

95. In the Collaborative Initial Glaucoma Treatment Study which of the following was shown?

A. Quality of life was worse in the surgical group.

B. Intraocular pressure was lower in the medically treated group.

C. Visual field outcomes were similar between the surgically and the medically treated groups.

D. Early visual acuity loss was greater in the medically treated group.

96. A 64-year-old woman brought into the operating room for cataract surgery develops an anterior-chamber hemorrhage upon your initial incision. Which of the following conditions is most likely present?

A. Fuchs' heterochromic iridocyclitis

B. Pigmentary glaucoma

C. Pseudoexfoliation glaucoma

D. Traumatic glaucoma

97. Which of the following is an appropriate management for this patient 5 years status post trabeculectomy?

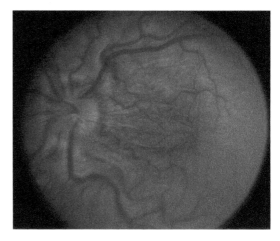

A. Brimonidine

B. Trabeculectomy revision

C. Frequent lubrication

D. Careful observation

98. Which of the following is a possible cause of elevated episcleral venous pressure?

A. The Valsalva maneuver

B. Thyroid eye disease

C. Iris neovascularization

D. primary open-angle glaucoma

99. A 50-year-old man was hit in the eye with a bottle cap. Subsequently, he developed a hyphema and an intraocular pressure of 5 mm Hg. His hyphema was self-resolved, and the decision was made to monitor his eye pressure. Two weeks later, he returns to the ER with extreme eye pain and an intraocular pressure of 45 mm Hg. What is the most likely diagnosis?

A. Recurrent hyphema

B. Late-onset ocular inflammation

C. Spontaneous closure of a cyclodialysis cleft

D. Corneal abrasion

100. Which of the following descriptions of visual field artifacts is incorrect?

A. Lens rim artifact—patient's prescription vision lens is placed too far from her eye.

B. False positive—patient does not respond to visual field stimulus in an area she previously has seen.

C. Cloverleaf artifact—patient loses attention and stops responding as the test progresses.

D. Fixation loss—patient's eye loses the fixation target and shifts during test.

2.2 Answers and Explanations

Easy	Medium	Hard

1. Correct: Asking the patient to look up or tilting the mirror down (B)

When the view of the desired angle is not clear, a better view can be achieved by either asking the patient to look into the mirror used to visualize the desired area of the angle or by tilting the gonioscopy mirror toward the angle being examined. (**A**) Would be helpful when asking the patient to look up, but tilting the mirror up would facilitate view of the superior angle (not inferior). Similarly, asking the patient to look down (**C and D**) would facilitate examination of the superior angle, not the inferior angle.

2. Correct: A patient who has a history of episodic eye pain (C)

This histologic image shows a patient with a history of acute angle-closure glaucoma, evidenced by adhesions involving the trabecular meshwork; this disease process is best correlated with episodic eye pain due to intermittent angle closure. It is possible for patients with a history of acute angle-closure glaucoma to have an extensive family history of glacuoma (**A**), but that is not the most specific answer here as that can be true of other forms of glaucoma. Poorly controlled diabetic patients (**B**) would more likely develop neovascular glaucoma. A history of trauma from a baseball injury (**D**) would be best correlated with angle-recession glaucoma.

3. Correct: conjunctival blood vessels (D)

LOXL1 mutations are single gene mutations associated strongly with the development of pseudoexfoliation syndrome or glaucoma. Deposits of pseudoexfoliatory material are found in various locations in the eye and in the body, including the lens epithelium, iris stroma, and iris blood vessels (**A–C**) but are not found in the conjunctival blood vessels (**D**).

4. Correct: Transient intraocular pressure increase (A)

The most commonly reported complication of SLT is transient increase in intraocular pressure, reported to occur in approximately 20% of patients. Iritis, synechiae, and pain (**B–D**) are all reported complications but occur less frequently than a transient intraocular pressure increase.

5. Correct: Start atropine eye drops in this eye (D)

This patient's presentation is suggestive of malignant glaucoma (also termed aqueous misdirection). Elevated intraocular pressure in the setting of a shallow anterior chamber and an elevated bleb is the typical presentation of this condition. If the bleb were not elevated, underfiltration may be the more likely etiology, in which case laser suture lysis might be performed during the early postoperative period (**C**). Starting timolol or acetazolamide (**A or B**) may improve the intraocular pressure but would not treat the etiology of this condition directly and likely would not be sufficient to control intraocular pressure.

6. Correct: Has a refraction of −4.00 diopters (C)

The image above shows a classic bowed iris configuration and dense pigmentation of the angle structures, characteristic of pigment dispersion syndrome or pigmentary glaucoma. This condition is most common in male patients with moderate myopia. Recent blunt trauma to the eye (**A**) would be associated with angle recession. Pigment dispersion syndrome is not typically associated with low intraocular pressure (**B**). Uveitis and/or steroid use (**D**), are not associated with a posteriorly bowed iris. Uveitis can be associated with heavy pigmentation of angle structures, but this is typically associated with peripheral anterior synechiae and not with a more regular appearance to the pigment as seen here.

7. Correct: Trabeculectomy with mitomycin C (B)

Of the presented options, trabeculectomy with mitomycin C can necessitate multiple postoperative visits and require frequent eye drop adminstration to allow proper postoperative recovery. It is important to discuss these needs with the patient and develop a treatment plan with which he or she is able to comply. Improper postoperative regimen after a trabeculectomy can result in severe complications. If a patient has difficulty with postoperative expectations (in this case, risk factors include advanced age, arthritis causing barriers to eye drop use, living alone), it may not be in his best interest to pursue the procedure. Glaucoma drainage device, selective laser trabeculoplasty, and transscleral diode cyclophotocoagulation (**A, C, D**) all require less demanding postoperative regimens and may prove better choices for this patient.

8. Correct: 4 (B)

The prevalence of glaucoma is up to four times greater in the black population when compared to the white population.

9. Correct: Bicarbonate (C)

There is proportionately less bicarbonate in the aqueous humor when compared to plasma. Aqueous humor has higher levels of hydrogen, chloride, and ascorbate (**A, B, D**), when compared to plasma.

10   Correct: Miotic drugs (A)

Uveoscleral outflow is decreased by miotics. Cycloplegic drugs and beta blocker drugs (**B, C**) increase uveoscleral outflow. Trauma does not have a direct relationship to uveoscleral outflow; however, a trauma that causes a cyclodialysis cleft can increase uveoscleral outflow through the cleft.

11.   Correct: Alcohol (C)

Alcohol has been shown to decrease intraocular pressure. The other answer choices here have all been shown to increase eye pressure.

12.   Correct: 33% (B)

About 33% of glaucoma patients may develop nerve fiber layer hemorrhages over time.

13.   Correct: Careful observation with repeat visual field testing (C)

In the absence of any other clinical signs of glaucoma in this otherwise healthy young man, a discussion of the challenges of monitoring for glaucoma in the myopic patient as well as careful observation with routine repeat visual field testing is most appropriate. The patient presents with a copy of an ocular coherence tomography scan showing diffuse segmentation failure or artifact, most likely from a myopic, tilted nerve. In myopic patients, tilted optic nerves can cause a failure of the optical coherence tomography (OCT) algorithm in which the OCT cannot properly identify the borders of the retinal nerve fiber layer. This can have the appearance on the retinal nerve fiber layer analysis of diffuse thinning (also termed "red disease"). Planning for laser trabeculoplasty (**A**) or initiation of latanoprost (**D**) would be inappropriate as there are no clinical signs of glaucoma. Neuroimaging (**B**) is also inappropriate in this otherwise healthy eye examination.

14.   Correct: Laser peripheral iridotomy alone (A)

In a patient with plateau iris configuration, as shown in this anterior-segment optical coherence tomography image, laser peripheral iridotomy alone is not an appropriate treatment plan. Laser peripheral iridotomy can alleviate any component of pupillary block but would not be sufficient to treat the anteriorly rotated ciliary processes that narrow the angle in plateau iris configuration. Phacoemulsification with intraocular lens implantation (**B**) is an appropriate treatment, as removal of the cataract debulks the angle anatomy, thus opening the angle. Initiation of timolol (**C**) is appropriate to lower the mildly elevated intraocular pressure. A series of two laser procedures for each eye (**D**) would be appropriate—first, laser peripheral iridotomy to alleviate pupillary block,

followed by laser gonioplasty, which can open the angle anatomy by shrinking peripheral iris tissue crowding the angle.

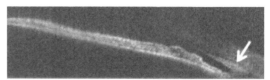

15.   Correct: Referral to her cardiologist to ensure adequate blood pressure control (B)

Low blood pressures have been associated with worsening visual field depressions. For patients on systemic antihypertensives with noted glaucomatous progression at "low" eye pressures, an evaluation to ensure the patient is not intermittently hypotensive is appropriate. There are no concerning signs for neurologic disease on this visual field and the patient's optic nerve description is consistent with this visual field (**A**). Timolol would not be the second-line therapy in a patient with asthma (**C**). This visual field is not suggestive of macular degeneration (**D**).

16.   Correct: Encapsulation of the extraocular reservoir surrounding the implant (C)

This is the leading theory to explain why some patients experience a "hypertensive phase" or higher intraocular pressure several weeks postoperatively from a valved glaucoma drainage device. Steroid-related intraocular pressure rise (**A**) is a possibility, although patients are typcally weaned off steroids by postoperative week 8. Prolonged inflammation and scarring are not thought to be reasons for higher eye pressure in this setting (**B**). While progressive glaucoma (**D**) is possible, it is much less likely than the above answer.

17.   Correct: Fatty liver disease (D)

The other answer choices are all potential adverse reactions to acetazolamide.

18.   Correct: 20% (C)

The long-term incidence of intolerance to brimonidine due to blepharoconjunctivitis is reported at 20%. This is often reversible with discontinuation of the medication.

19   Correct: Decreases HDL cholesterol levels (B)

Topical beta blockers have been shown to reduce serum HDL cholesterol, although that has not been shown to affect overall cardiovascular outcomes.

20.   Correct: Trabeculotomy ab externo (B)

In the setting of a cloudy cornea, trabeculotomy ab externo is the best approach surgically in primary congenital glaucoma; this utilizes an external approach in order to treat the angle structures. Goniotomy (**A**) is the first choice for surgical treatment if the view to the angle is clear; the trabecular meshwork can be incised using a blade or needle via an internal approach. Glaucoma drainage device and transscleral diode cyclophotocoagulation are not the first-line treatments in this setting (**C, D**).

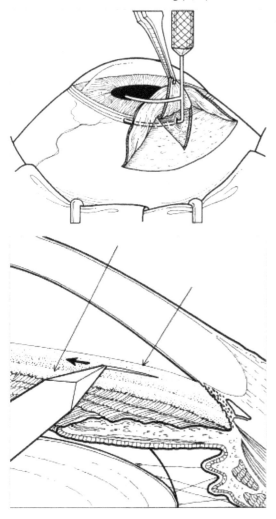

21. Correct: Low teens (B)

The typical intraocular pressure in the newborn is in the low teens.

22. Correct: Rotation of the iris stump toward the angle, leading to synechial angle closure (A)

This is the most common mechanism behind glaucoma in aniridia, which is the condition shown in the figure. While some patients do have abnormal development of the trabecular meshwork or angle structures (**B**), this is less common than (**A**). There is no evidence to support (**C**) and (**D**).

23. Correct: Choroidal hemorrhage (A)

This patient exhibits Sturge–Weber syndrome (encephalotrigeminal angiomatosis), a phakomatosis in which patients present with facial cutaneous hemangioma, choroidal hemangioma, and leptomeningeal angioma. The presence of choroidal hemangioma makes these patients more susceptible to choroidal hemorrhage when undergoing intraocular surgery. Hyphema (**B**) is not at increased risk in these patients as the hemangioma is located in the choroid, away from the anterior chamber. Neovascularization and prolonged inflammation (**C, D**) are not associated with this condition.

24. Correct: Photoreceptor segments clogging the trabecular meshwork (C)

This is the leading theory to explain this phenomenon, also termed Schwartz–Matsuo syndrome, which can be seen in patients with chronic rhegmatogenous retinal detachment (described in this clinical scenario as decreased vision in setting of flashing lights and three retinal tears). The photoreceptor outer segments are thought to travel through the retinal tear into the vitreous and subsequently the aqueous humor, clogging the drainage angle. There is no evidence the retinal pigment epithelial layer plays a role in this process (**A**). Photoreceptors rather than pigment (B) are thought to be the offending agent in clogging the trabecular meshwork. There is no evidence the detached retina causes anterior iris rotation (**D**).

25. Correct: Brimonidine (A)

Brimonidine has a pregnancy category B rating by the U.S. Food and Drug Adminstration for use during pregnancy. The other agents listed above (**B–D**) all have category C ratings. Category B signifies the presence of animal studies showing use is safe for the fetus.

26. Correct: Inuit (B)

The Inuit population has the highest prevalence of primary angle closure, thought to be greater than 20 times the incidence in Caucasians (represented by **C**). Asian populations (represented by **A**) are thought to have a prevelance of primary angle closure higher than that of Caucasians but lower than that of Inuits. East African (**D**) populations have a lower incidence of primary angle closure than the Inuit population.

27. Correct: A 33-year-old woman with history of open-angle glaucoma and elevated intraocular pressures, now controlled by trabeculectomy in both eyes (B)

(**B**) represents juvenile open-angle glaucoma (JOAG). The *TIGR/MYOC* gene, which codes for the TIGR protein within the trabecular meshwork, is located on chromosome 1 and is associated with JOAG. The 85-year-old woman with scleral spur identified on gonioscopy 360 degrees and history of maximal intraocular pressure of 35 mm Hg OU (**A**) represents primary open-angle glaucoma (POAG). POAG is thought to have a complex inheritence. The 65-year old woman with history of elevated intraocular pressure and moth-eaten pupillary border (**C**) represents pseudoexfoliation, which is linked to LOXL1 on chromosome 15. The 54-year-old man with posterior embryotoxon and history of elevated intraocular pressure (**D**) describes Axenfeld-Rieger syndrome, which is linked to PITX2, on chromosome 4.

28. Correct: Inner nonpigmented epithelial cells of ciliary processes (C)

Aqueous humor is produced by the ciliary processes, most specifically in the inner nonpigmented epithelial cells (**C**). It is not produced in the other anatomic locations presented here (**A, B, D**).

29. Correct: Tonography (B)

Tonography is performed by exposing the eye to fluorescein and then measuring its concentration in the anterior chamber; these data are used to extrapolate aqueous humor formation rate. Tonometry (**A**) is used to measure intraocular pressure. Fluorophotometry (**C**) is used to measure aqueous flow. Angiography (**D**) is used to map blood or vascular flow, as in fluorescein angiography to image the retinal blood vessels.

30. Correct: Juxtacanalicular meshwork (D)

The area of greaest resistance to outflow is the juxtacanalicular meshwork. Uveal meshwork (**A**), corneoscleral meshwork (**B**), and scleral spur (**C**) all exhibit lower resistance to outflow than the juxtacanalicular meshwork.

31. Correct: 15% (B)

In healthy adult eyes, approximatley 15% of the total aqueous humor outflow is attributable to the uveoscleral outflow pathway.

32. Correct: Low; high (A)

Corneal edema can cause falsely low pressure readings (**A and B**). Too much fluorescein during applanation can cause excessively wide mires and an overestimation of the true intraocular pressure (**A and C**). Notably, corneal scarring can lead to falsely elevated intraocular pressure readings due to lack of calibration of the tonometer for more rigid and irregular scarred corneal surfaces.

33. Correct: Ocular Hypertension Treatment Study (C)

In this study, thinner central corneal thickness was associated with increased risk of glaucoma development. This relationship remained even when controlling for intraocular pressure. The Blue Mountain Eye Study (**A**) was a large population-based study performed in Australia; it examined the prevelance of glaucoma in this population but did not examine central corneal thickness. The Collaborative Initial Glaucoma Treatment Study (CIGTS) examined if early trabeculectomy versus medication was a better treatment for glaucoma; they found that visual field progression was not significantly different between the two groups despite significantly lower intraocular pressure in the surgical group. The Early Manifest Glaucoma Trial (EGMT) studied treatment versus observation in early primary open-angle glaucoma; EGMT found that lowering IOP resulted in less progression of glaucoma.

34. Correct: Wiping the prism with 1:10 sodium hypochlorite (D)

This is not a validated method of cleaning the Goldmann applanation prism. The other methods listed (**A, B, C**) are all valid methods to clean the applanation prism.

35. Correct: 1.95 mm (D)

When using a 90 **D** lens for ophthalmoscopy, the disc height should be multipled by 1.3 (here, 1.5 mm × 1.3 = 1.95 mm). When using a 60 D lens, there is no conversion needed. When using a 78 **D** lens, the measured height should be multiplied by 1.1.

36. Correct: 1% (B)

Asymmetrical optic nerves with the degree of asymmetry greater than 0.3 is found in less than 1% of the normal population. This is supported by data from the Blue Mountains Eye Study.

37. Correct: 2.5 mm (B)

Patients with pupils smaller than 2.5 mm may have artificially constricted or depressed visual fields due to small pupil size.

38. Correct: Early glaucoma, M cells (B)

FDT testing can be especially useful in screening for early visual field depressions. In frequency doubling, a low-frequency sinusoidal grating is put through high-frequency counterphase flicker; this results in twice as many light and dark bars being seen than are actually present (or, frequency doubling). FDT technology mostly stimulates the mangocellular (**M**) cells of the visual pathway, which are responsible for the detection of motion. This is particularly useful in the diagnosis of glaucoma, as it is thought that M cells may be the earliest cells to be impaired in glaucoma.

39. Correct: Iridocorneal endothelial syndrome (D)

This syndrome is unilateral as are the clinical findings of glaucoma in this patient. Iridocorneal endothelial syndrome is also most common in women. The other conditions can often present bilaterally (**A–C**).

40. Correct: Shorter, lower (D)

Patients with pigmentary glaucoma may respond well to selective laser trabeculoplasty, although the duration of the treatment effect may be shorter than the average patient (**C and D**). They are also at a higher risk of postoperative intraocular pressure spikes. Since the trabecular pigmentation absorbs laser energy, the expected energy settings would be lower than the average patient (**B and D**).

41. Correct: Macrophages (D)

This patient presents with a clinical scenario classic for phacolytic glaucoma, a condition in which a mature cataract releases lens proteins through an intact lens capsule, stimulating an inflammatory response. In this condition, macrophages clog the trabecular meshwork, leading to elevated intraocular pressure. Basophils (**A**) are not associated with lens-related glaucomas. Neutrophils (**B**) are associated with infection and not phacolytic glaucoma. Eosinophils (**C**) are most associated with allergic conditions and not lens-related glaucomas.

42. Correct: HLA B27-associated uveitis (D)

HLA B27-associated uveitis is not associated with elevated intraocular pressure, as seen in this case scenario. All other answer choices are uveitic conditions associated with elevated intraocular pressures.

43. Correct: Superior vena cava syndrome (A)

Superior vena cava syndrome can cause downstream effects that, in chronic cases, lead to blood vessel changes and elevated filling pressures, which in turn can lead to engorged episcleral vessels. The other conditions noted above do not cause this phenomenon.

44. Correct: 8–10 mm Hg (C)

Normal episcleral venous pressure (EVP) is between 8 and 10 mm Hg. EVP is typically not measured clinically, as its measurement is often invasive. The only direct method to measure EVP is via direct cannulation of the vein.

45. Correct: Girl hit by tree branch leading to corneal abrasion (B)

An ocular injury from a baseball hit (**A**) can lead to angle recession, which is strongly associated with glaucoma development. A metal grinding injury (**C**) leading to intraocular metallic foreign body can lead to glaucoma, as both siderosis or chalcosis can cause glaucoma. Bleach (**D**) is an alkaline substance that can cause inflammation and damage to the drainage angle leading to glaucoma. Of these injuries, only tree branch leading to corneal abrasion (**B**) has no clear association with glaucoma.

46. Correct: Oxybutynin (C)

The image above shows an anatomic narrow angle; oxybutynin can lead to angle closure in this setting due to its anticholinergic properties. The other medications are not associated with angle closure. Although fluticasone (**D**) can be associated with elevated eye pressures with chronic use, as any steroid, there is not any specific reason to avoid this medication in this patient over any other person.

47. Correct: Is a woman (B)

The figure shows essential iris atrophy, a form of iridocorneal endothelial (ICE) syndrome, which is most common in women. It is typically a unilateral condition (**A**) found in younger adults (**C**). There is no known association with ocular trauma (**D**). ICE syndrome is a condition characterized by abnormal corneal endothelium; it can affect the eye in various ways and to varying degrees, and is comprised of three subtypes: Chandler's syndrome, Cogan–Reese syndrome, and essential iris atrophy. Chandler's syndrome is responsible for approximately 50% of ICE syndromes; it is recognized as corneal edema with minimal to no iris changes. Cogan–Reese syndrome (or iris nevus syndrome) is recognized by pigmented nodules on the iris surface. Essential iris atrophy is characterized by irregular iris holes, corectopia, ectropion uveae, and iris atrophy.

48. Correct: Transscleral diode cyclophotocoagulation (D)

In eyes with a history of ocular melanoma, there is the concern that incisional surgical procedures could spread tumor cells to the rest of the body, leading to remote, metastatic disease spread. In these eyes, nonincisional transscleral diode cyclophotocoagulation is the most reasonable surgical glaucoma intervention. Since the intraocular pressure is 40 mm Hg in an eye with 20/100 vision, monitoring the eye on the current treatment (**A**) would put the patient at significant risk of vision loss. Incisional procedures, such as trabeculectomy (**B**) or glaucoma drainage device (**C**), as noted above, carry the possibility of spreading tumor cells to the rest of the body and are typically avoided.

49. Correct: Tuberous sclerosis (D)

Tuberous sclerosis is not associated with glaucoma. The other phakomatoses seen here (**A–C**) are all associated with glaucoma.

50. Correct: Occurs in males (A)

The symptoms of blepharospasm ("grimacing" facial movements), tearing, and photophobia are classic for primary congenital glaucoma, which is more common in males. This disease is most often diagnosed by 1 year of age (**B**). It is bilateral in approximately two-thirds of patients (**C**). Primary congenital glaucoma has a worse prognosis if diagnosed as a newborn (**D**).

51. Correct: Ischemia (C)

The figure shows glaukomflecken, a sequelae thought to be related to ischemia from angle closure. These anterior subcapsular opacities appear white or gray as seen here. They are not thought to be related to inflammation (**A**) or iris pigment (**B**). There is no known association with regressed neovascularization (**D**).

52. Correct: Brimonidine and pilocarpine 2% (A)

Brimonidine can be used topically to assist in lowering the elevated intraocular pressure seen during acute angle closure (most often in conjunction with other topical, oral, or IV ocular antihypertensives). Apraclonidine should be avoided in angle closure due to its potential to dilate the pupil and worsen the angle closure (**C and D**). Pilocarpine in lower concentrations (2% or lower) can be useful in acute angle closure by constricting the pupil and opening the angle. However, higher powers of pilocarpine (4%, seen in B and D), can rotate the lens anteriorly, worsening angle closure, and should be avoided.

53. Correct: Pilocarpine (C)

In Marfan's syndrome with ectopia lentis, as seen here, the etiology of angle closure is pupillary block from the displaced crystalline lens. In this situation, cycloplegia (as with atropine, **B**) can help relieve the angle closure by moving the lens interface posteriorly. Conversely, miotics like pilocarpine (**C**) can worsen the pupillary block by rotating the lens interface or ciliary body forward. Laser iridotomy can be useful in relieving pupillary block (**A**). Acetazolamide, given either orally or intravenously, can help lower the elevated intraocular pressure seen in this condition (**D**).

54. Correct: Sudden onset of decreased vision in the upper half of the visual field (C)

The clinical vignette describes elevated intraocular pressure in the setting of a mid-dilated pupil and abnormal blood vessels at the anterior-chamber angle (neovascularization of the angle); this is a classic description of neovascular glaucoma. Any vascular disease involving the eye may lead to chronic ischemia and subsequent neovascular glaucoma. (**C**) describes sudden onset of decreased vision in the upper half of the visual field, which would be suggestive of branch retinal vein occlusion. Neovascular glaucoma is very rare in branch retinal vein occlusion, likely due to the limited level of ischemia seen in this condition. Sudden onset of diffusely decreased

vision (**A**) is suggestive of central retinal vein occlusion, which is one of the most common etiologies of neovascular glaucoma. History of panretinal photocoagulation (**B**) is consistent with either central retinal vein occlusion or diabetic retinopathy, another leading cause of neovascular glaucoma. Episodes of dark vision that self-resolve (**D**) is suggestive of ocular ischemic syndrome, also one of the top three most common etiologies of neovascular glaucoma, along with diabetes and central retinal vein occlusion.

55. Correct: 10% (B)

56. Correct: Nd:YAG laser treatment (A)

This clinical scenario is most consistent with malignant glaucoma (also known as aqueous misdirection). The mechanism of this condition is poorly understood but may result from misdirected flow of the aqueous fluid posteriorly. In this condition, Nd:YAG laser can be used in the pseudophakic patient to treat the anterior hyaloid face and return normal fluid flow within the eye. Cycloplegia (not represted in the answer choices) is also an appropriate treament for malignant glaucoma. Pilocarpine would not help the condition and may exacerbate the aqueous misdirection (**B**). (**C**) and (**D**) would treat a wound leak leading to a shallow anterior chamber. That is unlikely in this scenario as the intraocular pressure is noted to be high; in the setting of a wound leak, the intraocular pressure would be low.

57. Correct: Argon laser (C)

Argon laser treatment can be useful in the diagnosis of epithelial ingrowth, as seen in the figure. Epithelial ingrowth is most commonly seen after complex surgery or trauma, or in any condition in which the ocular wound is not well sealed. Epithelial tissue grows within the eye causing, as seen here, overlying corneal edema. The edge of epithelial tissue is seen as a white, prominent edge. Argon laser can be used to treat areas of affected iris—iris with overlying epithelial ingrowth will respond to argon laser treatment by creating white burns (while normal iris shows typical shrinkage from argon laser). Diagnosis of epithelial ingrowth can also be aided by biopsy of affected tissues or testing of aqueous humor or vitreous samples. Ultrasound biomicroscopy (**A**), CT scan (**B**), or pachymetry (**D**) are not helpful in this diagnosis.

58. Correct: Chronic angle closure (B)

The case scenario of leukocoria (white pupillary reflex) caused by a retrolental membrane describes persistent fetal vasculature (PFV), a condition in which the fetal hyaloid vascular complex does not regress. In PFV, the PFV tissue can slowly contract over time, leading to a narrow-angle and angle-closure glaucoma. There is no reason to suspect inflammatory glaucoma (**A**) in PFV. Open-angle glaucoma would not be the most likely etiology in PFV (**C**). Steroids are not typically a treatment on PFV patients (**D**).

59. Correct: Immediate laser peripheral iridotomy (C)

This case vignette describes topiramate-induced angle closure in this young woman using topiramate for migraine headache. Since topiramate-induced angle closure is typically related to choroidal effusions, and not pupillary block, iridotomy is not indicated. Topiramate should be immediately discontinued in these cases (**B**) and the glaucoma often self-resolves shortly thereafter. Acetazolamide (**A**) can be used to lower intraocular pressure in the acute setting, although, interestingly, acetazolamide has been associated with secondary angle-closure glaucoma from choroidal effusion. Atropine (**D**) can help relieve the angle closure via cycloplegia depending on the anterior chamber angle.

60. Correct: Descemet's membrane (C)

Haab's striae are irregularities in Descemet's membrane, seen in primary congenital glaucoma.

61. Correct: Sporadic (D)

This image of a corneal leukoma represents Peters' anomaly. In this condition, affecting the corneal endothelium, Descemet's membrane, and stroma, nearly 50% of people develop glaucoma. This is primarily due to deformation of the angle structures. Peters' anomaly can be inherited via autosomal recessive (**A**) or autosomal dominant (**B**) inheritance but is most frequently sporadic.

62. Correct: Nephrologist (B)

Aniridia, as seen in this image, is associated with the WAGR syndrome (Wilms' tumor, aniridia, genitourinary disease, and mental retardation). An infant with aniridia would benefit from referral to nephrology to evaluate for Wilms' tumor. Notably, aniridia is also associated with Gillespie's syndrome (aniridia, cerebellar ataxia, mental retardation).

63. Correct: Small corneal diameter (B)

Infants receiving cataract surgery are typically left aphakic following surgery; the risk of developing glaucoma when aphakic may be as high as 50%. Smaller corneal diameter has been associated with increased risk of aphakic glaucoma. Cataract surgery before age of 1 year (vs. **A**) and surgical complicatons (vs. **C**) are associated with increased risk. There is no reported association of cataract density with risk of aphakic glaucoma.

64. Correct: 10 mm (C)

The average normal corneal diameter in the newborn is approximately 10 mm. This distinction is important when screening for congenital glaucoma, which can lead to increased corneal diameter. By the age of 1 year, the cornea typically increases in size up to 11.5 mm.

65. Correct: 50 minutes (C)

The normal rate of aqueous formation is approximately 2 µL per minute. If 100 µL is withdrawn from the anterior chamber, it would take approximately 50 minutes for the fluid to be reproduced.

66. Correct: 10 (C)

There is a normal variation in intraocular pressure over the course of the day; this is thought to be between 2 and 6 mm Hg in the normal individual without glaucoma. A variation greater than 10 mm Hg is thought to be suggestive of glaucoma.

67. Correct: Pregnancy (D)

During pregnancy, most people experience lower intraocular pressure. The other answers are all correlated with higher eye pressures, at least at the time of activity. Playing a wind instrument (**A**) causes higher eye pressure due to straining. Prolonged head down positions in yoga (**B**) can contribute to higher eye pressurs during that moment. Chronic constipation (**C**) can lead to straining or Valsalva, which also leads to higher eye pressures at that time.

68. Correct: Younger age (A)

Older age is associated with glaucoma progression in multiple studies, including Advanced Glaucoma Intervention Study, Collaborative Initial Glaucoma Treatment Study, and Early Manifest Glaucoma Trial. By contrast, larger cup to disc ratio (**B**) has been associated with glaucoma progression. Higher intraocular pressure is a clear risk factor for glaucoma progression (**C**). Race, most notably for people of African descent, is correlated with glaucoma progression.

69. Correct: *GLC1A* (A)

The trabecular meshwork-induced glucocorticoid response protein (*TIGR*) gene or myocilin (*MYOC*) gene at locus *GLC1A* is associated with juvenile open-angle glaucoma. *GLC1B* (**B**), *GLC1C* (**C**), and *GLC1E* (**D**) are all associated with primary open-angle glaucoma.

70. Correct: External ocular examination (D)

This visual field shows sudden and deep superior field loss, not in the arcuate pattern most typical of glaucoma; this should prompt examination for ptosis or visually significant dermatochalasis. If the patient's eyelids are getting in the way of her visual field testing, the lids should be held or taped out of the patient's vision for repeat testing, and upper eyelid surgery considered for visually significant lid changes. Starting brimonidine (**A**) may be appropriate if a visual field with no artifacts from the eyelids confirm glaucomatous progression. Close observation alone (**B**) would not be appropriate if there is new visual field depression. The visual field depression here is not consistent with a neurologic condition (**C**).

71. Correct: Thin, avascular bleb (D)

The case vignette describes bleb-related infection, indicated by 1 day of eye pain and decreased vision associated with injection surrounding the trabeculectomy and hypopyon. This could signify blebitis versus endophthalmitis, the latter being diagnosed if there is posterior segment inflammation as well. Thin, avascular trabeculectomy blebs are associated with an increased risk of infection, thought to be most likely related to their potential for intermittent leaking. An eye shield at night (**A**) should be protective against eye rubbing or bleb trauma, leading to lower risk of infection. Moderate weight lifting (**B**) should not affect a bleb. While swimming without goggles would be a risk factor for bleb infection, watertight goggles (**C**) should guard against this.

72. Correct: Delayed laser suture lysis (D)

Young, myopic patients (myopia is commonly associated with pigmentary glaucoma) are at risk of hypotony with filtering surgery. Because of the risk of hypotony, laser suture lysis (**D**) should be done with caution and often is avoided in the early postoperative period. There is no indication to increase wear of the eye shield at night (**A**), topical antibiotic use (**B**), or ocular lubrication (**C**) in these patients.

73. Correct: Increased aqueous humor outflow due to changes in matrix metalloproteinases in the trabecular meshwork (D)

The mechanism of action of selective laser trabeculoplasty is not fully understood. However, the leading thought is that the laser treatment changes the expression of matrix metalloproteinases within the trabecular meshwork, leading to increased outflow. There is no evidence of thermal or other damage or openings in the trabecular meshwork leading to increased outflow (**A, B, and C**).

74. Correct: Tinnitus (D)

Mannitol is a hyperosmotic drug that can be used to treat elevated intraocular pressure, but it can cause a myriad of side effects. Some of the most concerning of these side effects include subdural hemorrhage (**A**), subarachnoid hemorrhage (**B**), and worsening of congestive heart failure (**C**). It can also cause headache, confusion, dehydration, and myocardial infarction. Tinnitus is not a side effect from mannitol and, in some cases, mannitol can be used in the treatment of tinnitus.

75. Correct: Blebitis (D)

Postoperative 5-FU is given to help prevent excessive scarring that can lead to bleb failure. There are a number of potential side effects from this medication, including wound leak, corneal epithelial irritation, hypotony, and suprachoroidal hemorrhage. Blebitis (**D**) is a potential risk in any leaking bleb or in any thin, avascular bleb (as can form with 5-FU). There is no association with 5-FU and cataract or retinal tear formation (**A and B**). 5-FU is associated with corneal epithelial disease (not endothelial) (**C**).

76. Correct: High-viscosity viscoelastic (A)

In patients with an anatomic narrow angle, using a high-viscosity viscoelastic can be helpful in deepening the anterior chamber and allowing safer phacoemulsification. Because of the shallow anterior chamber, the cataract should not be removed by phacoemulsification above the iris plane (**B**), as this can predispose to excessive corneal edema due to the proximity of the phacoemulsification energy to the corneal endothelium. Increasing the bottle height (vs. decreasing, **C**) can help deepen the anterior chamber. Creation of a larger main incision (**D**) may allow more viscoelastic to escape the eye, making the anterior chamber shallower and the surgery more difficult.

77. Correct: Discussion of a low-vision evaluation (B)

This patient has best corrected visual acuity of 20/40 in one eye and 20/200 in the other eye; at this level of vision, his depth perception is likely impaired. Patients with lower vision may benefit from discussion of a low-vision or vision rehabilitation evaluation (**B**) to try to improve any vision-related difficulties in their activities of daily living. Discussion of the treatment plan with a family member is not necessary if the patient is able to manage his own care (**A**). Discussion of insurance coverage of medication, while not inappropriate, does not appear to be needed here as the patient notes compliance with his medications (**C**). Asssitance with transportation costs to/from clinic is not unreasonable (**D**), if such resources are available, but does not appear pressing at this time as the patient is noted to be adherent to his visits and treatment plan.

78. Correct: High, low (D)

Excessive fluorescein instilled into the eye leads to thicker than desired mires, which leads to overestimation of intraocular pressure (IOP) when the mires are lined up (**C or D**). See the figure. Because of lower scleral rigidity, IOP can be underestimated in high myopia (**A or D**).

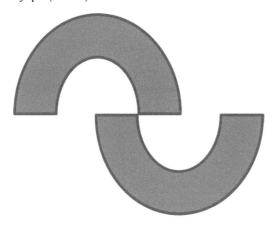

79. Correct: Posner's lens (D)

To correctly perform gonioscopy, the procedure seen here, an upright view of the angle structures is necessary; this is achieved via direct gonioscopy, in which the angle is viewed directly with the applied light beam. The Koeppe lens (**A**), Barkan's lens (**B**), and the Swan–Jacob lens (**C**) are all tools that can be used to perform direct gonioscopy. The Posner lens (**D**) is used to perform indirect gonioscopy, which is more common in the ophthalmology clinic. In indirect gonioscopy, light shone into the anterior-chamber angle is reflected into a lens mirror, allowing a view of the anterior-chamber angle.

80. Correct: Cataract extraction (A)

The patient is shown to have plateau iris, with the classic "double hump" sign. The "double hump" sign is seen on indentation gonioscopy—one hump shows the iris resting on the lens and a second hump closer to the angle showing the anteriorly rotated ciliary body. In this condition, laser peripheral iridotomy (**B**) improves any pupillary block component but cannot sufficiently deepen the angle due to the anteriorly rotated ciliary processes. Either cataract extraction or the combination of laser peripheral iridotomy and argon laser iridoplasty can sufficiently open the angle anatomy. Brimonidine (**C**) may control the intraocular pressure but will not ultimately improve the underlying anatomic issue. There is no role for panretinal photocoagulation (**D**).

81. Correct: Hypospadias (A)

This photograph of posterior embryotoxon signifies Axenfeld's anomaly, which is associated with

Axenfeld–Rieger syndrome. In this syndrome, patients have Axenfeld's anomaly and dental anomalies, facial bone anomalies, redundant periumbilical skin, pituitary disease, and/or hypospadias (**A**). Enlarged molars (**B**) are not associated with the disease (microdontia, instead, is). Mottled skin pigmentation (**C**) and ataxia (**D**) are not associated with this condition.

82. Correct: The circle of Zinn–Haller (A)

The lamina cribrosa region of the optic nerve is supplied by the circle of Zinn–Haller, an anastomosis of typically four short posterior ciliary arteries surrounding the optic nerve. The anterior optic nerve is typically supplied by the posterior ciliary arteries. The nerve fiber layer is supplied by arterioles from the central retinal artery (**B**). The temporal region of the nerve fiber layer may be supplied by the cilioretinal artery (**D**) in people in whom this artery exists. The prelaminar region, like the lamina cribrosa region of the optic nerve, is also supplied by the circle of Zinn–Haller (and other short posterior ciliary arteries). Retinal capillaries (**C**) do not supply the laminar region of the optic nerve.

83. Correct: 4 mm² (C)

The standard size for the visual field stimulus on a Humphrey perimeter is 4 mm². This is the same size as the Goldmann perimeter size III stimulus.

84. Correct: A patient requiring an in-the-bag lens implant +28 diopters for emmetropia (B)

A most likely requires this strong lens power due to short axial length. People with short axial lengths are more likely to develop malignant glaucoma, a condition characterized by elevated intraocular pressure in the presence of a shallow anterior chamber (when this is not due to pupillary block, i.e., with a patent peripheral iridotomy). Patients with pigmentary glaucoma (**A**) typically are myopic with longer axial length. A patient with an average to long axial length (**C**) would not be at increased risk of malignant glaucoma over a high hyperopia. The number of intraocular medications used to control intraocular pressure (**D**) is not correlated with risk of malignant glaucoma.

85. Correct: Sixteen times larger (D)

A Goldmann size I stimulus is ¼ mm² in size, while a Goldmann size III stimulus is 4 mm² in size; therefore, the Goldmann size III stimulus is 16 times larger than the Goldmann size I stimulus. With each increase in the Goldmann stimulus size, the size increases fourfold, that is, the Goldmann stimulus I is sized ¼ mm² and the next larger stimulus, size II, is sized 1 mm².

86. Correct: Iritis (D)

Pilocarpine is a cholinergic agonist, which decreases intraocular pressure by increasing aqueous fluid outflow by contracting the longitudinal ciliary muscle and opening the trabecular meshwork. The other answer choices listed (**A–C**) are all known potential side effects of pilocarpine. Other potential side effects include brow ache or headache, pupillary constriction, ocular irritation or allergy, cicatricial pemphigoid, and a shallow anterior chamber.

87. Correct: Observation (A)

This photograph shows a trabeculectomy leak, using Seidel's testing with sodium fluorescein. Bleb leaks can put patients at risk of vision loss due to hypotony or hypotony maculopathy. Most importantly, they are a risk for infection. For these reasons, observation (**A**) is not an appropriate treatment course. Autologous blood injection (**B**) has been used as a treatment for bleb leaks. Some bleb leaks heal with use of lubricants, such as antibiotic ointment (**C**), or with bandage contact lens placement. Timolol (**D**), for its aqueous suppressant properties, may be useful in bleb leak—by allowing less fluid to flow through the leak, potentially promoting wound healing.

88. Correct: Image B (B)

Patients with pseudoexfoliation glaucoma can benefit from large decreases in intraocular pressure from selective laser trabeculoplasty. Primary open-angle glaucoma (Image A, illustrated here with a normal anterior-chamber angle on gonioscopy) can also greatly benefit from selective laser trabeculoplasty, but classically pseudoexfoliation can benefit more. Angle-recession and uveitic glaucoma (Image C and Image D, respectively) are conditions for which selective laser trabeculoplasty is relatively contraindicated, due to risk for inflammation and/or intraocular pressure spike.

89. Correct: Dorzolamide (D)

In treating a black hyphema patient with unknown past medical history, the care team should avoid carbonic anhydrase inhibitors (CAIs) to be cautious about the possibility of sickle cell anemia or sickle cell trait, which is asymptomatic. CAIs, such as dorzolamide and systemic acetazolamide, are typically not used in controlling intraocular pressure in hyphema patients with sickle cell anemia or sickle cell trait; CAIs can increase aqueous acidity, leading to greater red blood cell sickling that makes the hyphema more difficult to clear. Latanoprost, brimonidine, and timolol (**A–C**) do not cause this complication.

90. Correct: Intraocular pressure of 35 mm Hg for 3 days (B)

In the absence of sickle cell trait or anemia (i.e., normal blood work), elevated intraocular pressure it typically tolerated for up to 5 days prior to surgical intervention, as most hyphemas clear without complication with medical interventions only. Corneal blood staining (**A**) can be permanent, and this is a reason to proceed with surgery to preserve vision. In patients with sickle cell trait or sickle cell anemia, intraocular pressure should be treated more aggressively, due to increased risk of intraocular pressure spikes and persistently elevated intraocular pressure due to difficulty clearing sickled cells from the anterior chamber. Patients with sickle cell are typically treated surgically if they sustain an intraocular pressure of greater than or equal to 25 mm Hg for more than or equal to 24 hours (**C and D**).

91. Correct: Central retinal artery (A)

The central retinal artery has arterioles that supply the blood to the superficial nerve fiber layer of the optic nerve. The lamina cribrosa region of the optic nerve is supplied by the cricle of Zinn–Haller (**C**), an anastomosis of typically four short posterior ciliary arteries surrounding the optic nerve. The anterior optic nerve is typically supplied by the posterior ciliary arteries (**B**). The temporal region of the nerve fiber layer may be supplied by the cilioretinal artery in people in whom this artery exists. The prelaminar region, like the lamina cribrosa region of the optic nerve, is also supplied by the circle of Zinn–Haller (and other short posterior ciliary arteries).

92. Correct: Brimonidine (B)

Brimonidine can cause several serious side effects in infants and children, including respiratory depression, lethargy, and central nervous system depression. This drug should be avoided in this age group. Timolol (**A**), dorzolamide (**C**), and latanoprost (**D**) are not known to have this effect.

93. Correct: *Streptococcus* (A)

Streptococcus bacteria are the most common pathogen identified in bleb-related endophthalmitis, likely causing more than half of these infections. *Staphylococcus* and *Haemophilus influenzae* are less common bacterial pathogens (**B and C**). Fungi (**D**) are also less common pathogens.

94. Correct: Central corneal thickness (A)

The Ocular Hypertension Treatment Study found a strong correlation with central corneal thickness and risk of glaucoma development. Even when correcting for intraocular pressure, thicker central cornea was found to be protective against glaucoma.

95. Correct: Intraocular pressure was lower in the medically treated group

The ultimate visual field outcomes were similar between the medically and surgically treated groups in this trial. Quality of life was similar between the medically and surgically treated groups (**A**). The intraocular pressure was lower in the surgically treated group (**B**), although the visual field outcomes did not appear different despite this. Early visual acuity loss was greater in the surgically treated group (**D**), possibly related to cataract formation.

96. Correct: Fuchs' heterochromic iridocyclitis (A)

In Fuchs' heterochromic iridocyclitis, small blood vessels can grow across the trabecular meshwork; upon entering the eye with a wound during cataract surgery, these blood vessels may break and cause an anterior-chamber hemorrhage. This phenomenon is not seen in the other conditions listed here.

97. Correct: Trabeculectomy revision (B)

This patient is seen to have hypotony maculopathy with prominent macular folds, which can cause significant decrease in vision; the recommended treatment for this condition is reversal of the hypotony, most likely by bleb revision. If there is no bleb leak to be repaired, a short trial of medications, such as steroids and cycloplegia, can also be tried. Brimonidine (**A**) would not be appropriate, as this would likely further lower the intraocular pressure and worsen the hypotony. Frequent lubrication (**C**) would not help the hypotony. Careful observation (**D**) would not be advised in the prescence of macular folds as these can become permanent and cause permanent vision loss if not reversed in a reasonable time frame.

98. Correct: Thyroid eye disease (B)

Thyroid eye disease can cause increased episcleral venous pressure due to orbital congestion; this can lead to obstruction of venous outflow and increased episcleral venous pressure. There is neither any known association with the Valsalva maneuver and chronic elevation in episcleral venous pressure (**A**) nor with iris neovascularization (**C**) or primary open-angle glaucoma (**D**).

99. Correct: Spontaneous closure of a cyclodialysis cleft (C)

After blunt ocular trauma, a cyclodialysis cleft (rupture of the ciliary body from the scleral spur) can cause ocular hypotony; these clefts can self-resolve and the intraocular pressure can spike much higher with this resolution. This increase in eye pressure can be transient and may be related to the need for the trabecular meshwork to readjust its function following cleft closure. Two weeks would be out of the usual window for recurrent hyphema (**A**) and/or late-onset ocular inflammation (**B**). A corneal abrasion would not become symptomatic 2 weeks after the initial incident (**D**).

100. Correct: False positive—patient does not respond to visual field stimulus in an area she previously has seen (B)

The above description illustrates a false negative; false positive exists when the patient presses the visual field response button when no stimulus was been presented. Lens rim artifact (**A**) occurs when the patient's prescription vision lens is decentered on her eye or placed too far away from her eye, getting in the way of her peripheral vision. Cloverleaf artifact occurs when the patient stops responding midway through the visual field testing (**C**), resulting in a characteristic cloverleaf pattern; this can also be a sign of nonorganic vision loss. Fixation losses (**D**) are seen when the patient's eye loses site of the fixation target (or the patient generally loses attention), rendering the visual field test unreliable.

The patient presents with a concern for worsening visual fields. The visual field test shown above demonstrates a classic "cloverleaf" artifact. The most reasonable approach would be to discuss with the patient visual field testing strategies and then repeat visual field testing. Laser trabeculoplasty would be indicated if the patient's examination and testing support true progression of his glaucoma (**A**). There is no evidence here for a neurological problem leading to visual field depression (**B**). Observation is not appropriate if there is concern of progressive glaucoma (**C**).

Chapter 3

Lens and Cataract

Christian Song, Grace Sun, Viral Juthani, Lisa Park

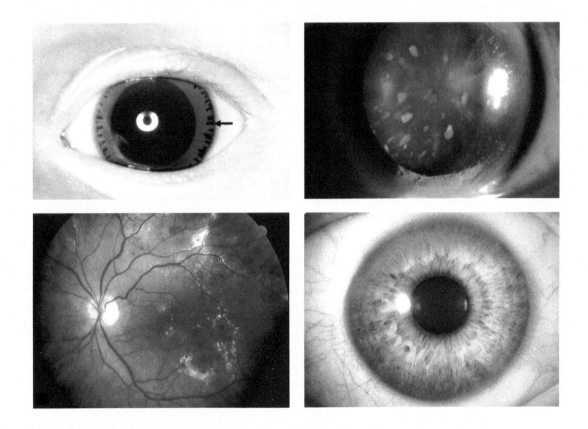

3.1 Questions

Easy	Medium	Hard

1. A medical student is preparing to travel with you on a medical mission and asks you what is the most likely cause of blindness in the patients you encounter. You answer as follows:

A. Glaucoma

B. Cataract

C. Macular degeneration

D. Trachoma

2. Which of the following was the first known risk factor for the development of cataracts?

A. Smoking

B. UV light exposure

C. High myopia

D. Topical corticosteroid use

3. The adult crystalline lens normally lacks a blood supply and innervation after fetal development. Where does it derive nutrients required for metabolic function?

A. Lens capsule

B. Zonules of Zinn

C. Aqueous humor

D. Vitreous humor

4. You have followed a patient over the past 20 years for routine eye care. The patient brings up the topic of cataract surgery—"my friend's having it"—and wants to know how his lens has changed with time. Which of the following would you not expect with aging of the crystalline lens?

A. The relative thickness of the cortex increases.

B. The lens adopts an increasingly curved shape.

C. The index of refraction increases with age.

D. The eye may become either more hyperopic or myopic as the lens ages.

5. The lens capsule is comprised of _____ collagen, and is thinnest at the _____.

A. Type I, anterior pole

B. Type IV, anterior pole

C. Type I, posterior pole

D. Type IV, posterior pole

6. As lens epithelial cells elongate to form lens fiber cells, which of the following is true?

A. There is a significant increase in the mass of cellular proteins in the fiber cell membrane.

B. Cells gain organelles including nuclei, mitochondria, and ribosomes.

C. Metabolic functional capacity increases.

D. Light passing through the cells is scattered at an increasing rate.

7. The oldest layers of the lens, the embryonic and fetal lens nuclei, exist at which of the following?

A. At the posterior pole of the lens

B. At the center of the lens

C. Toward the equator of the lens

D. At the anterior pole of the lens

8. The Y-shaped sutures of the lens appear as which of the following?

A. Erect anteriorly and posteriorly

B. Inverted anteriorly and posteriorly

C. Erect anteriorly and inverted posteriorly

D. Inverted anteriorly and erect posteriorly

9. Which of the following is the largest group of lens proteins by molecular mass?

A. α-Crystallins

B. β-Crystallins

C. βL-Crystallins

D. γ-Crystallins

10. You diagnose a 75-year-old woman with visually significant cataracts. She has read about this condition online and asks you if everything she has read is accurate. Which of the following is false?

A. Proteins aggregate to form large particles which become water insoluble.

B. An increase in water insoluble proteins correlates with the degree of lens opacification in advanced cataracts.

C. Increased levels of glutathione and decreased levels of glutathione disulfide in the cytoplasm of nuclear fiber cells lead to increased protein aggregation.

D. Nuclear proteins are highly cross-linked by disulfide and non-disulfide bonds.

11. Which of the following is false regarding accommodation?

A. Most of the accommodative change in lens shape occurs at the central anterior lens surface.

B. The curvature of the posterior surface of the lens does not significantly change with accommodation.

C. Zonular tension increases with accommodation.

D. Lens equatorial diameter decreases with accommodation.

12. The majority of adenosine triphosphate (ATP) responsible for metabolic function in the lens is generated by which of the following?

A. Citric acid cycle

B. Anaerobic glycolysis

C. Hexose monophosphate shunt

D. Sorbitol pathway

13. Which of the following is the key enzyme in the sorbitol pathway responsible for the conversion of glucose to sorbitol?

A. Phosphofructokinase

B. Aldose reductase

C. Hexokinase

D. Polyol dehydrogenase

14. You are asked to see an inpatient admitted for diabetic ketoacidosis, now complaining of decreased vision. Which of the following is likely true of his lens metabolism upon admission?

A. Sorbitol is metabolized to fructose by the enzyme polyol dehydrogenase, which has a low affinity for sorbitol.

B. In addition to sorbitol, fructose accumulates in the lens due to activation of the hexose monophosphate (HMP) and sorbitol pathway.

C. Fructose and sorbitol increase the osmotic pressure in the lens, drawing in water.

D. All of the above.

15. A 45-year-old man is status post pars plana vitrectomy and membrane peel for an epiretinal membrane. He develops a nuclear sclerotic cataract shortly after his retinal surgery. What is the most likely mechanism of his cataract formation?

A. Inadvertent trauma to the lens capsule during infusion cannula placement

B. Inadvertent trauma to the lens capsule during vitrectomy

C. Inadvertent trauma to the lens capsule during creation of sclerotomies

D. Reduced protection from oxidative damage to the lens due to the removal of the vitreous

16. The lens cells with the highest metabolic rates are found in which of the following?

A. Epithelium and outer cortex

B. Nucleus

C. Inner cortex

D. Posterior pole

17. The lens vesicle, a single layer of cuboidal cells, forms at approximately _____ days of gestation.

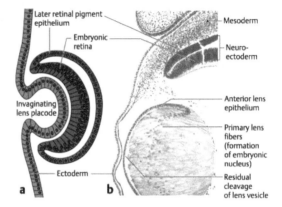

A. 10

B. 20

C. 30

D. 40

18. A fetal remnant of the tunica vasculosa lentis sometimes persists as a small opacity or strand on the posterior lens capsule called a _____.

A. Mittendorf's dot

B. Lens coloboma

C. Bergmeister's papilla

D. Posterior polar cataract

19. A 2-year-old boy is brought by his parents after the pediatrician notes an abnormal light reflex OD. You find a unilateral cataract. Which of the following conditions is most commonly associated with this?

A. Down's syndrome

B. Rubella

C. Persistent fetal vasculature

D. Aniridia

20. The condition seen in the figure is most commonly associated with loss of one allele in the _____ gene.

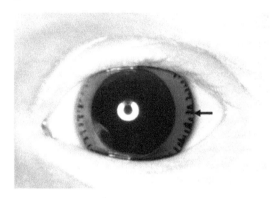

A. *PITX2*
B. *FOXC1*
C. *CYP1B1*
D. *PAX6*

21. The condition seen in the figure is associated with which of the following systemic features?

1. Small stature
2. Short and stubby fingers
3. Reduced joint mobility
4. Dilation of the aortic root

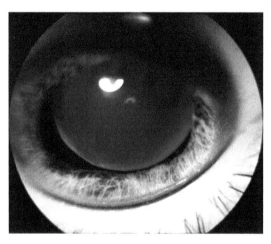

A. 1 and 2
B. 3 and 4
C. 1 and 3
D. All of the above

22. The condition seen in the figure is most classically associated with which of the following systemic features?

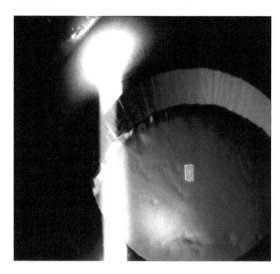

A. Seizures
B. Mitral valve prolapse
C. Sensorineural deafness
D. Cardiac conduction abnormalities

23. The image shown is most commonly associated with which of the following?

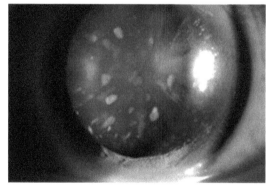

A. Diabetes
B. Myotonic dystrophy
C. No association
D. Congenital cataract

24. Bladder cells are associated with what type of cataract?

A. Morgagnian cataract
B. Cortical cataract
C. Nuclear cataract
D. Posterior subcapsular cataract

25. A 60-year-old patient presents for a dilated examination and is found to have cortical cataracts. This is often associated with which of the following?

A. Symmetric visual complaints

B. A local disruption of lens fiber cells

C. Increase in the refractive index of the lens leading to a myopic shift

D. Greater disruption of visual symptoms at near

26. When coupled with erythromycin, concomitant use of which of the following drugs may increase the risk of cataract?

A. Simvastatin

B. Prednisone

C. Pilocarpine

D. Chlorpromazine

27. A 50-year-old patient has had type 2 diabetes for 10 years. Which of the following is true regarding cataracts for this specific patient?

A. An increase in sorbitol in the lens may result in swelling of the lens fibers.

B. Increased amplitude of accommodation.

C. Given the swelling of the lens, presbyopia can occur later in patients with diabetes than those without diabetes.

D. A sunflower cataract is a typical cataract of a diabetic patient.

28. A 17-year-old male patient has periocular dermatitis. You notice lichenification on the flexural surface of his arms. Which of the following is the most likely associated lens change?

A. Polychromatic iridescent crystals in the lens cortex

B. Posterior synechiae and posterior subcapsular cataract

C. Have an "oil droplet" appearance on retroillumination, which can progress to total opacification of the lens

D. An anterior subcapsular shield-like cataract that typically develops in the early adult years

29. A 3-week-old newborn has symptoms of jaundice, hepatomegaly, and mental deficiency has been found to have an inherited metabolic condition that may be treated by diet modifications. In this condition, the ocular examination may reveal which of the following lenses?

A. Have inferior colobomas.

B. Are dislocated into the anterior chamber due to their small size.

C. Have an "oil droplet" appearance on retroillumination, which can progress to total opacification of the lens.

D. Have been dislocated inferiorly and temporally given the zonular laxity.

30. You are examining the patient with the condition shown. Her best corrected visual acuity of 20/80 and is interested in cataract surgery.

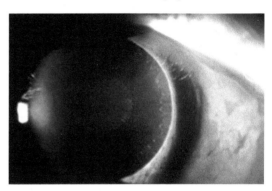

Which of the following may the patient be at higher risk for?

A. Suprachoroidal hemorrhage

B. Zonular dehiscence

C. Aqueous misdirection

D. Endophthalmitis

31. A 27-year-old man presents in your office with visual loss in the left eye status post assault a few months prior. On examination, his best corrected visual acuity of 20/80, which you determine is due to a focal cortical cataract. You also notice which of the following signs of trauma?

A. A fibrillogranular white material deposited on the lens and trabecular meshwork

B. Polychromatic iridescent crystals in the lens cortex

C. Vossius' ring

D. Soemmering's ring

32. A 30-year-old male construction worker presents to your office and on examination is found to have a small foreign body embedded in the lens. The cornea is Seidel negative, the anterior lens capsule appears to have sealed the perforation site, and the eye is quiet with no anterior chamber inflammation. Which of the following materials must be removed?

A. Glass

B. Titanium

C. Iron

D. Stone

33. A 52-year-old woman comes to your office for a follow-up visit. On examination, her vision is 20/40, the eye is white and quiet, the cornea is clear, and intraocular pressure (IOP) is 18. On her lens, you note gray–white epithelial and anterior cortical lens opacities. These opacities are associated with which of her recent episodes?

A. Phacoantigenic uveitis

B. Phacolytic glaucoma

C. Angle closure glaucoma

D. Lens particle glaucoma

34. Which of the following ocular treatments does not lead to the formation of cataract?

A. Hyperbaric oxygen

B. Scleral buckle

C. Pars plana vitrectomy

D. Topical steroids on the eyelids

35. A 55-year-old man presents with complaint of difficulty reading. Which of the following indicates cataracts are unlikely to be a contributing factor?

A. History of being on a college boxing team

B. Diagnosis of a skin disorder, currently being treated by a dermatologist

C. Complaint of glare and halos while driving at night

D. History of never wearing glasses

36. An 85-year-old man presents with pain and redness for the last few days. He has had decreased vision for over 10 years. Which of the following is the cause for his presenting complaint?

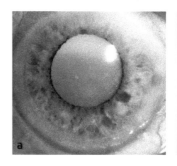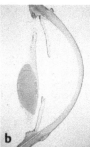

A. Phacolytic glaucoma

B. Primary angle closure glaucoma

C. Lens particle glaucoma

D. Phacomorphic glaucoma

37. A 73-year-old woman with hypertension, hyperlipidemia, and thyroid eye disease presents decreased vision for 7 years. She has a previous 40-pack-year history of smoking and a remote history of IV drug abuse. Your examination is normal except for nuclear sclerotic cataracts and early age-related macular degeneration. Which of the following risk factors is most likely associated with the development of cataracts?

A. Lack of age-related eye disease study (AREDS) multivitamin use

B. Hyperlipidemia

C. IV drug use

D. Smoking

38. A 28-year-old man presents to your office for recent decrease in vision. His previous ocular history is significant for high myopia, astigmatism, and a laser retinopexy for a retinal tear in his right eye. On examination, you see the following, which you suspect accounts for the decrease in vision. The rest of the ophthalmic examination is stable.

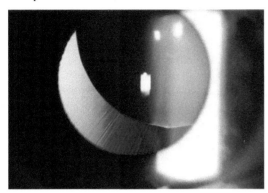

Which of the following is associated with this condition:

A. Short stature

B. Mental retardation

C. Abnormal metabolites in the urine

D. Aortic enlargement

39. A 32-year-old man with mild mental retardation, ataxia, and tremor presents to your office with recent decrease in vision. On examination, vision is decreased to 20/30 but refracts to 20/25+2. Examination is significant for a cataract and the findings demonstrated.

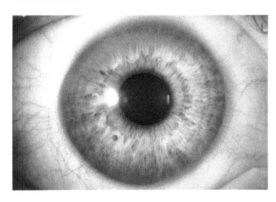

Which of the following may not associated with this condition?

A. Sunflower cataract

B. Portal hypertension

C. Hepatocellular carcinoma

D. Hepatic encephalopathy

40. A 72-year-old man has reduced visual acuity of 20/70. This has affected his ability to drive, read, and watch television. Upon review of his medical history, you find that he is currently taking tamsulosin for benign prostate hypertrophy. Prior to his cataract surgery, which of the following would you not consider?

A. Review with the patient the associated risks of tamsulosin with cataract surgery

B. Have the patient stop tamsulosin the day before surgery

C. Use of pupil expansion devices during cataract surgery

D. Utilize different parameters during phacoemulsification

41. You are evaluating macular function in a patient with a limited view of the retina. Which of the following may not be helpful to determine macular function?

A. Photostress recovery time

B. The Maddox rod

C. Blue-light entoptoscopy

D. Humphrey visual field testing

42. During the preoperative appointment prior to performing cataract surgery, you note that the patient has good dilation of the pupil and guttatA. Corneal edema after cataract surgery is associated with a central corneal thickness greater than which of the following?

A. 500 µm

B. 540 µm

C. 600 µm

D. 640 µm

43. A patient with medical history significant for hypertension, diabetes, and coronary artery disease with a cardiac stent is brought to the operating room for cataract surgery. IV sedation and a retrobulbar block are given. Upon sterile draping, it is noted that the orbit is taut with ecchymosis of the eyelids and conjunctiva. The eye is extremely firm to palpation. What is the most appropriate course of action?

A. Perform digital massage.

B. Request the anesthesiologist to decrease sedation.

C. Examine the fundus with indirect ophthalmoscopy to check for globe penetration.

D. Perform a lateral canthotomy and cantholysis.

44. During phacoemulsification of the lens nucleus, a tear is identified in the posterior lens capsule. Which of the following is the most appropriate next step?

A. Remove the phacoemulsification probe from the eye immediately.

B. Inject a dispersive ophthalmic viscosurgical device (OVD) over the tear.

C. Proceed with anterior vitrectomy using a bimanual technique.

D. Inject diluted triamcinolone to determine whether vitreous has prolapsed anteriorly.

45. A 72-year-old woman presents for preoperative evaluation for cataract surgery in her right eye. Her refraction measures +0.50 −2.25 ×140 with 20/50 visual acuity. Biometry reveals an axial length of 24.10 mm and keratometry readings of 42.25 and 42.37 at 84 degrees. Which of the following is the most appropriate method for treating her astigmatism at the time of cataract surgery?

A. Limbal relaxing incision

B. Astigmatic keratotomy

C. Toric intraocular lens implantation

D. None of the above

46. A colleague presents wondering which of four medications he should choose for his benign prostatic hyperplasia (BPH). You know that he will likely need cataract extraction in the upcoming year. Which of the following would be the worst choice?

A. Alfuzosin

B. Doxazosin

C. Tamsulosin

D. Terazosin

47. Proposed methods for the management of intraoperative floppy iris syndrome include all of the following except which one?

A. The use of iris retractors

B. Injection of epinephrine into the anterior chamber

C. Mechanical stretching of the pupil

D. Lowering flow settings

48. You are asked to perform cataract surgery on a veteran treated with prazosin for posttraumatic stress disorder (PTSD). What might his medication result in?

A. Increased iris sphincter tone

B. Iris stromal atrophy

C. Pupillary mydriasis

D. Decrease aqueous humor secretion

49. A 61-year-old man undergoes cataract surgery of his left eye without complication. He is seen again 18 hours later complaining of mild pain, photosensitivity, and worsening vision. His visual acuity is 20/200 and shows diffuse corneal edema with dense cells in the anterior chamber and a small hypopyon. The therapy most likely to lead to resolution of this condition is which of the following?

A. Intensive topical corticosteroid therapy in conjunction with a brief course of systemic corticosteroids

B. Vitreous tap and injection of broad-spectrum antibiotic

C. Fortified broad-spectrum antibiotic drops given every hour

D. Broad-spectrum antibiotics given intravenously followed by an extended course of oral antibiotics

50. A day after undergoing cataract surgery complicated by posterior capsular rupture and vitreous loss, a small strand of vitreous is observed extending through a paracentesis incision to the ocular surface. Which of the following is the most appropriate management for this?

A. Nd:YAG laser vitreolysis.

B. Return to the operating room for vitrectomy.

C. Extended course of topical corticosteroid and nonsteroidal anti-inflammatory drug.

D. Increase dosage frequency of broad-spectrum topical antibiotic until the wound has fully epithelialized.

51. An angulated intraocular lens (IOL) is designed such that the optic is vaulted posteriorly relative to the haptics. Insertion of such a lens upside down in the capsular bag may result in which of the following?

A. Hyperopic refractive surprise

B. Zonular instability

C. Corneal decompensation

D. Pupillary block glaucoma

52. A 53-year-old man with a visually significant cataract and history of rigid gas-permeable contact lens wear wishes to achieve spectacle independence with cataract surgery. His corneal topography is shown below.

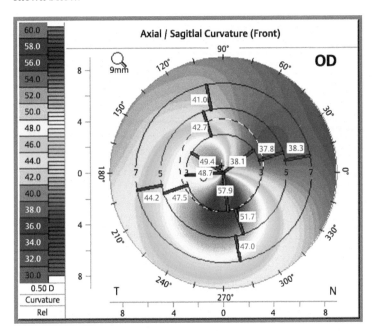

Which of the following would be the best intraocular lens (IOL) option to achieve this goal?

A. Single-piece monofocal intraocular lens (IOL)

B. Toric IOL

C. Multifocal IOL with limbal relaxing incisions

D. Multifocal toric IOL

53. A 65-year-old woman undergoes uncomplicated cataract surgery with insertion of a toric intraocular lens (IOL). At her 1-month postoperative visit, her uncorrected visual acuity is 20/80. Based on the information below, which of the following is the most likely cause?

Preoperative keratometry:

- 42.00 @ 180
- 45.00 @ 90

Postoperative refraction:

- +1.50 −3.00 × 180

Postoperative keratometry:

- 42.00 @ 180
- 45.00 @ 90

A. The lens has rotated off axis by approximately 30 degrees.

B. The lens has been implanted erroneously 90 degrees away from the correct axis.

C. The estimated surgically induced astigmatism of the main incision was too low.

D. The estimated surgically induced astigmatism of the main incision was too high.

54. You are performing an uncomplicated cataract extraction, and have started hydrodissection. The globe suddenly becomes firm, and there is marked shallowing of the anterior chamber. Which of the following is the most appropriate course of action?

A. Attempt to depressurize the globe by "burping" a paracentesis.

B. Administer mannitol intravenously.

C. Inject a cohesive ophthalmic viscosurgical device to reform the anterior chamber.

D. Inject a dispersive ophthalmic viscosurgical device to reform the anterior chamber.

55. A 71-year-old man with no significant past medical history presents 3 months after uneventful cataract surgery complaining of mildly reduced vision. Slit-lamp biomicroscopy reveals low-grade anterior chamber cell and flare, mild keratic precipitates, and normal fundoscopy except for trace vitreous cell. His best corrected visual acuity is 20/40.

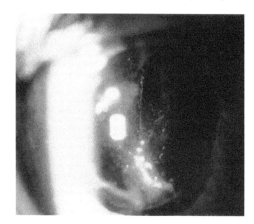

Which of the following is the most definitive management for this condition?

A. Injection of intravitreal antibiotics with capsulectomy

B. Topical corticosteroids with slow tapering

C. Nd:YAG laser capsulotomy

D. Systemic evaluation for autoimmune disease with appropriate therapy for the underlying condition

56. Cataract surgery with topical anesthesia would be most appropriate for which of the following patients?

A. A 67-year-old man with severe hearing impairment and grade 2+ nuclear sclerosis cataract

B. An 88-year-old man with a hypermature, brunescent nuclear sclerosis cataract, limiting visualization of the fundus

C. A 75-year-old woman with pseudoexfoliation, grade 3+ nuclear sclerosis cataract, and mild subluxation

D. A 45-year-old woman with trace nuclear sclerosis, dense cortical spokes, and 1 clock hour of posterior synechiae obscuring the red reflex

57. Compared to scleral tunnel incisions, which of the following regarding clear corneal incisions is not true?

A. Has little to no effect on astigmatism.

B. More efficient construction.

C. Reduces the risk of endophthalmitis.

D. Permits use of topical anesthesia.

58. Compared to a cohesive ophthalmic viscosurgical device (OVD), advantages of a dispersive OVD include all of the following except which one?

A. Protection of the corneal endothelium from phacoemulsification energy

B. Partitioning of the eye during capsular rupture

C. Minimal risk of postoperative ocular hypertension if retained in the eye

D. Suppression of vitreous prolapse through a posterior capsular tear

59. During phacoemulsification of a dense nuclear sclerotic cataract, the cornea at the main incision suddenly turns white and excessive egress of fluid is observed through this wound around the phaco probe.

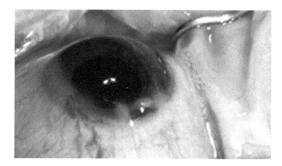

Methods that could have prevented this complication include all of the following except which one?

A. Using pulse or burst mode phacoemulsification

B. Lowering the aspiration flow rate

C. Ensuring the incision is constructed to the appropriate width

D. Converting to a nuclear expression technique (e.g., extracapsular cataract extraction)

60. A 37-year-old man has a history of traumatic injury resulting in angle recession glaucoma and lens dislocation, which required a complete lensectomy. Which of the following is the most appropriate intraocular lens (IOL) implant option to correct his aphakia?

A. Anterior chamber IOL (ACIOL)

B. Three-piece IOL secured to the iris with 9–0 nylon sutures

C. One-piece acrylic IOL secured to the sclera with 9–0 polypropylene sutures

D. Three-piece IOL with haptics externalized and secured via scleral tunnels

61. Conditions associated with the finding shown in the image include all of the following except which one:

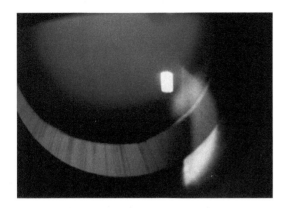

A. Pseudoexfoliation syndrome

B. Homocystinuria

C. Axenfeld–Reiger syndrome

D. Blunt force trauma

62. Cataract surgery is performed on a subluxated lens and a radial tear develops in the anterior capsule during phacoemulsification. Which of the following should be avoided?

A. Continue phacoemulsification in the capsular bag

B. Insertion of capsule tension ring

C. Use of iris hooks

D. Insertion of anterior chamber intraocular lens (ACIOL)

63. A 65-year-old patient with history of prior pars plana vitrectomy for nonclearing vitreous hemorrhage presents for cataract surgery. Which of the following should be avoided?

A. Lowering the irrigating bottle before placing the phaco tip in the eye

B. Filling the entire anterior chamber with ophthalmic viscosurgical device (OVD) to maintain positive pressure

C. Placing a second instrument between the iris and the anterior capsule prior to turning on the infusion

D. Creating a large capsulorrhexis to prolapse the lens nucleus

64. During cataract surgery, severe zonular instability has resulted in posterior dislocation of the lens with presentation of vitreous into the anterior chamber. Prior to the insertion of an anterior chamber intraocular lens (ACIOL), which of the following is the most appropriate sequence of steps?

A. Vitrectomy, inject acetylcholine, create peripheral iridectomy, inject ophthalmic viscosurgical device (OVD), enlarge wound.

B. Enlarge wound, vitrectomy, create peripheral iridectomy, inject acetylcholine, inject OVD.

C. Create peripheral iridectomy, vitrectomy, inject OVD, enlarge wound, inject acetylcholine.

D. Inject OVD, enlarge wound, vitrectomy, inject acetylcholine, create peripheral iridectomy.

65. During phacoemulsification, significant post-occlusion surge is detected. Modifications that help to reduce surge include any of the following except which one?

A. Limiting the amount of vacuum applied with the foot pedal when on the linear setting

B. Lowering the height of the irrigation bottle

C. Use of rigid, low-compliance tubing

D. Decreasing the vacuum setting

66. After the cataractous lens has been divided into quadrants during cataract surgery, the surgeon struggles to attract nuclear fragments to the phaco tip for removal. Adjustments that may help to improve followability include all of the following except which one?

A. Increase the aspiration flow rate on a peristatic pump machine.

B. Increase the vacuum on a Venturi-based system.

C. Decrease longitudinal phaco power.

D. Switch from pulse mode to continuous phacoemulsification.

67. A 72-year-old man with diabetes presents 8 weeks after uncomplicated phacoemulsification cataract surgery complaining of blurry vision. His visual acuity was previously 20/20 but has now decreased to 20/50. Examination reveals the following finding.

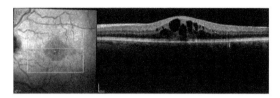

Which of the following is the most appropriate initial therapy?

A. Subtenon injection of triamcinolone acetonide

B. Intravitreal injection of triamcinolone acetonide and oral acetazolamide

C. Intravitreal injection of antivascular endothelial growth factor (anti-VEGF) agent

D. Topical ketorolac and topical prednisolone acetate

68. An 80-year-old nondiabetic patient develops decreased vision and cystoid macular edema (CME) after cataract surgery. Which of the following is true?

A. Most cases of uncomplicated CME resolve without treatment.

B. The use of preoperative corticosteroids reduces the risk of CME.

C. Anterior chamber (open-loop design) intraocular lenses (IOLs) increase the risk of persistent CME.

D. There is a higher incidence of CME with acrylic IOLs than with silicone IOLs.

69. Which of the following scenarios is least likely to result in a postoperative myopic refractive surprise?

A. Placement of an intraocular lens (IOL) in the sulcus

B. Inverted placement of an IOL

C. Choroidal effusions

D. History of myopia treated with laser in situ keratomileusis (LASIK)

70. A 55-year-old man with uncontrolled diabetes and proliferative diabetic retinopathy with isolated areas of tractional retinal detachment presents with a dense posterior subcapsular cataract.

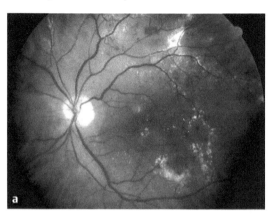

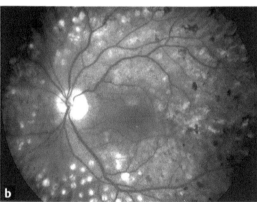

All of the following statements are true except which one?

A. A silicone intraocular lens (IOL) is the preferred type of lens implant.

B. The risk of postoperative cystoid macular edema is increased.

C. Oral hypoglycemic medications should be withheld on the morning of surgery.

D. Multifocal IOLs should be discouraged.

3.2 Answers and Explanations

Easy	Medium	Hard

1. Correct: Cataract (B)

Cataract is considered the leading cause of blindness worldwide defined by the World Health Organization (WHO) as visual acuity less than 3/60 (20/400). WHO data from 2002 estimated cataracts to be responsible for 48% of blindness worldwide prompting Vision2020, a global initiative to address reversible world blindness. Progress has been made in the last decade, and more recent data from 2015 attribute global causes of blindness in all ages to cataract 34%, glaucoma 8%, macular degeneration 6%, and trachoma less than 1%. The incidence of trachoma has decreased significantly in the last 25 years. The percentage of blind from uncorrected refractive error is believed to be 20% and from other or unknown causes is 25%.

2. Correct: Smoking (A)

The Beaver Dam Eye Study and the Blue Mountains Eye Study were among the earliest studies to conclude that there is a dose-related risk of visually significant nuclear sclerosis among smokers (**A**). Since then, numerous studies have demonstrated that UV light exposure (**B**), high myopia (**C**), and topical (along with inhaled and oral) corticosteroid use (**D**) are also risk factors for the development of cataract.

3. Correct: Aqueous humor (C)

The lens depends entirely on the aqueous humor (**C**) to meet its metabolic and nutritional demands. The lens capsule (**A**) is a basement membrane consisting primarily of collagen that encapsulates the lens, forming a barrier to large molecules from entering the lens. The zonules of Zinn (**B**) are a ring of fibrous strands that connects the ciliary body with the crystalline lens of the eye, acting as suspensory ligaments of the lens. The vitreous humor (**D**) is a relatively stagnant fluid, unlike the aqueous which is continuously replenished and metabolically active. The vitreous has a gel-like consistency with very few cells and low metabolic exchange with the systemic circulation.

4. Correct: The index of refraction increases with age (C)

As the lens ages, the relative thickness of the cortex increases (**A**), and the lens has an increasingly curved shape (**B**), resulting in more refractive power and a progressive myopic shift (**D**). However, the index of refraction of the lens *decreases* with age, likely related to the increased presence of insoluble protein particles, which can result in a hyperopic shift (**D**).

5. Correct: Type IV, posterior pole (D)

The lens capsule is synthesized by the lens epithelium and mainly composed of type IV collagen and sulfated glycosaminoglycans. It is thickest in the pre-equatorial zones and thinnest at the central posterior pole, where it may measure only 2–4 μm. The anterior capsule is considerably thicker and increases throughout life.

6. Correct: There is a significant increase in the mass of cellular proteins in the fiber cell membrane (A)

Under the anterior lens capsule, there is a single layer of lens epithelial cells that are metabolically active, generating adenosine triphosphate (ATP) to meet the energy needs of the lens. These epithelial cells undergo mitosis and migrate toward the equator, where they differentiate into lens fibers. As they elongate, there is an increase in the mass of cellular proteins in the fiber cell membrane (**A**). At the same time, they lose their organelles (**B**) as well as their metabolic function (**C**) becoming dependent on glycolysis for energy production. This morphological change allows for enhanced optical clarity and reduction of light absorption and scatter (**D**).

7. Correct: At the center of the lens (B)

As the new lens fibers are laid down, they crowd and compact the previously formed fibers, so that the oldest layers are located in the center of the lens. The outermost fibers are the most recently formed and make up the cortex of the lens.

8. Correct: Erect anteriorly and inverted posteriorly (C)

The lens sutures are formed by the interdigitation of the anterior and posterior tips of the spindle-shaped fibers. These Y-shaped sutures can be observed with biomicroscopy and appear erect anteriorly and inverted posteriorly.

9. Correct: α-Crystallins (A)

α-Crystallins are the largest group of lens proteins with a molecular mass of 600 to 800 kDA. β-Crystallins (**B**) have a molecular mass of 23 to 32 kDa, and βL-crystallins (**C**) are a subset of β-crystallins. γ-Crystallins (**D**) have a molecular mass of 20 kDa or less.

10. Correct: Increased levels of glutathione and decreased levels of glutathione disulfide in cytoplasm of nuclear fiber cells lead to increased protein aggregation (C)

As the lens ages, its proteins aggregate to form large particles, which become water-insoluble and scatter light, increasing the opacity of the lens (**A and B**). Oxidative changes occur, leading to *decreased* levels of glutathione and *increased* levels of glutathione disulfide (**C**) in the cytoplasm of nuclear fiber cells, resulting in increased disulfide bonds, protein cross-linking (**D**), and cataract formation.

11. Correct: Zonular tension increases with accommodation (C)

When the ciliary muscle contracts, the zonular tension decreases so that the axial thickness of the lens increases, and the equatorial diameter decreases (**D**). This change is most significant at the anterior lens surface (**A**), while the posterior surface curvature does not change significantly (**B**).

12. Correct: Anaerobic glycolysis (B)

Although less efficient than other pathways, the majority of high phosphate bonds required for cellular metabolism in the lens is provided by anaerobic glycolysis. The lens is therefore not dependent on oxygen and can sustain normal metabolism and remain transparent even in an anoxic state. However, when deprived of glucose, the lens can become hazy within several hours.

13. Correct: Aldose reductase (B)

Aldose reductase is responsible for the conversion of glucose to sorbitol.

14. Correct: All of the above (D)

In hyperglycemia, three glucose metabolism pathways are activated: anaerobic glycolysis, which is the most active pathway, the hexose monophosphate shunt, which on average metabolizes 5% of lens glucose, and the sorbitol pathway, which becomes activated under severe hyperglycemic states. When the sorbitol pathway is activated, sorbitol accumulates along with fructose, increasing osmotic pressure and drawing in water within the lens. This causes swelling of the lens fibers, disruption of the normal cytoskeletal architecture, and opacification of the lens, known as "sugar" cataracts.

15. Correct: Reduced protection from oxidative damage to the lens due to the removal of the vitreous (D)

Choices (**A, B, and C**) may lead to cataract formation; however, these are more commonly posterior subcapsular cataracts. The leading hypothesis regarding the progression of nuclear cataracts after vitrectomy is that the lens undergoes more oxidative damage acutely during vitrectomy and chronically after vitreous removal.

16. Correct: Epithelium and outer cortex (A)

The lens cells with the highest metabolic rate are found at in the epithelium and outer cortex.

17. Correct: 30 (C)

At 25 days of gestation, the optic vesicles form from the forebrain or diencephalon and become adherent to the surface ectoderm, forming a lens placode. An indentation or invagination of this placode leads to a sphere of cells, which separates and becomes a lens vesicle at approximately 30 days of gestation.

18. Correct: Mittendorf's dot (A)

A Mittendorf dot (**A**) can be commonly found as a small, dense white spot inferonasally, a remnant of the posterior pupillary membrane of the tunica vasculosa lentis, where the hyaloid artery came into contact with the posterior surface of the lens. A lens coloboma (**B**) is an anomaly of lens shape, seen primarily as a wedge-shaped defect or indentation of the lens periphery. Bergmeister's papilla (**C**) is a remnant of the hyaloid artery in which glial tissue is seen on the disc in association with avascular prepapillary veils and epipapillary membranes. Posterior polar cataracts (**D**) are lens opacities involving the subcapsular cortex and capsule of the lens, often associated with capsular fragility.

19. Correct: Persistent fetal vasculature (C)

Down's syndrome (**A**) and aniridia (**D**) are most commonly associated with bilateral cataracts. Rubella (**B**) is commonly associated with both unilateral and bilateral cataracts, which may also be associated with retinopathy, microspherophakia, and glaucoma. Mothers who contract the rubella virus during the first trimester are at the highest risk for the fetus to develop congenital rubella syndrome whose classic triad includes sensorineural deafness, congenital heart disease, as well as the above eye abnormalities.

20. Correct: *PAX6* (D)

The figure demonstrates aniridiA. *PAX6* is associated with aniridia and Peters' anomaly. *PITX2* (**A**) and *FOXC1* (**B**) are associated with Peters' anomaly and Axenfeld–Rieger syndrome. *CYP1B1* (**C**) is associated with congenital glaucoma and Peters' anomaly.

21. Correct: All of the above (D)

The anomaly seen in the figure is microspherophakia, which is a developmental anomaly in which the lens is small and spherical. The lens equator can be visualized through the dilated pupil. Small stature, short stubby fingers, and reduced joint mobility are seen in Weill–Marchesani syndrome, which is the most common association with microspherophakia.

Dilation of the aortic root is seen in Marfan's syndrome, which is also associated with microsphero-phakia. Other associations include Peters' anomaly, Lowe's syndrome, Alport's syndrome, and congenital rubella.

22. Correct: Seizures (A)

The photo shows an inferonasal lens subluxation, which is a classic condition in homocystinuria. Homocystinuria is associated with seizures, osteoporosis, cognitive impairment, and thromboembolic episodes. It is an autosomal recessive inborn error of methionine metabolism. Mitral valve prolapse (**B**) is associated with Marfan's syndrome, in which ectopia lentis is classically superotemporal. Sensorineural deafness (**C**) is associated with Alport's syndrome and congenital rubella syndrome. Cardiac conduction abnormalities (**D**) are associated with myotonic dystrophy.

23. Correct: No association (C)

Cerulean cataracts or blue-dot cataracts are small bluish opacities in the lens cortex, and are not usually visually significant. Snowflake cataracts (**A**) are gray–white subcapsular opacities typically associated with diabetes. Christmas tree cataracts (**B**) are polychromatic, reflective, needle-shaped opacities associated with myotonic dystrophy. Lamellar cataracts (**D**) are the most common form of congenital cataract and often have a disc-shaped configuration.

24. Correct: Posterior subcapsular cataract (D)

Bladder, or Wedl, cells are associated with posterior subcapsular cataracts. Lens epithelial cells that have migrated posteriorly from the lens equator to the inner, posterior aspect of the lens capsule undergo an aberrant swelling and enlargement. The cells are called bladder cells.

25. Correct: A local disruption of lens fiber cells (B)

Cortical cataracts are typically bilateral, but often are asymmetric. Histopathologically, cortical cataracts are due to the local disruption of the structure of mature lens fiber cells. Cortical "spokes" or wedge-like opacities most commonly lead to symptoms such as glare from focal light sources such as oncoming headlights. In nuclear cataracts, an increase in the refractive index occurs with hardening of the lens, leading to generally symmetric visual complaints (**A**) and a myopic shift (**C**). Posterior subcapsular cataracts generally cause greater disruption of visual symptoms at near (**D**).

26. Correct: Simvastatin (A)

Corticosteroids, miotics, and phenothiazines have been associated with drug-induced lens changes. Statins alone have not been shown to increase cataract risk in humans. However, simvastatin has been associated with a nearly twofold increased risk of cataract with concomitant use of erythromycin, which increases the circulating levels of statin in the body.

27. Correct: An increase in sorbitol in the lens may result in swelling of the lens fibers (A)

An increase in blood glucose will increase the glucose level in the aqueous humor and the lens by diffusion. Some of the glucose will be converted by the enzyme aldose reductase to sorbitol, which in turn will accumulate in the lens cell cytoplasm along with its subsequent by-product, fructose. This increase in osmotic pressure may lead the lens fibers to swell (**A**). Given the swelling of the lens, presbyopia can occur earlier in patients with diabetes than those without diabetes (**C**), and decrease amplitude of accommodation (**B**). A snowflake cataract is a typical cataract of a diabetic patient. A sunflower cataract is associated copper in the lens capsule (**D**).

28. Correct: An anterior subcapsular shield-like cataract that typically develops in the early adult years (D)

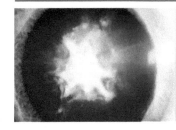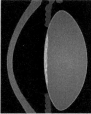

This question describes a patient with atopic dermatitis. These patients can present with an anterior subcapsular shield-like cataract. Polychromatic iridescent crystals in the lens cortex are associated with myotonic dystrophy (**A**). Posterior synechiae and posterior subcapsular cataract are associated with uveitis (**B**). Cataracts associated with galactosemia have an "oil droplet" appearance on retroillumination, which can progress to total opacification of the lens (**C**).

29. Correct: "Oil droplet" appearance on retroillumination, which can progress to total opacification of the lens (C)

The question refers to galactosemia, an autosomal recessive condition. In the most common and severe form, there is a defect in galactose-1-phosphate uridyltransferase (Gal-1-PUT), one of the enzymes involved in the metabolic conversion of galactose to glucose. These patients can present with hepatomegaly, jaundice, malnutrition, and mental deficiency in the first weeks of life. About 75% of these patients will have early bilateral cataracts, which typically have an "oil droplet" appearance on retroillumination and can result in total opacification of the lens. Diagnosis can be made with detection of galactose in the urine. Treatment can include dietary restriction of milk products (**A**). Lens colobomas are embryological anomalies that can be associated with colobomas of the iris, optic nerve, or retina (**B**). With microspherophakia, the lens may be dislocated in the anterior chamber due to small size (**D**). Ectopia lentis can occur in many conditions but also can occur as an isolated anomaly with autosomal dominance.

30. Correct: Zonular dehiscence (B)

The question refers to pseudoexfoliation. These patients are at increased risk for poor dilation, increased vitreous loss, and zonular dehiscence (**B**) during cataract surgery. Suprachoroidal hemorrhage (**A**) is caused by sudden surgical decompression resulting in transient hypotony, which increases choroidal venous pressure with an effusion in the suprachoroidal space that stretches the posterior ciliary vessels which rupture. This complication is associated with high myopia, glaucoma, diabetes, and hypertension. Aqueous misdirection (**C**) is generally believed to result from a diversion of aqueous flow into the posterior segment that results from an abnormal relationship between the ciliary body processes, lens, and anterior vitreous. Acute postoperative endophthalmitis (**D**) is associated with clear corneal incisions, posterior capsular rupture, and intraoperative complications.

31. Correct: Vossius' ring (C)

Vossius' ring refers to the pigment from the pupillary ruff of the iris imprinting on the anterior capsule of the lens and can serve as an indicator of previous blunt trauma. A fibrillogranular white material deposited on the lens, and trabecular meshwork is seen in pseudoexfoliation (**A**). Polychromatic iridescent crystals in the lens cortex (**B**) are commonly called a Christmas tree cataract associated with myotonic dystrophy. Soemmering's ring (**D**) is sometimes observed postcataract surgery with peripheral deposition of white material from lens epithelial cells in the lens capsule.

32. Correct: Iron (C)

Iron intraocular foreign bodies can result in siderosis bulbi, a condition characterized by deposition of iron molecules in the trabecular meshwork, lens epithelium, iris, and retina. The epithelium and cortical fibers of the affected lens at first show a yellowish tinge, followed by a rusty brown discoloration, and then complete cortical cataract formation and retinal dysfunction. In rare cases, an inert foreign body may remain in the lens without significant complication; lens opacification and cataract formation may be anticipated, but does not always occur.

33. Correct: Angle closure glaucoma (C)

The patient is presenting for follow-up after having an emergent peripheral iridotomy after an acute angle closure attack, where her presenting eye pressure was 55. The opacities noted are glaukomflecken, composed of necrotic lens epithelial cells and degenerated subepithelial cortex. Phacoantigenic uveitis (**A**) typically occurs days to weeks after traumatic rupture of the lens capsule or following cataract surgery, when retained cortical material is retained within the eye, triggering a severe inflammatory reaction. Phacolytic glaucoma (**B**) occurs with a hypermature cataract, where the liquefied lens proteins leak through an intact lens capsule. The trabecular meshwork can be obstructed by the swollen macrophages, which ingest these lens proteins leading to increased intraocular pressure (IOP), inflammation, eye pain and redness, and poor vision. Lens particle glaucoma (**D**) refers to particles of retained lens cortex after cataract surgery or YAG capsulotomy, which can clog the trabecular meshwork and lead to increased IOP.

34. Correct: Scleral buckle (B)

Posterior subcapsular formation have been reported in long-term use of cortico steroids (**D**) via several routes of administration including topical, nasal, subconjunctival, and inhaled. Vitrectomy (**C**) can cause nuclear sclerotic cataracts within 2 years in 60 to 90% of patients. Retinal surgery such as scleral buckles without vitrectomy is not associated with cataract formation. Hyperbaric oxygen therapy (**A**) has been noted to cause a myopic shift due to increased nuclear sclerosis.

35. Correct: History of never wearing glasses (D)

Choices (**A, B, and C**) may lead to cataract formation, most commonly posterior subcapsular or traumatic cataracts, which may have a greater impact on near vision (**A**). Repeated blunt trauma to the head may lead to traumatic cataracts (**B**). A history of dermatologic care should include a discussion about chronic topical steroid use, which may be associated with posterior subcapsular cataracts (**C**). The complaint of glare and halos while driving at night is a classic symptom of posterior subcapsular cataracts that requires a close examination of the lens (**D**). A history of never wearing glasses should lead one to consider refractive error and treatment of presbyopia to address this patient's symptoms.

36. Correct: Phacolytic glaucoma (A)

Phacolytic glaucoma occurs with a hypermature cataract where the liquefied lens proteins leak through an intact lens capsule. The trabecular meshwork can be obstructed by the swollen macrophages ingesting these lens proteins leading to increased intraocular pressure (IOP), inflammation, eye pain and redness, and poor vision. Primary angle closure glaucoma (**B**) can be caused by relative pupillary block. Typically, patients present with acute vision loss, pain, red eye, nausea, and vomiting from increased IOP and a narrow angle on examination. Lens particle glaucoma (**C**) refers to particles of retained lens cortex after cataract surgery or YAG capsulotomy, which can be clogged and lead to increased IOP. Phacomorphic glaucoma (**D**) is caused by an intumescent lens pushing the iris forward with a shallowing of the anterior chamber to induce secondary angle closure.

37. Correct: Smoking (D)

Smoking (**D**) is the most significant modifiable risk factor associated with the development of cataracts. The age-related eye disease study (AERDS) was designed to determine if daily intake of certain vitamins and minerals could reduce the risk of cataract and advanced age-related macular degeneration (AMD). Neither omega-3 fatty acids nor lutein/zeaxanthin, when added to the original AREDS formulation (**A**), had any overall effect on the need for cataract surgery. However, supplementation with lutein/zeaxanthin appeared to make a difference for 20% of patients with the lowest dietary levels and was associated with a 32% reduction in progression to cataract surgery. Hypertension, but not hyperlipidemia (**B**), is considered a risk factor for cataracts. IV drug use (**C**) has not been shown to be a risk factor for cataract formation.

38. Correct: Aortic enlargement (D)

The photo demonstrates a superotemporal dislocation of the lens, which is associated with Marfan's syndrome. Marfan's syndrome is an autosomal dominant genetic disorder characterized by a mutation in the gene that makes fibrillin. Patients are typically tall, have flexible joints, and can have severe cardiac abnormalities. Intelligence is not affected (**B**), and there are no abnormal metabolites found in the urine (**C**), unlike homocystinuria. Visual symptoms in Marfan's syndrome are commonly related to changes in the lens due to partial lens dislocation due to weak zonules.

39. Correct: Hepatocellular carcinoma (C)

The image depicts a Kayser–Fleischer ring associated with Wilson's disease. Wilson's disease is an autosomal recessive disorder due to a mutation in the Wilson disease protein gene, allowing for accumulation of copper in various tissues. Wilson's patients can demonstrate ophthalmic findings such as copper in Descemet's membrane (Kayser–Fleischer ring) and a sunflower cataract (**A**) with petal-shaped deposition of yellow or brown pigmentation in the lens capsule radiating from the anterior axial pole of the lens to the equator. These cataracts may cause a minimal decrease in vision. Associated liver disease may manifest as portal hypertension (**B**), hepatic encephalopathy (**D**), and esophageal varices. Hepatocellular carcinoma (**C**) is a relatively low risk in patients with Wilson's disease. Approximately half of the patients with Wilson's disease demonstrate neuropsychiatric symptoms.

40. Correct: Have the patient stop tamsulosin the day before surgery (B)

Intraocular floppy iris syndrome (IFIS) has been associated with tamsulosin as well as other alpha-antagonist medications. Alpha antagonists can bind to the postsynaptic nerve endings of the iris dilator muscle indefinitely and can cause excess iris mobility during cataract surgery. The effect of the drug can persist permanently even after stopping the medication and can also affect the muscle even after a single use. Techniques such as pupil expansion devices (**C**), lowering flow rates during phaco (**D**), the use of viscoelastic and intracameral mydriatics can stabilize the iris and reduce complications during surgery. This increased risk of complications with tamsulosin should be discussed with the patient (**A**) as part of the informed consent process.

41. Correct: Humphrey visual field testing (D)

Normal photostress recovery time is 27 seconds with a standard deviation of 11 seconds. Prolonged photostress recovery time of greater than 50 seconds is an indication of macular disease (**A**). The Maddox rod testing can aid in macular function by asking the patients if they note a loss of the red line of the Maddox rod in their view (**B**). Blue-light entoptoscopy can also aid in testing macular function (**C**). During this examination, the patient views an intense homogenous blue-light background. In this setting, the patient should see shadows produced by the white blood cells coursing through the perifoveal capillaries, indicating an intact macular function. Dense cataracts resulting in a limited view of the retina would likely cause a generalized depression on Humphrey's visual field (HVF) testing, limiting the utility of this method in testing for macular function.

42. Correct: 640 μm (D)

Corneal guttata with a central corneal thickness (CCT) greater than 640 μm may indicate difficulty in recovering corneal clarity after cataract surgery.

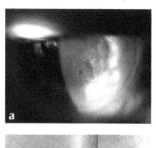
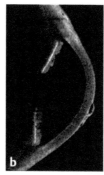

This figure shows bullous keratopathy; corneal edema is due to failure of endothelial cells and results in blister (bullous) elevation of the epithelium. The possibility of corneal surgery (descemet stripping automated endothelial keratoplasty [DSAEK], penetrating keratoplasty [PKP]) should be discussed as part of the informed consent process.

43. Correct: Perform a lateral canthotomy and cantholysis (D)

Complications of retrobulbar anesthesia include retrobulbar hemorrhage (**D**), which should be addressed with immediate lateral canthotomy and cantholysis. It is generally advised to cancel cataract surgery until the hemorrhage has resolved. Other complications of retrobulbar injection include globe penetration, which may be determined on fundus examination (**C**) and toxicity to extraocular muscles, which may result in permanent necrosis and strabismus. Intravenous injection may result in cardiac arrythmia and intradural injection with respiratory arrest and brainstem anesthesia, requiring immediate intervention by the anesthesiologist (**B**). Digital massage (**A**) may be applied after a routine retrobulbar injection to lower intraocular pressure.

44. Correct: Inject a dispersive ophthalmic viscosurgical device (OVD) over the tear (B)

Once a tear in the posterior capsule has been identified, the most important initial step is to limit the prolapse of vitreous anteriorly and the dislocation of lens material posteriorly. Injecting a dispersive OVD over the tear will help to tamponade the vitreous and elevate nuclear fragments, which may allow the surgeon to proceed carefully to remove remaining lens material. A dispersive OVD is preferred because of its better retention, unlike a cohesive OVD that would have a greater tendency to be aspirated out of the eye as the case proceeds (**A**). As vitreous may already be entrapped at the phaco tip, immediately removing the phaco probe may risk pulling on the vitreous creating traction on the retina, and may cause shallowing of the anterior chamber allowing more vitreous to come forward (**C**). Once the eye is stabilized with OVD in the eye, if vitreous is suspected in the anterior segment, vitrectomy should be performed (**D**). Triamcinolone may be injected at this point to help visualize the vitreous if there is uncertainty.

45. Correct: None of the above (D)

The patient's refraction measures moderate astigmatism; however, the keratometry reveals only 0.12 D of corneal astigmatism, which suggests that the source of most of the refractive astigmatism is the lens (**A, B, and C**). Once the cataract is surgically removed, the cornea alone becomes the source of refractive astigmatism, which is insignificant in this case and would not warrant surgical treatment.

46. Correct: Tamsulosin (C)

Tamsulosin is a selective α-1a adrenergic antagonist, commonly used to treat urinary symptoms associated with benign prostatic hypertrophy. Selective antagonists have a greater effect on the iris than nonselective agents which include alfuzosin (**A**), doxazosin (**B**), and terazosin (**D**). Doxazosin and terazosin are also used to treat hypertension in addition to benign prostatic hyperplasia (BPH).

47. Correct: Mechanical stretching of the pupil (C)

Intraoperative floppy iris syndrome is characterized by a triad of iris billowing, progressive intraoperative miosis, and a propensity for the iris to prolapse out of the cornea wounds. Turbulence created by irrigation fluid and manipulation of the iris may induce progressive miosis (**A**). When pupillary dilation is inadequate, iris retractors or pupil expansion rings can aid in maintaining dilation and stabilization of the iris (**B**). Diluted epinephrine (bisulfite-free and preservative-free) injected into the anterior chamber may help improve iris tone and pupillary dilation (**D**). Additionally, minimizing turbulence in the anterior chamber by lowering irrigation, flow, and vacuum settings reduces the risk of iris billowing and prolapse (**C**). Mechanical stretching of the pupil may improve dilation under certain circumstances but would be ineffective with a floppy iris and, in fact, may worsen the situation.

48. Correct: Iris stromal atrophy (B)

Prazosin is a nonselective α-1 adrenergic receptor inhibitor. Blockage of α-1a adrenergic receptors leads to a relaxation of the iris dilator smooth muscles within the iris stroma. Over time, this chronic loss of tone results in atrophy of the iris stroma. In this setting, (**C**) pupillary miosis results from unopposed iris sphincter constriction, (**A**) not a direct increase in iris sphincter tone (**D**). Topical α-2 agonists are used in the treatment of glaucoma and act by decreasing aqueous humor secretion and increasing uveoscleral outflow.

49. Correct: Intensive topical corticosteroid therapy in conjunction with a brief course of systemic corticosteroids (A)

Toxic anterior segment syndrome (TASS) is an acute form of sterile endophthalmitis that occurs when a toxic material, such as a preservative or inadequately sterilized instrument, is introduced into the anterior chamber. This may mimic an infectious endophthalmitis, but typically presents within 12 to 24 hours after surgery. Acute infectious endophthalmitis generally develops 2 to 7 days after surgery, a function of the time it takes for bacteria to replicate and mount an infection. Other differentiating features of TASS include limbus-to-limbus cornea edema, pain that tends to be remarkably mild in spite of the intense intraocular inflammation, poorly reactive pupil, and increased intraocular pressure (IOP). The definitive treatment of TASS is an intensive course of topical corticosteroid therapy, and a short course of systemic corticosteroids given concomitantly may help to hasten resolution (**A**). As a precaution, clinicians may be inclined to perform a vitreous tap and administer intravitreal antibiotics (**B**) and topical fortified antibiotics (**C**) until culture results are confirmed to be negative. Intravenous antibiotics have no role in the treatment of acute infectious endophthalmitis (**D**), as intraocular penetration is poor.

50. Correct: Return to the operating room for vitrectomy (B)

Vitreous wick syndrome occurs with protrusion of vitreous through a corneal wound, which prevents the wound from closing allowing the entry of microorganisms leading to endophthalmitis (**D**). The wound would not be expected to epithelialize as long as vitreous is protruding through it (**B**). The patient should be taken back to the operating room and, with sterile prep and draping, clear the prolapsed vitreous with vitrectomy. In many cases after a complicated surgery, vitreous may adhere to the cornea without external prolapse. In the absence of further sequelae, this may be observed (**C**). However, due to an increased risk of cystoid macular edema, it may be prudent to treat with a prolonged course of topical nonsteroidal anti-inflammatory drug (NSAID) and steroid (**A**). In the presence of cystoid macular edema (CME) refractory to topical medications, it may be necessary to lyse the offending vitreous strand by Nd:YAG laser.

51. Correct: Pupillary block glaucoma (D)

(**A**) If an angulated intraocular lens (IOL) is implanted upside down, this would cause the optic to be vaulted anteriorly, which would lead to a more myopic refractive result than intended (**D**). Additionally, the proximity of the optic to the pupillary margin in this more anterior position may cause a pupillary block glaucoma (**B, C**). Zonular instability and corneal decompensation would not directly result from an upside-down lens in the capsular bag, however an upside-down anterior chamber intraocular lens (ACIOL) would increase the risk of corneal endothelial cell loss and secondary decompensation.

52. Correct: Single-piece monofocal intraocular lens (IOL) (A)

The topography reveals irregular astigmatism with inferior steepening that is consistent with keratoconus (**C, D**). Multifocal IOLs are ideally suited for patients with healthy corneas and, if present, lower amounts of astigmatism that is regular and readily treatable at the time of surgery if necessary. Higher-order aberrations induced by the irregular cornea increases the risk of dysphotopsias such as glare and halos, and further reduces contrast sensitivity with multifocal IOLs (**C**). Limbal relaxing incisions should be reserved for the treatment of regular astigmatism and would be ineffective in a keratoconus patient (**B**). A toric IOL may be acceptable in select patients with stable keratoconus when part of the astigmatism appears regular over the pupil but is unlikely to be adequately effective with a more distorted cornea. Independence from spectacles (or contact lenses) is an unrealistic goal with cataract surgery in this case, and the patient should be counseled as such (**A**). A monofocal IOL would be the best option to avoid further compromising visual quality. The patient may subsequently continue rigid gas-permeable (RGP) lens wear to optimize his vision.

53. Correct: The lens has rotated off axis by approximately 30 degrees (A)

The keratometry reveals that there is 3 D of corneal astigmatism with the steep axis at 90 degrees both preoperatively and postoperatively. Postoperatively, there is 3 D of refractive astigmatism that coincides with the corneal astigmatism. This would imply that the orientation of the toric intraocular lens (IOL) is such that it is having a negligible effect on the refractive astigmatism. For every degree, the toric IOL is rotated off axis, 3.3% of its astigmatic correction is lost (**A**). Thus, if the toric IOL is off axis by 30 degrees, it would have no effect on the refractive astigmatism (**B**). A toric IOL that is implanted 90 degrees away from the correct axis would result in refractive astigmatism that is double the amount of corneal astigmatism.

Surgically induced astigmatism (SIA) from the main corneal incision is an important element to factor in preoperative calculations for the toric IOL power and is typically estimated based on a surgeon's past results (**C, D**). While there is often a small amount of astigmatism induced by small-incision clear corneal incisions, typically ranging from 0 to 0.50 D, an underestimation or overestimation is unlikely to have been significant enough to account for the 3 D of residual astigmatism. Of note, in this case, the SIA is zero as the keratometry remained unchanged postoperatively.

54. Correct: Administer mannitol intravenously (B)

The scenario most likely described here is posterior infusion syndrome. Fluid that is injected too forcefully during hydrodissection may become misdirected and accumulate posteriorly in the vitreous cavity causing the anterior chamber to shallow. Applying gentle pressure on the lens may alleviate this, but if unsuccessful, (**B**) intravenous mannitol may be administered to reduce the vitreous volume (**A**). When there is excessive posterior pressure, burping a corneal wound will risk causing prolapse of iris tissue (**C, D**). Attempting to deepen the anterior chamber by injecting ophthalmic viscoelastic device (OVD) is likely to be ineffective when the globe is already tense, and would cause OVD to be expelled back out a corneal wound or potentially cause the iris to prolapse.

55. Correct: Injection of intravitreal antibiotics with capsulectomy (A)

Chronic postoperative endophthalmitis is an indolent infection caused by less virulent microorganisms that typically manifests more than 6 weeks after surgery. Propionibacterium acnes is the most commonly implicated pathogen, but others include *Staphylococcus epidermidis* and *Candida parapsilosis*. Inflammation may initially respond to topical corticosteroids, but persistence particularly in the presence of a white intracapsular plaque that does not resolve with a slow corticosteroid taper (**B**) should raise suspicion for a low-grade infections endophthalmitis. Definitive therapy to eradicate the organism is likely to require pars plana vitrectomy with intravitreal antibiotics and partial or total capsulectomy (with intraocular lens [IOL] exchange) (**A**). An otherwise healthy patient is less likely to present with a new systemic autoimmune disease at this age (**D**). Nd:YAG laser capsulotomy would risk releasing the pathogen into the vitreous and is not advised in this setting (**C**).

56. Correct: A 45-year-old woman with trace nuclear sclerosis, dense cortical spokes, and 1 clock hour of posterior synechiae obscuring the red reflex (D)

Topical anesthesia should be reserved for cases in which the patient is expected to be cooperative with relatively low risk of complication (**D**). In a case such as this, posterior synechiae may be lysed and capsular dye may be used to enhance visualization of the capsulorrhexis, after which the case should be expected to proceed in routine fashion (**B**). A hypermature cataract may require extracapsular cataract extraction (ECCE) for which a block would be more appropriate (**C**). A mildly subluxated lens in an eye with pseudoexfoliation suggests severe zonular laxity, which may portend a more difficult surgery with increased risk of intraoperative lens dislocation and vitreous loss prolonging the operative time (**A**). Finally, patients who may have difficulty following instructions during surgery should be considered candidates for general anesthesia.

57. Correct: Reduces the risk of endophthalmitis (C)

There have been reports of an increased incidence of endophthalmitis associated with clear corneal incisions compared to scleral tunnel incisions. Meticulous construction of the clear corneal incision such that the length closely approximates the width is necessary to ensure the wound is self-sealing. Additionally, adequate pressurization of the globe at the conclusion of the case is required, as hypotony may allow ingress of fluid and microorganisms from the ocular surface. Because there may be greater discomfort or pain with incisions into the conjunctiva and sclera and the use of cautery for hemostasis, retrobulbar or peribulbar anesthesia is typically given when a scleral tunnel incision is planned (**B, D**). Clear corneal incisions require fewer steps to create with less manipulation of ocular tissues, enabling the surgery to be performed with greater ease under topical anesthesia (**A**). When properly constructed, both small scleral tunnel incisions and clear cornea incisions induce minimal astigmatism. However, a clear corneal incision that is placed too anteriorly has a greater likelihood of inducing more astigmatism.

58. Correct: Minimal risk of postoperative ocular hypertension if retained in the eye (C)

Ophthalmic viscosurgical devices (OVDs) of any type can obstruct the trabecular meshwork and reduce aqueous outflow leading to increased intraocular pressure (IOP). Because dispersive OVDs have lower self-adherence, special care must be taken to evacuate it thoroughly from the eye at the conclusion of the case to avoid a postoperative IOP spike. However, this property also enables (**B**) partitioning of space in the event of a posterior capsular rupture, and (**D**) reduces the risk or amount of vitreous prolapse through the defect (**A**). Dispersive OVDs have lower surface tension than cohesive OVDs, which enhances their ability to coat and protect the corneal endothelium.

59. Correct: Lowering the aspiration flow rate (B)

Thermal injury to the cornea during phacoemulsification results from excessive heat produced by friction generated by the oscillating phaco probe. This may cause contraction of corneal collagen leading to distortion and gaping of the wound. Significant astigmatism may result, and such a wound may be difficult to close often requiring the placement of several tight sutures. The flow of fluid down the irrigation sleeve around the phaco probe and subsequently through the probe via aspiration help cool the probe by convection (**C**). A wound that is too tight may impede the flow of irrigation fluid and also increase friction against the probe. Reduction of flow through the probe due to occlusion, such as with lens material or ophthalmic viscosurgical device (OVD), or by (**B**) decreasing the aspiration flow rate, may cause the probe to overheat (**A**). Limiting phaco power with judicious foot pedal control and/or by employing pulse or burst mode phaco are additional preventative measures. (**D**) Finally, when it appears, an excessive amount of phaco power is being required with limited progress in nuclear disassembly, converting to nuclear expression technique should be strongly considered.

60. Correct: Three-piece IOL with haptics externalized and secured via scleral tunnels (D)

(**A**) Anterior chamber IOL (ACIOL) can provide excellent visual outcomes. However, they are associated with an increased rate of endothelial loss. Over many years, this may lead to corneal decompensation with persistent corneal edema, and uveitis-glaucoma-hyphema (UGH) syndrome in which chafing from IOL implants leading to iris transillumination defects, pigment dispersion, and hyphema with elevated intraocular pressure (IOP). Thus, in younger patients, an IOL fixated posterior to the iris would be the preferred choice. Additionally, an ACIOL may risk further compromising the angle that has already sustained some damage from the traumatic injury (**D**). Scleral fixation of a three-piece IOL with the haptics externalized and secured via scleral tunnels enables excellent stability and centration of the IOL. Alternatively, the lens may be fixated to the sclera or iris with 9–0 polypropylene sutures (**B**). Nylon sutures are more susceptible to degrading

over time, which may result in late lens dislocation (**C**). The haptics of a one-piece acrylic IOL are thicker with sharper edges, which can more easily chafe against the iris and cause suture breakage. Moreover, the high flexibility of these IOLs can make centration and avoidance of tilting more difficult.

61. Correct: Axenfeld–Reiger syndrome (C)

(**A, B, and D**) Zonular weakness and lens subluxation are findings associated with pseudoexfoliation syndrome, homocystinuria, and traumatic eye injury. (**C**) Axenfeld–Reiger syndrome is characterized by developmental abnormalities of the anterior chamber angle, iris, and trabecular meshwork, which may lead to glaucoma. However, lens subluxation is not a feature of this condition.

62. Correct: Insertion of capsule tension ring (B)

Capsule tension rings (CTRs) may be used to stabilize and maintain centration of the capsular bag when there is zonular weakness. When there is significant zonulopathy resulting in lens subluxation, a CTR with eyelets may be inserted and fixated to the sclera with sutures (**B**). However, inserting a CTR in the presence of a radial anterior capsular tear may cause further extension of the tear posteriorly and should be avoided (**C**). There is no contraindication to using iris hooks, if necessary, in this setting, and in fact may be useful to retract the iris to confirm whether the tear has extended posteriorly. If placed after the capsulorrhexis has been completed, care should be taken to avoid capturing the edge of the anterior capsule within the hook (**A**). The surgeon may continue phacoemulsification within the capsular bag paying special attention to minimize tension on the capsule. Because of the lack of adequate capsular support and the inability to place a CTR, a posterior chamber intraocular lens (IOL) should not be placed in the capsular bag or sulcus (**D**). Instead, acceptable IOL options include an anterior chamber IOL (ACIOL) or posterior chamber IOL (PCIOL) fixated to the iris or sclera.

63. Correct: Filling the entire anterior chamber with ophthalmic viscosurgical device (OVD) to maintain positive pressure (B)

Cataract surgery after pars plana vitrectomy is a challenge, because the surgeon must pay careful attention to fluctuations in anterior chamber depth without a vitreous cushion (**A**). Lowering the irrigating bottle can prevent sudden deepening of the anterior chamber and also decreases patient pain. These cases are susceptible to lens–iris diaphragm retropulsion syndrome (LIDRS) where iridocapsular contact can result in reverse pupillary block (**C**). Manually separating the iris from the anterior capsule rim using a second instrument can prevent this problem (**B**). Overfilling the anterior chamber with OVD should be avoided to prevent zonular stretch and breakage.

64. Correct: Vitrectomy, inject acetylcholine, create peripheral iridectomy, inject ophthalmic viscosurgical device (OVD), enlarge wound (A)

Vitrectomy should be the initial step performed to thoroughly clear vitreous from the anterior chamber. In preparation for ACIOL insertion, acetylcholine is injected to pharmacologically constrict the pupil. At this stage, the peripheral iris is on stretch and more easily accessed for iridectomy. OVD is then placed to maintain a formed anterior chamber prior to enlarging the wound to accommodate the insertion of the lens (**B, C, and D**). All of the aforementioned steps are best performed with greater safety prior to enlarging the wound.

65. Correct: Lowering the height of the irrigation bottle (B)

Postocclusion surge occurs when excessive vacuum builds within the aspiration tubing causing it to collapse, while there is an occlusion at the aspiration port. When the occlusion suddenly breaks, rebound of the tubing results in a brief and abrupt increase of fluid outflow from the anterior chamber through the aspiration port. This may cause the anterior chamber to shallow momentarily with risk of injury to the iris and lens capsule from the phaco tip. Increasing inflow pressure or reducing the amount of negative pressure buildup within the aspiration tubing during occlusion can help to reduce surge (**B**). This can be accomplished by raising the bottle height (or increasing the intraocular pressure [IOP] setting on newer phaco machines) and (**A, D**) decreasing vacuum by foot pedal control or with the machine settings, respectively (**C**). Low-compliance tubing with thicker and more rigid walls resist collapse during occlusion. Modern phaco machines are generally engineered with the minimal compliance possible within the fluidics circuit that does not restrict the pumping mechanism.

66. Correct: Switch from pulse mode to continuous phacoemulsification (D)

Followability refers to the ability of the aspiration port of the phaco tip to attract and hold lens fragments. This is a function of the aspiration flow rate, which can be adjusted directly on a peristaltic pump machine (**A**) and indirectly by increasing the vacuum setting on a Venturi-based system (**B**). Traditional longitudinal phacoemulsification power can be likened to jackhammer, causing the probe to oscillate forward and backward, and has a tendency to repel nuclear fragments resulting in chatter. Vacuum is necessary to hold and evacuate lens fragments at the aspiration port and must be sufficiently high

to overcome the repulsive forces of the ultrasonic energy. Thus, reducing phaco power (**C**) can diminish chatter and improve followability. Finally, phaco power can be modulated by employing pulse mode that alternates automatically between periods of "power on" and "power off." This enables the aspiration port to reengage with nuclear fragments during the "off" cycles. Remaining on continuous phaco will limit this ability (**D**).

67. Correct: Topical ketorolac and topical prednisolone acetate (D)

Treatment of cystoid macular edema after cataract surgery is generally approached in a stepwise manner (**D**). Therapy with a combination of topical nonsteroidal anti-inflammatory drug (NSAID) and topical corticosteroid appears to hasten resolution and leads to improved visual outcomes compared to monotherapy with either agent (**A, C**). If this is unsuccessful, subtenon or intravitreal injection of triamcinolone or intravitreal injection of an antivascular endothelial growth factor (anti-VEGF) agent may be considered (**B**). Treatment with oral carbonic anhydrase inhibitors such as acetazolamide has shown limited success in cases of cystoid macular edema (CME).

68. Correct: Most cases of uncomplicated cystoid macular edema (CME) resolve without treatment (A)

Approximately 95% of cases of CME uncomplicated by other precipitating factors, such as chronic inflammation or vitreous adhesions, resolve spontaneously (**A**). The risk of CME is not greater with any particular type of intraocular lens (IOL) material whether it is acrylic, silicone, or polymethyl methacrylate (**D**). A properly positioned open-loop anterior chamber IOL does not appear to increase the risk of CME. Conversely, any type of IOL that is malpositioned and chafing against intraocular structures is associated with a higher incidence of CME (**C**). Preoperative treatment with topical nonsteroidal anti-inflammatory drugs (NSAIDs), but not corticosteroids, has been demonstrated to reduce the risk of CME, though combined treatment with both medications postoperatively is beneficial (**B**).

69. Correct: History of myopia treated with laser in situ keratomileusis (LASIK) (D)

Anterior displacement of an intraocular lens (IOL) increases its effective power resulting in a more myopic result. (**A**) This may occur with an IOL originally intended for placement in the capsular bag that is instead placed in the sulcus. (**B**) In addition, some commonly used posterior chamber intraocular lenses (PCIOLs) are designed with the optic offset posteriorly relative to the haptics. Thus, inverting the IOL may result in a more anterior position of the optic. (**C**) Choroidal effusions may cause anterior displacement of the lens–iris diaphragm and shallowing of the anterior chamber resulting in myopic shift. LASIK alters the curvature of the cornea and reduces the accuracy of keratometric measurements used with traditional IOL power calculations. (**D**) In eyes that have undergone LASIK for treatment of myopia, this tends to result in a suggested IOL power that is underpowered for the eye causing a hyperopic surprise. In eyes that have previously undergone hyperopic LASIK, the opposite effect may occur. Modifications to these formulas and instruments that more accurately calculate or measure the refractive power of the cornea have helped to mitigate these effects.

70. Correct: A silicone intraocular lens (IOL) is the preferred type of lens implant (A)

There is a greater likelihood that this patient may require pars plana vitrectomy with silicone oil in the future for repair of tractional retinal detachment. Silicone oil may condense and adhere to the surface of a silicone IOL with resultant visual disturbances. Thus, an acrylic IOL (or other non-silicone IOL) would be preferred in this situation. (**D**) Multifocal IOLs may lead to minor loss of contrast sensitivity and scotopic vision, which may be further compounded by macular disease and are generally not recommended when maculopathy is present or is more likely to develop. (**B**) Diabetes is a risk factor for the development of postoperative cystoid macular edema (CME). (**C**) Because surgical patients are expected to fast after midnight on the day of surgery, oral hypoglycemic medications are typically withheld to avoid excessive hypoglycemia.

Chapter 4

Neuro-Ophthalmology

Alberto Giuseppe Distefano

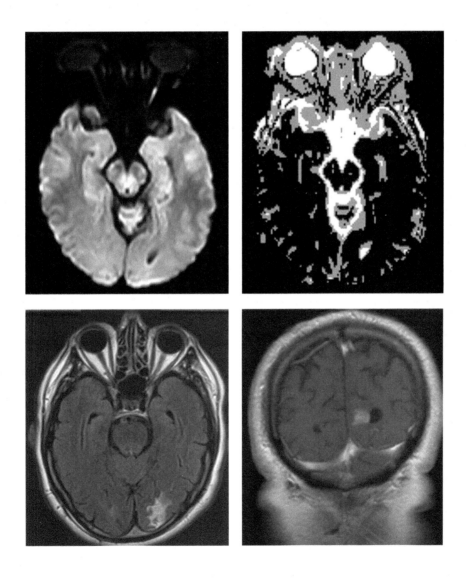

4 Neuro-Ophthalmology

Easy	Medium	Hard

1. A 43-year-old woman complains of blurred vision over the past month. Best corrected visual acuity is 20/50 in the right eye and 20/25 in the left eye. Photostress recovery test was found to be prolonged in the right eye at 50 seconds. What is the best next test?

A. Humphrey's visual field 30–2

B. MRI of the brain and orbits

C. Retinal nerve fiber layer analysis

D. Optical coherence tomography (OCT) of the macula

2. A 13-year-old adolescent girl is seen urgently for sudden vision loss. She was at school when she experienced painless loss of vision in both eyes. She states she can only see a bright light when it is shown in each eye. The pupils are equal, round, and reactive to light without afferent pupillary defect. Intraocular pressures are normal, as is the remainder of the anterior and posterior dilated examination. What test should be performed next?

A. Optokinetic testing

B. MRI of the brain and orbits

C. Fluorescein angiography

D. The Amsler grid testing

3. A 32-year-old woman with past medical history of multiple sclerosis presents with blurred vision on her left side. Confrontation visual fields reveal a left homonymous hemianopia. MRI is obtained and reveals a right optic tract demyelinating lesion. Examination may have shown what other finding?

A. Right relative afferent pupillary defect

B. Left relative afferent pupillary defect

C. Right optic nerve head edema

D. Left optic nerve head edema

4. A 63-year-old man is sent to you for preoperative evaluation of a known left parietal meningioma causing chronic headaches. What findings may be noted on examination?

A. An incongruous left homonymous hemianopia

B. A right superior quadrantanopia

C. An abnormal optokinetic response with the drum rotated to the right

D. An abnormal optokinetic response with the drum rotated to the left

5. A 72-year-old man complains of right-sided vision loss after a cardiac surgery. Humphrey's visual field is performed with the results shown below. An embolus to which artery most likely explains the findings?

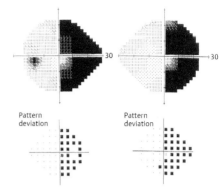

A. Right middle cerebral artery

B. Right posterior cerebral artery

C. Left middle cerebral artery

D. Left posterior cerebral artery

6. A 42-year-old man presents with the complaint that his vision being "off." His visual acuity is 20/20 in both eyes. Pupils are equal, round, reactive to light, and without relative afferent pupillary defect. Intraocular pressures are normal. The anterior and dilated fundus examinations are within normal limits. Optical coherence tomography of the macula is performed and found to be normal. The patient is reassured that his eyes and vision are normal. The patient returns 6 months later with progressive vision loss in both eyes over the past few weeks. Examination shows a visual acuity of 20/60 in both eyes and a dense bitemporal hemianopia. MRI reveals a 15-cm sellar mass compressing the optic nerve chiasm. The mass is resected, but the patient is unable to recover his vision. What steps should have been taken to avoid this missed diagnosis?

A. Check color vision.

B. Check red desaturation.

C. Visual field testing.

D. All of the above.

7. A 23-year-old woman presents to the emergency department with 2 days of blurred vision in the left eye. She has pain when performing extraocular movements. There is a 1+ relative afferent pupillary defect on the left. MRI is shown below. The remainder of the MRI is within normal limits. What is this patient's risk of developing multiple sclerosis within the next 15 years?

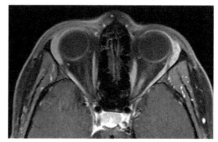

A. 23%

B. 56%

C. 74%

D. Cannot be determined from the given information

8. A 34-year-old woman presents to the emergency department with 2 days of blurred vision in the right eye. She has pain when performing extraocular movements. There is a 1+ relative afferent pupillary defect on the right. Orbital MRI shows enhancement of the right optic nerve. Fluid-attenuated inversion recovery (FLAIR) sequence is shown below. What is this patient's risk of developing multiple sclerosis by 15 years?

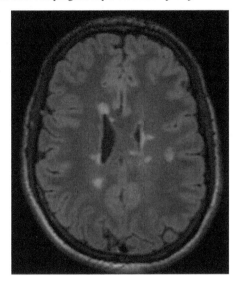

A. 23%

B. 56%

C. 74%

D. Cannot be determined from the given information

9. A 72-year-old hypertensive man presents to the emergency department with acute vision loss in the right eye upon awakening in the morning. He denies any headaches, jaw claudication, night sweats, fevers, or unintentional weight loss. Examination shows visual acuity of counting fingers in the right eye with a relative afferent pupillary defect. The optic nerve is diffusely edematous. The left eye has visual acuity of 20/25 with a healthy, cupless optic nerve. Which of the following is the next best step in this patient's management?

A. Start topical brimonidine for neuroprotection.

B. Obtain complete blood count (CBC), erythrocyte sedimentation rate (ESR), and C-reactive protein (CRP).

C. Start oral prednisone 20 mg daily.

D. Reassure the patient with outpatient follow-up for automated visual field testing.

10. A 58-year-old woman with past medical history of hypertension, diabetes mellitus type 2, and obstructive sleep apnea awoke with blurred vision in her inferior visual field from the right eye. Examination found a relative afferent pupillary defect in the right eye, superior segmental optic nerve edema with few peripapillary hemorrhages, and automated perimetry as shown below. Which of the following is not indicated for this patient?

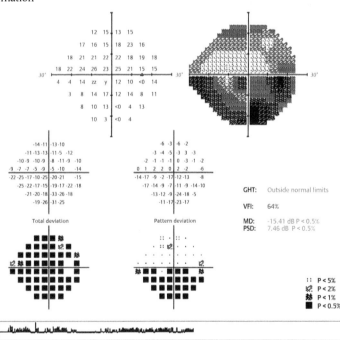

A. Ensure blood pressure medication is not taken at night.

B. Obtain carotid Doppler ultrasound.

C. Order sleep study.

D. Control blood sugar level.

11. A 54-year-old man complains of painless loss of vision from the right eye. He is in the postanesthesia care unit after having undergone a spinal fusion. Ophthalmic examination shows no light perception vision in the right eye with relative afferent pupillary defect on the right and otherwise normal examination. The below MRI is urgently obtained. What is the cause of this patient's vision loss?

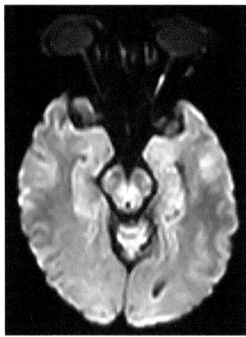

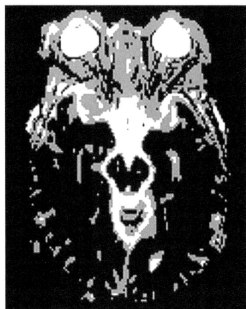

A. Ischemic infarction of the posterior orbital optic nerve

B. Embolic ophthalmic artery occlusion

C. Compressive retrobulbar hemorrhage

D. None of the above

12. A 26-year-old man presents with blurred vision in both eyes. He states it began 2 weeks ago in the right eye, and 2 days ago in his left eye. Examination shows mild optic nerve edema bilaterally with multiple fine tortuous peripapillary vessels. After diagnosis, the patient should be referred for which of the following tests?

A. Carotid Doppler ultrasound

B. Echocardiogram

C. Chest CT

D. Electrocardiogram

13. A 45-year-old man with past medical history of diabetes mellitus type 2, hypertension, and tuberculosis is seen for slowly progressive blurred vision in both eyes. Symptoms began 1 week ago. Color vision is decreased in both eyes. Visual acuity is 20/60 on the right and 20/50 on the left. Which of the following should be the next step?

A. MRI of orbits and brain.

B. Perform automated perimetry.

C. Review medications.

D. Check color vision.

14. A 5-year-old child is seen for slowly progressive proptosis of the left eye. A relative afferent pupillary defect is noted. Imaging is obtained as shown below. Examination may also demonstrate which one of the following?

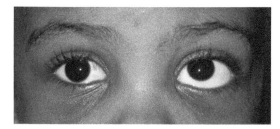

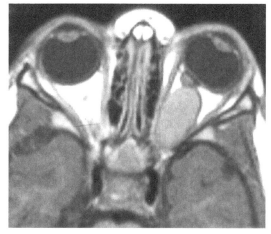

A. Flat hyperpigmented skin lesions

B. Hearing loss

C. Hypopigmented skin lesions

D. Facial capillary malformation

15. A 46-year-old woman presents with progressive vision loss in the right eye. A trace relative afferent pupillary defect is noted. Imaging is obtained as shown below. Visual acuity is 20/30 in the affected eye. Humphrey's visual field shows nonspecific changes. What is the best next step?

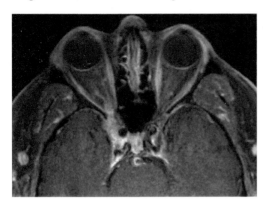

A. Biopsy
B. Surgical resection
C. Radiotherapy
D. Observation

16. A 15-year-old adolescent boy is referred for optic nerve edema. Examination findings are shown in the images below. What is the most likely recommended treatment plan?

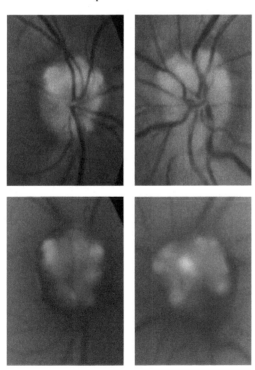

A. Obtain QuantiFERON gold and chest X-ray.
B. Order orbital MRI.
C. Reassurance.
D. Refer for genetic testing.

17. A 6-month-old female infant is brought in as the parents do not feel their child is tracking objects well. A dilated fundus examination reveals bilateral optic nerve hypoplasia. MRI is obtained and shown below. What should be further evaluated in this patient?

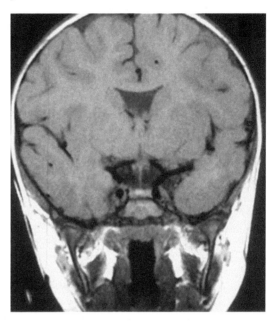

A. CT chest
B. Electrocardiogram
C. Urinalysis
D. Endocrine evaluation

18. A patient is found to have a serous macular detachment secondary to an optic pit. Management options include all of the following except which one?

A. Observation
B. Corticosteroids
C. Pars plana vitrectomy
D. Laser photocoagulation

19. A 56-year-old overweight woman complains of worsening headaches over the past month. Examination demonstrates bilateral optic nerve edema. Imaging findings are shown below. What is the best treatment?

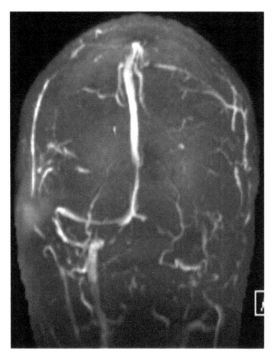

A. Intravenous antibiotics
B. Intravenous steroids
C. Anticoagulation
D. Diuresis

20. A 34-year-old woman is sent to the emergency room for worsening headache and bilateral optic nerve edema. Imaging is obtained and shown. Lumbar puncture is performed with opening pressure of 32 cm H_2O and normal cerebrospinal fluid analysis. What is the next best step in management?

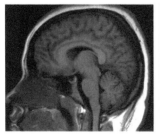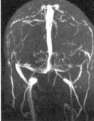

A. Intravenous antibiotics
B. Intravenous corticosteroids
C. Anticoagulation
D. Diuresis

21. A patient with Balint's syndrome shows all of the following clinical signs except which one?

A. Simultagnosia
B. Hemineglect
C. Ocular apraxia
D. Optic ataxia

22. You are seeing a 22-year-old woman with suspected right optic neuritis. A pocket watch is swung from its chain back in forth in a horizontal plane. The patient states the watch is moving in an elliptical path. What is this perception called?

A. Prosopagnosia
B. Ocular apraxia
C. The Pulfrich phenomenon
D. The Riddoch phenomenon

23. A patient is blind due to bilateral occipital lesions. However, she insists that she is able to see the room. What is this patient exhibiting?

A. Anton's syndrome
B. Charles Bonnet syndrome
C. Visual allesthesia
D. Metamorphopsia

24. A 43-year-old woman is noted to have a relative afferent pupillary defect on the right side. The remainder of her ophthalmic examination is within normal limits, including visual field testing. Where is the lesion located?

A. Right optic nerve tract
B. Left optic nerve tract
C. Right pretectal nucleus
D. Left pretectal nucleus

25. A 62-year-old man presents with double vision over the past week. Examination shows −4 abduction of the right eye. Also noted is anisocoria with the right pupil 2 mm smaller than the left, and margin to reflex distance 1 of 2 mm on the right and 4 mm on the left. Dilation lag of the right pupil in the dark is noted. There is no anhidrosis. Which one of the following is most likely the possible diagnosis?

A. Demyelinating brainstem lesion
B. Apical lung tumor
C. Internal carotid artery dissection
D. Intracavernous carotid aneurysm

26. A 6-month-old female infant is seen for a droopy eyelid for the past week. You note a mild ptosis on the right along with anisocoria—the right pupil is smaller than the left. What is the next best step?

A. Discuss the likely benign etiology, and follow-up in 1 month.

B. Order an MRI of the brain, orbits, neck, and chest.

C. Order an MRI of the abdomen.

D. None of the above.

27. A 46-year-old woman hospitalized for chronic obstructive pulmonary disease (COPD) exacerbation is seen for anisocoria. She has insulin-dependent diabetes mellitus and hypertension controlled with amlodipine. Her COPD has been under improved control on nebulizers. Examination shows visual acuity at near 20/20 on the right and 20/60 on the left. Pupils are round with the right pupil 4 mm in dark and 2 mm in light. The left pupil is 8 mm and nonreactive to both light and accommodation. Extraocular motilities are full, and the patient is orthophoric. Anterior examination is within normal limits. What is the most likely cause of anisocoria?

A. Pharmacological

B. Adie's tonic pupil

C. Third cranial nerve palsy

D. Traumatic mydriasis

28. A 34-year-old 30-week gravid woman with history only significant for headaches comes to the emergency room for sudden onset of severe headache this morning. She also states she has double vision. Examination shows anisocoria with the left pupil larger than the right, and a bigger difference in light than dark. There is left ptosis and limited adduction, supraduction, and infraduction. Which of the following is the next best step?

A. Pharmacological pupil testing

B. Lumbar puncture

C. MRI of the brain

D. Intravenous corticosteroids

29. A 62-year-old man presents with diplopia for the past month. Examination demonstrates a right hypertropia consistent with right fourth cranial nerve palsy. Which of the following is most consistent with the diagnosis?

A. Right hypertropia worse in right gaze and right head tilt

B. Right hypertropia worse in right gaze and left head tilt

C. Right hypertropia worse in left gaze and right head tilt

D. Right hypertropia worse in left gaze and left head tilt

30. A 43-year-old woman presents with proptosis and double vision that began 2 months ago. MRI was performed as seen below. What is the most likely diagnosis?

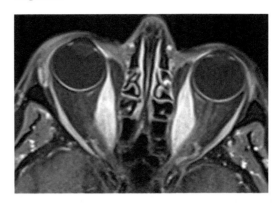

A. Inflammatory myositis

B. Thyroid eye disease

C. Orbital cellulitis

D. None of the above

31. A 35-year-old man presents with acute-onset right eye pain with vertical diplopia, worse in left gaze. Examination shows poor elevation of the right eye when looking up and to the left. Inflammation of which muscle's tendon is responsible for these findings?

A. Superior rectus

B. Inferior rectus

C. Superior oblique

D. Inferior oblique

32. A 73-year-old woman presents with 2 weeks of double vision that comes and goes. Examination shows normal visual acuity, full extraocular motilities, and orthophoria. There is mild keratopathy. You recommend artificial tears and a follow-up in 1 month. She returns in 1 week with count finger vision in the right eye. What testing should have been performed at the initial visit?

A. Acetylcholine receptor antibodies

B. C-reactive protein

C. Thyroid-stimulating immunoglobulin

D. Antineutrophil cytoplasmic antibody

33. A 46-year-old man presents with 1 month of slowly developing enophthalmos on the right. What is the most likely finding on imaging?

A. Agenesis of the sphenoid wing

B. Hypertrophied extraocular muscles

C. Atrophy of the maxillary sinus

D. Orbital fat stranding

34. A 56-year-old man complains of difficulty with reading. When he attempts to read the newspaper, everything appears doubled. Examination shows bilateral ptosis and severely decreased extraocular movements in all directions. What testing must be obtained in this patient?

A. MRI of the brain and orbits

B. CT chest

C. Renal ultrasound

D. Electrocardiogram

35. A 43-year-old man presents with blurred vision in both eyes. You note the patient has frontal balding, a long face, and temporal wasting. You shake his hand, but he is unable to immediately release. Examination reveals bilateral ptosis and reduced extraocular motility. Slit lamp examination reveals a cataract. What type of cataract is likely in this patient?

A. Oil droplet

B. Christmas tree

C. Sunflower

D. Cerulean

36. A 72-year-old French Canadian woman presents with progressive droopy eyelids. Examination reveals bilateral ptosis and severely restricted extraocular movements. This patient should undergo what type of testing?

A. Sleep study

B. Barium swallow

C. Urinalysis

D. Lumbar puncture

37. A 46-year-old woman presents for evaluation of droopy eyelids. She states it started about 1 year ago and is worse in the evening. Examination shows ptosis with margin to reflex distance 1 of 1 mm on the right and 2 mm on the left. When the patient is asked to maintain upgaze, the eyelids begin to descend around 30 seconds. When looking down and looking straight ahead, the eyelids appear to overshoot before settling back in their prior position. Myasthenia gravis is suspected. You note no systemic signs or symptoms. Acetylcholine receptor antibodies are ordered, but all return negative. What should the patient be told?

A. Acetylcholine receptor antibodies are positive in up to 90% of patients. There is a small chance you have myasthenia gravis.

B. Your acetylcholine receptor antibodies are normal; you may proceed with ptosis surgery.

C. Acetylcholine receptor antibodies are positive in up to 50% of patients. There is still a chance you have myasthenia gravis.

D. None of the above.

38. What additional testing should a patient with ocular or systemic myasthenia gravis undergo?

A. CT chest

B. MRI of the brain and orbits

C. Urinalysis

D. Electrocardiogram

39. A 34-year-old man complains of double vision over the past week worse in left gaze. He also complains of headaches over the past month and intermittent graying out of his vision when he bends over. What would you expect to find on further testing?

A. Ischemic lesion in posterior midbrain

B. Elevated erythrocyte sedimentation rate (ESR) and C-reactive protein (CRP)

C. Elevated intracranial pressure

D. Thickened left lateral rectus

40. A 20-year-old woman presents for double vision in both left and right gaze since childhood. She has no other complaints. Examination shows decreased abduction of the right eye in right gaze and decreased abduction of the left eye in left gaze. Examination additionally reveals decreased orbicularis strength and a flattened smile bilaterally. What other finding may be discovered on examination?

A. Eyelid ptosis

B. Light-near dissociation

C. Papilledema

D. Difficulty hearing

41. A 43-year-old woman states she has difficulty focusing and pain. The episodes started 2 weeks ago and are intermittent. You ask the patient to follow an object. As you move to the left, you note her left eye does not abduct, rather moves toward her nose along with the right eye. What finding hints toward a nonorganic disorder?

A. Retraction during convergence

B. Miosis during convergence

C. Limitation in upgaze

D. Tonic medial deviation of the left eye

42. Which of the following is true about the fourth cranial nerve?

A. Exits the midbrain ventrally, stays ipsilateral, and enters the orbit outside the annulus of Zinn.

B. Exits the midbrain dorsally, stays ipsilateral, and enters the orbit outside the annulus of Zinn.

C. Exits the midbrain dorsally, crosses contralaterally, and enters the orbit outside the annulus of Zinn.

D. Exits the pons dorsally, crosses contralaterally, and enters the orbit inside the annulus of Zinn.

43. A 76-year-old hypertensive man presents with acute onset of double vision. MRI is performed and shows an area of restricted diffusion in the right midbrain at the level of the superior colliculus. What examination findings may be noted?

A. Compensatory right head tilt

B. Compensatory left head tilt

C. Right limitation in supraduction, infraduction and adduction, and bilateral ptosis

D. Right limitation in infraduction and adduction, bilateral ptosis, and supraduction deficit

44. A 68-year-old diabetic woman complains of double vision over the past 3 days with left-sided headache. Examination demonstrates left-sided ptosis with decreased supraduction. All other extra-ocular movements appear intact. Pupils are equal, round, and reactive to light and accommodation. What is the next best step?

A. Obtain contrasted MRI of the brain and orbits and MRA.

B. Reassure of likely ischemic nature, and follow-up in 1 month.

C. Reassure of likely ischemic nature, and follow-up in 1 day.

D. Either A or C.

45. An 86-year-old man complains of double vision. Examination is consistent with a right complete third nerve palsy. Complete neuro-ophthalmic examination also reveals left-sided tremor. The patient states this is new since the double vision started. MRI reveals ischemia in the right midbrain. Which syndrome does this patient have?

A. Weber's syndrome

B. Benedikt's syndrome

C. Claude's syndrome

D. Nothnagel's syndrome

46. A 54-year-old woman comes to the emergency room with sudden onset of double vision and severe right-sided eye pain. Examination reveals a right dilated and poorly reactive pupil, right-sided ptosis, and decreased supraduction, infraduction, and adduction on the right. MRI and MRA are found to be negative. What is the next best step?

A. Conventional angiography

B. Erythrocyte sedimentation rate (ESR) and C-reactive protein (CRP)

C. Lumbar puncture

D. Acetylcholine receptor antibodies

47. A 46-year-old woman develops severe right-sided pain and double vision. Examination shows complete right ophthalmoplegia and ptosis with a dilated pupil. Imaging should be directed to which of the following?

A. Orbital apex

B. Cavernous sinus

C. Brainstem

D. None of the above

48. A 7-year-old girl complains of sudden-onset double vision. Examination demonstrates a right-sided pupil-involving third nerve palsy. MRI is found to be normal. What is the next best step?

A. MRA

B. CTA

C. Conventional angiography

D. Lumbar puncture

49. A 36-year-old man is hospitalized for ataxia and double vision. Examination shows bilateral ophthalmoplegia with dilated and poorly reactive pupils. The facial muscles are bilaterally weak. Deep tendon reflexes are absent. What will testing show?

A. Elevated cerebrospinal fluid (CSF) protein

B. CSF pleocytosis

C. Decreased CSF glucose

D. All of the above

50. A 50-year-old man presents to the emergency room after being found on the ground outside. The patient is unkempt. He is unsure of where he is, and needs to be told that he is at the hospital after collapsing multiple times. Examination shows a bilateral vertical ophthalmoplegia and horizontal gaze-evoked nystagmus. Upon having the patient stand up and walk, he is noted to be profoundly ataxic. MRI is performed and finds increased T2 signal in bilateral mammillary bodies. What is the most appropriate treatment?

A. Intravenous antibiotics

B. Intravenous steroids

C. Vitamin B1

D. Vitamin B12

51. A 36-year-old woman presents with difficulty looking to the left for the past few days. Examination shows normal extraocular movements in all fields of gaze when the patient is asked to follow a finger. However, the patient is unable to look from the examiner to a stationary finger to the patient's left. Looking at a finger in other fields of gaze is normal. MRI is consistent with an inflammatory lesion. Where is the lesion located?

A. Left sixth nerve nucleus

B. Left paramedian pontine reticular formation

C. Right medial longitudinal fasciculus

D. Right third nerve nucleus

52. A 25-year-old woman presents with intermittent double vision over the past few days. Double vision only occurs when looking to the left. Examination finds a right hypertropia that is worse in right gaze and right head tilt. Gaze to the right is full. Gaze to the left finds a slowed saccade of the right eye with mild limitation, as well as a horizontal-beating nystagmus of the left eye. Where is the patient's lesion located?

A. Left frontal lobe

B. Right fourth nerve nucleus

C. Left paramedian pontine reticular formation

D. Right medial longitudinal fasciculus

53. A 76-year-old man presents with decreased eye movements since the morning. Examination demonstrates an inability to perform saccades or smooth pursuit to the right. In left gaze, the right eye slowly adducts while the left eye has an abducting nystagmus. MRI finds a hemorrhage involving which area?

A. Right sixth nerve nucleus

B. Right paramedian pontine reticular formation

C. Right medial longitudinal fasciculus

D. Both A and C

54. A 70-year-old man complains of difficulty reading. Examination shows an increased near point of convergence. What other findings might be seen on examination?

A. Internuclear ophthalmoplegia

B. Movement-related tremor

C. Decreased vertical eye movements

D. None of the above

55. A 54-year-old woman presents with trouble seeing with her glasses. She has seen multiple eye doctors, and had multiple pairs of glasses prescriptions filled. Examination finds mild presbyopia with her current glasses. Her corrected visual acuity is 20/20 in each eye. She states that with both eyes images seem to be doubled. Extraocular motility is normal. There is a comitant 12 prism diopter esotropia at distance. She is orthophoric at near. What is the next best step?

A. Reassurance to likely benign and idiopathic etiology.

B. Prescribe prism glasses.

C. Order MRI brain.

D. All of the above.

56. An 86-year-old hypertensive woman is seen with her eyes deviated to the left. She has no other complaints or findings. MRI would most likely show an ischemic focus in which of the following?

A. Right frontal cortex

B. Left frontal cortex

C. Right brainstem

D. Left brainstem

57. A 46-year-old man is referred for neuro-ophthalmic evaluation for a known mass compressing the dorsal midbrain. Which finding is not likely to be seen on examination?

A. Supranuclear upward gaze palsy

B. Convergence-retraction nystagmus on attempted upgaze

C. Bilateral ptosis

D. Light-near dissociation on pupillary examination

58. A 26-year-old man is seen in the hospital 1 week after having suffered a massive trauma. He has been unable to move his limbs or speak. He is able to look up and down, but unable to look laterally. Eyelid function is normal. MRI shows a large area of ischemia in which of the following?

A. Frontal cortex

B. Thalamus

C. Midbrain

D. Pons

59. A 36-year-old woman is found to have a carotid-cavernous fistula (CCF) on MRI. Which of the following is expected on examination?

A. "Corkscrew" dilated conjunctival vessels

B. Elevated intraocular pressure

C. Proptosis

D. All of the above

60. A 42-year-old man presents with 2 weeks of intermittent eye bulging. He works as a mail carrier, and states his eye bulges when he picks up heavy packages. It goes away as soon as the activity stops. What is expected to be seen on further testing?

A. An audible periorbital bruit

B. Pulsatile proptosis

C. Dilated orbital varix on CT during the Valsalva maneuver

D. Dilation and thrombosis of the cavernous sinus

61. A 3-month-old female infant is brought in by her parents after noting shaking eyes for the past week. Examination shows a horizontal nystagmus with a mixed rotary and pendular nystagmus. Nystagmus appears to dampen the most in left gaze. You diagnose an infantile nystagmus. Which of the following is not fitting with this diagnosis?

A. A normal optokinetic testing response

B. Abolished during sleep

C. Retinal dystrophy noted on examination

D. Diminished in convergence

62. A 56-year-old man presents with a droopy eyelid as seen in the figure below. Further testing is performed and shown in the following two panels of the figure. What is the next best step?

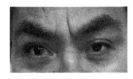

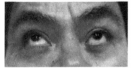 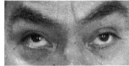

A. Obtain MRI of the brain and orbits.

B. Offer surgical repair of levator dehiscence.

C. Obtain MRA.

D. Check proximal muscle strength.

63. A 6-month-old male infant is found to have spasmus nutans. Which of the following is not true of this condition?

A. MRI is recommended for common anterior visual pathway gliomas.

B. It is benign and self-limiting with resolution in a few months.

C. Head nodding is typically seen.

D. Torticollis is present.

64. A 34-year-old woman with insulin-dependent diabetes mellitus, hypertension, and bipolar disorder is seen for a sensation of things moving around, especially when reading. Examination finds a downbeat nystagmus in primary position that is worse in downgaze and diminished in upgaze. Which step is most likely to help this patient?

A. Discontinuation of lithium

B. Discontinuation of atenolol

C. MRI of the midbrain

D. Base-up prisms in reading glasses

65. A 44-year-old woman with multiple sclerosis is seen with a right jerk horizontal nystagmus. Two minutes later, you notice she has a left jerk horizontal nystagmus. What will most likely help this patient?

A. Start clonazepam.

A. Start baclofen.

B. B12 supplementation.

C. Iron supplementation.

66. A 53-year-old man develops oscillopsia and vertigo over the past month. Nystagmus is noted on neuro-ophthalmic examination. MRI is obtained and shown below. What type of nystagmus is seen?

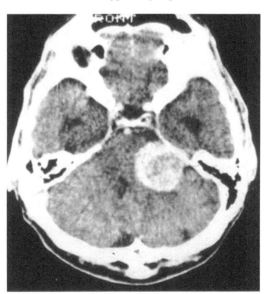

A. High frequency, low-amplitude nystagmus in left gaze

B. Low-frequency, high-amplitude nystagmus in left gaze

C. Periodic alternating nystagmus

D. Monocular horizontal jerk nystagmus in abduction with adduction deficit of the fellow eye

67. A 43-year-old woman is referred for nystagmus evaluation. An MRI is obtained and shown below. What type of nystagmus is expected?

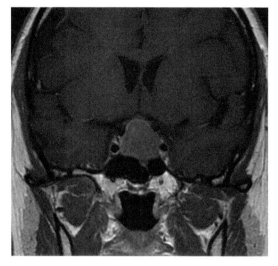

A. Brun's nystagmus

B. Periodic alternating nystagmus

C. Seesaw nystagmus

D. Dissociated jerk nystagmus

68. What type of lesion would be expected to cause the visual field defect shown below?

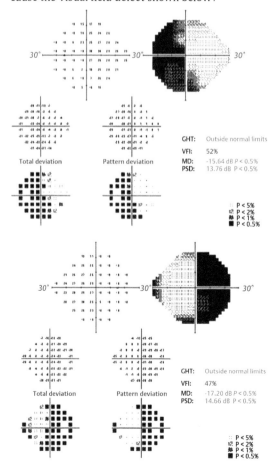

A. Left optic tract inflammation

B. Left occipital lobe ischemia

C. Sellar mass

D. Left temporal lobe mass

69. A 62-year-old man is seen with a vertical pendular nystagmus. MRI is performed and shows an old area of infarct at the inferior olivary nucleus. What else may be noted on examination?

A. Orthostatic hypotension

B. Internuclear ophthalmoplegia

C. Resting tremor of the upper extremities

D. Tremor of the palate

70. A 36-year-old man is seen in the emergency room after being found poorly responsive outside. The patient has become more responsive but is confused. Examination notes pendular convergence and divergence eye movements. Supraduction is limited bilaterally. A rhythmic motion of the jaw is also noted. What is the best treatment for this patient?

A. Intravenous corticosteroids

B. Intravenous mannitol

C. Intravenous ceftriaxone

D. Intravenous heparin

71. A 42-year-old woman complains of peripheral vision loss. She also feels uneasy when she is walking, especially down long corridors or aisles at the grocery store. The Goldmann visual field is obtained and shown below. What is the most likely cause of her loss in peripheral vision?

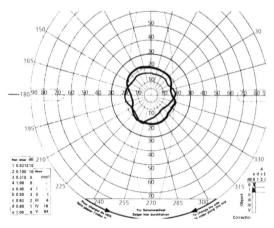

A. Glaucoma

B. Retinitis pigmentosa

C. Occipital lobe ischemia

D. Nonorganic vision loss

72. A 25-year-old man complains of blurred vision in the left eye. Fundus findings are shown below. The right eye is normal. What is the next best step?

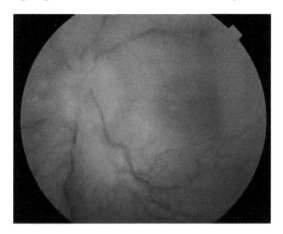

A. Obtain optical coherence tomography (OCT).

B. Perform B-scan ultrasound.

C. Obtain CT of the brain and orbits.

D. Obtain MRI of the brain and orbits.

73. A 36-year-old man is seen for glare when he is driving at night. A previous MRI is reviewed and shown below. What is the most likely cause for this patient's complaint?

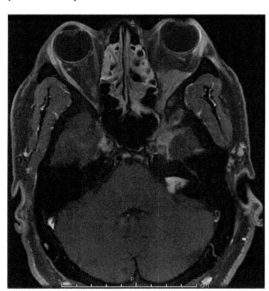

A. Exposure keratopathy

B. Anterior uveitis

C. Nuclear sclerotic cataracts

D. Posterior subcapsular cataracts

74. A 63-year-old woman presents with gradual proptosis and vision loss. MRI is performed and shown below. Which of the following is true regarding this type of lesion?

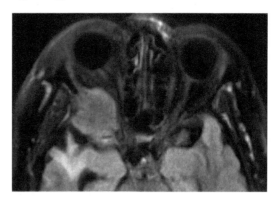

A. Incidence is higher in males than females.

B. They originate from arachnoid cells.

C. There is an increased risk of these lesions in patients with neurofibromatosis type 1.

D. Lesions are responsive to steroids, but tend to recur.

75. A 60-year-old woman presents with progressive prominence of the right eye over the last 6 months. Examination shows right-sided proptosis. Imaging is obtained and shown below. Which of the following statements is true regarding this lesion?

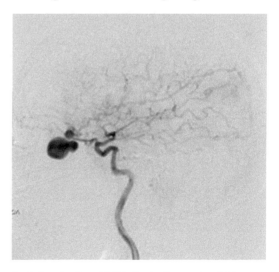

A. A dural tail on MRI helps in diagnosis of this lesion.

B. The lesion arises from a branch of the external carotid artery.

C. This is the most common location for presentation of these lesions.

D. The involved vessel is inferior to the optic nerve.

76. A 72-year-old man with diabetes mellitus type 2 and coronary artery disease complains of blurred vision that has not resolved after an episode of sudden-onset right-sided hemiparesis, dizziness, and blurred vision. MRI is obtained and shown below. What type of visual field deficit is expected?

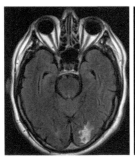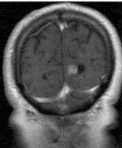

A. No visual field deficit

B. Complete right homonymous hemianopia

C. Right homonymous hemianopia sparing the vertical meridian

D. Right inferior quadrantanopia sparing the horizontal meridian

77. A 45-year-old man is seen for painless progressive vision loss in the left eye. MRI is obtained and shown below. Which feature would help to differentiate this lesion from meningioma?

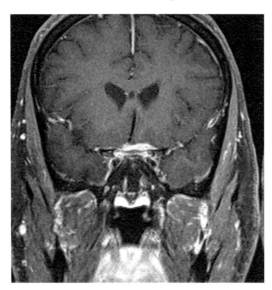

A. No dural tail compared to meningioma

B. Higher incidence in males compared to females for meningioma

C. Diffusely enhances with gadolinium compared to meningioma

D. None of the above

78. A brain mass was biopsied, and pathology is shown below. Which of the following is not true regarding this lesion?

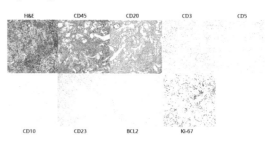

A. Composed of neoplastic small B-cell lymphocytes

B. Negative for markers CD5 and CD10, but positive for CD23

C. Associated with chronic inflammation

D. Associated with immunosuppression

79. A 63-year-old man presents with double vision. His extraocular movements are shown below. These findings are least consistent with which diagnosis?

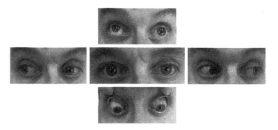

A. Ischemia

B. Aneurysmal compression

C. Myasthenia gravis

D. Idiopathic intracranial hypertension

80. A 56-year-old woman presents with 2 months of increased thirst, frequent urination, and bilateral proptosis. MRI is performed and shown below. What is the next best step in management?

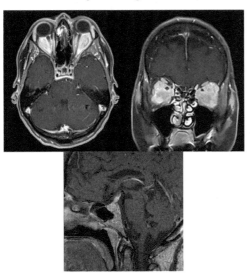

A. Intravenous corticosteroids.

B. Intravenous antibiotics.

C. Radiation therapy.

D. Obtain orbital biopsy.

81. An orbital mass was biopsied from the right side of a patient with bilateral proptosis. The pathology is shown below. What is the most accurate statement regarding this disorder?

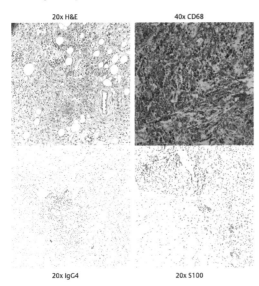

A. First-line therapy is surgical debulking with adjuvant radiotherapy.

B. The disease is curable with excellent long-term prognosis.

C. More than 50% are positive for the BRAF V600E mutation.

D. Tumors are composed of neoplastic Langerhans' cells.

82. A 53-year-old diabetic woman returns for follow-up 3 months after an episode of pupil-sparing third nerve palsy. You note miosis on adduction of the affected eye. Which of the following is the next best step?

A. Reassurance of ischemic cause secondary to diabetes.

B. Check acetylcholine receptor antibodies.

C. Order MRI or MRA.

D. Order carotid Doppler ultrasound.

83. A 36-year-old man presents with 3 months right-sided periocular and perioral twitching. Which of the following is the best next step?

A. Imaging

B. Chemodenervation

C. Reassurance to self-resolving course

D. None of the above

84. A 26-year-old woman presents for further evaluation of headaches that began a few years ago. Headaches start with a scintillating scotoma that resolves after 20 minutes and is followed by a severe headache that resolves after 10 hours. Which description would prompt further imaging?

A. Nausea and vomiting

B. Intense photophobia

C. Ptosis and miosis ipsilateral to headache

D. Sudden-onset headache after exercise

85. A 53-year-old man develops right-sided neck pain. Examination demonstrates right-sided ptosis with margin to reflex distance 1 of 1 mm on the right and 3 mm on the left. There is also anisocoria with the right pupil smaller than the left. The anisocoria is more prominent in dark than light. Imaging is obtained and shown below. What is the most appropriate treatment?

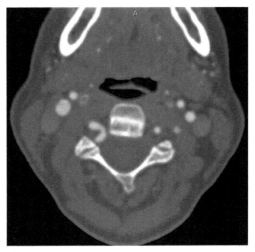

A. Resection of mass

B. Anticoagulation

C. Intravenous corticosteroids

D. Observation

117

86. A 62-year-old woman develops binocular double vision and difficulty closing her eye. Examination reveals a left-sided facial nerve palsy. MRI is obtained and shown below. What is causing the double vision?

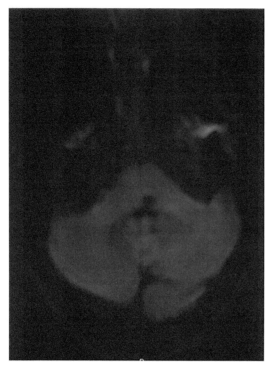

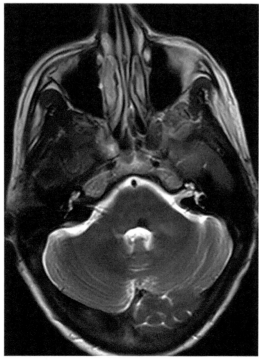

A. Severe exposure keratopathy

B. Third cranial nerve palsy

C. Internuclear ophthalmoplegia

D. Sixth cranial nerve palsy

87. A 26-year-old man suffers a motor vehicle accident with vision loss to light perception in the right eye. There is a right relative afferent pupillary defect. Examination is otherwise within normal limits. CT is performed and found to be normal. What is the best statement to tell the patient?

A. Surgical decompression of your optic canal is indicated and should lead to improved vision.

B. IV corticosteroids should be started and will improve your vision compared to observation.

C. No known treatment will definitely improve your vision. We will observe.

D. None of the above.

88. A 72-year-old man presents with right-sided proptosis, periorbital erythema, and ocular injection. Imaging is performed and shown below. Visual acuity is 20/20 and the remainder of the examination is within normal limits. A biopsy is performed with immunoglobulin G4 (IgG4) stain shown below. Which of the treatments is not appropriate for this patient?

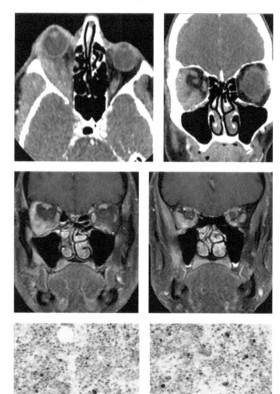

A. Orbitotomy for mass excision

B. Corticosteroids

C. Rituximab

D. Radiation therapy

89. A patient with optic neuritis should not be treated with which of the following modalities?

A. Oral prednisone dosed at 1 mg/kg

B. Intravenous methylprednisolone dosed at 1g/d

C. Rituximab

D. Intravenous immunoglobulin

90. A 34-year-old woman is seen with right facial paralysis and pain in her ear. Examination shows an erythematous vesicular rash involving the right pinna. What is the best management for this patient?

A. Obtain MRI of the brain and orbits with gadolinium.

B. Start oral antibiotics.

C. Obtain lumbar puncture.

D. Start steroids and antivirals.

91. A 36-year-old man complains of recent-onset double vision. The patient has a left head tilt. The double vision is worse when looking to the left. Which of the following would point to a more benign etiology for the patient's double vision?

A. Uncontrolled hypertension and diabetes

B. Large fusion amplitudes

C. New onset of headaches

D. No head tilt in old photographs

92. The patient below is seen for double vision. Which of the following tests will not help in determining the cause?

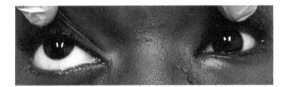

A. CT scan of the orbits

B. Acetylcholine receptor antibodies

C. Lumbar puncture for opening pressure

D. Thyroid-stimulating immunoglobulin

93. A 15-year-old adolescent boy has a CT scan for double vision in upgaze as shown below. What is the best treatment for this patient?

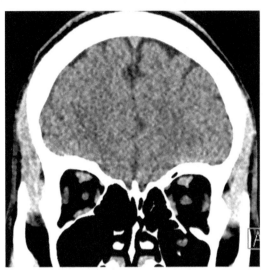

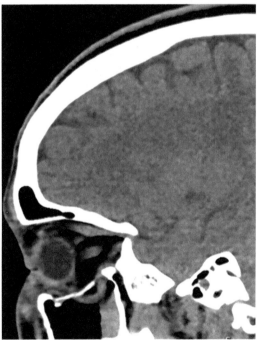

A. Corticosteroids

B. Thyroidectomy

C. Pyridostigmine

D. Orbital surgery

94. A 62-year-old woman complains of slowly darkening vision on the right side. She has no other complaints. Examination shows visual acuity of 20/60 on the right and 20/25 on the left. There is a trace relative afferent pupillary defect on the right. Examination demonstrates trace anterior chamber cell and flare. Fundus examination shows moderate dot blot hemorrhages and trace optic nerve edema. Lab studies show erythrocyte sedimentation rate (ESR) of 22 and C-reactive protein (CRP) of 1.0. Carotid Doppler ultrasound finds stenosis of 73% on the right. Blood pressure and serum glucose are within normal limits. What is the best management for this patient?

A. Start intravenous corticosteroids.

B. Refer for carotid endarterectomy.

C. MRI of the orbits with contrast.

D. None of the above.

95. A 10-year-old girl is seen for a failed vision screen at school. Examination demonstrates bilateral visual acuity of 20/200. Genetic testing finds a mutation of *OPA1*. All of the following are true of this disorder except which one?

A. Prognosis for final visual acuity ranges from 20/200 to 20/400.

B. Optic nerve examination will show bilateral temporal to diffuse atrophy.

C. Transmission is autosomal dominant.

D. Most patients present in the first decade of life.

96. A 12-year-old girl with insulin-dependent diabetes mellitus is seen for progressive vision loss. Ophthalmic examination is only significant for bilateral optic nerve atrophy. All of the following are true of this disorder except which one?

A. About 50% of patients also have diabetes insipidus.

B. About 10% of patients have sensorineural hearing loss.

C. Inheritance is autosomal recessive.

D. A mutation of *WFS1* or *WFS2* causes this condition.

97. A 15-year-old adolescent boy with worsening ataxia is seen with ophthalmic examination only revealing conjunctival telangiectasia. Imaging in this syndrome should reveal which of the following?

A. Midbrain atrophy

B. Cerebellar atrophy

C. Optic nerve atrophy

D. No atrophic changes

98. A 20-year-old woman with history of seizures since childhood is noted to have angiofibromas in the malar area. MRI shows bilateral subependymal nodules. Which of the following is not true of this syndrome?

A. Half of patients have learning difficulties.

B. Angiomyolipomas of the kidneys may cause hematuria.

C. Astrocytic hamartomas are the only ocular involvement.

D. Inheritance is in an autosomal dominant pattern.

99. An 18-year-old man with history of photocoagulation to a retinal angioma 1 year ago comes in for new headaches over the past month. Examination shows new bilateral optic disc edema. MRI of the brain and orbits shows a vascular cerebellar lesion. Which test is not indicated in this condition?

A. Abdominal ultrasound

B. Skin biopsy

C. Urinary catecholamine metabolites

D. MRI spinal cord

100. A 34-year-old woman presents with severe, shooting pain down the right side of her face. Examination reveals atrophy of the right side of the face with enophthalmos and a collapsed malar area. There is linear scar extending from the forehead to the midface on the right side. Which of the following statements regarding this syndrome is incorrect?

A. Trauma is the underlying mechanism.

B. It is considered to be a variant of scleroderma.

C. Horner's syndrome may be seen in some patients.

D. May be associated with ipsilateral body hemiatrophy.

4.2 Answers and Explanations

Easy	Medium	Hard

1. Correct: Optical coherence tomography OCT) of the macula (D)

The photostress test differentiates between macular disease and optic neuropathies. After initially measuring the best corrected visual acuity, a light is held in front of one eye for 10 seconds and the vision is rechecked. *Normal is considered recovery to within one line of the best corrected visual acuity* within 30 seconds, with symmetry. Abnormal photostress recovery test is associated with macular disease as recovery of photoreceptor pigments is compromised. Choices (**A**), (**B**), and (**C**) are tests for neural function.

2. Correct: Optokinetic testing (A)

Severe vision loss with a normal neuro-ophthalmic examination will make nonorganic vision loss rise on the differential. While it is important to rule out other serious causes of vision loss, some of the testing may be unnecessary to perform at this time. The optokinetic response is a normal type of jerk nystagmus best seen when tracking fast moving objects. It is difficult to suppress and useful in determining vision in nonorganic vision loss or in preverbal infants. In optokinetic testing, a striped rotating drum is rotated in front of a patient, and the eyes are noted to track the stripes in the direction of rotation with a jerk saccade in the opposite direction to track the next object. Intact optokinetic response confirms vision of at least 20/400. Testing can be performed monocularly. While MRI (**B**) may be useful in patients with acute vision loss, this would not be the next best test in this situation as other neuro-ophthalmic testing such as checking optokinetic responses and stereopsis are easily done in the office and can provide further information to the likely nonorganic cause in this case. Fluorescein angiography (**C**) is useful in evaluating retinal and choroidal pathology. The Amsler grid testing (**D**) is useful in evaluating the effect of macular disease on central vision.

3. Correct: Left relative afferent pupillary defect (B)

The right optic tract contains fibers from the ipsilateral temporal retina and contralateral nasal retina (including the nasal macula). The optic tract contains 55% crossed fibers and 45% uncrossed fibers. Pupillary examination in a patient with a right optic tract lesion would be expected to reveal a left relative afferent pupillary defect due to the greater percentage of crossed fibers. A right relative afferent pupillary defect (**A**) would not be expected in this case. Optic nerve edema of either side (**C**) and (**D**) would not be expected in retrochiasmal demyelinating disease.

4. Correct: An abnormal optokinetic response with the drum rotated to the left (D)

A left parietal mass would be expected to have an abnormal optokinetic nystagmus response with the drum or stimuli moving toward the side of the lesion. Foveal pursuit pathways pass from the occipitoparietal association area to the ipsilateral brainstem horizontal gaze center. Damage to the foveal pursuit pathways should result in disrupted slow pursuit to the ipsilateral side. Rotating the drum to the right should be normal in this case (**C**). A left parietal lesion would be expected to create an incongruous right homonymous hemianopia (**A and B**).

5. Correct: Left posterior cerebral artery (D)

Blood supply to the majority of the occipital cortex comes from the posterior cerebral artery. The most posterior portion subserving the central macula is brought by terminal branches of the middle cerebral artery. The patient has a right homonymous hemianopia with macular sparing. Ischemia to the occipital cortex in the territory of the left posterior cerebral artery would lead to this visual defect. Embolus to the right-sided vessels (**A and B**) would lead to a left-sided visual field defect. Embolus to the left middle cerebral artery (**C**) would cause a right homonymous scotomatous visual field defect (affecting the macula).

6. Correct: All of the above (D)

Patients who come in with a complaint should be worked up until all possible diagnoses are excluded. Some patients may have difficulty describing their symptoms, but the clinician should make every attempt to elucidate the problem. The patient was found to have an anatomically normal eye and 20/20 vision. Multiple tests may have picked up his early optic neuropathy, including all of the listed tests. Decreased color vision may be the first sign of an early optic neuropathy (**A**). Red desaturation may also be noted as an early change in the vision (**B**). It is ideal to check for red desaturation in all quadrants. An early bitemporal hemianopia may have been noted. Confrontation and formal visual field testing (**C**) should also have been performed, and may have demonstrated a visual field deficit.

7. Correct: 23% (A)

Although obtaining MRI is not necessary in diagnosing optic neuritis, it is helpful in determining a patient's risk of developing multiple sclerosis in the future. According to the Optic Neuritis Treatment Trial, a patient who has optic neuritis and a normal brain MRI has a 23% risk of developing MS by 15 years. If brain MRI demonstrates one T2-weighted (or fluid-attenuated inversion recovery) lesion greater than 3 mm in diameter, the 15-year risk increases to 56% (**B**). With more than six T2-weighted lesions, the risk increases further to 74% (**C**).

8. Correct: 74% (C)

This case shows a sagittal FLAIR with greater than six T2-weighted white matter lesions suggestive of multiple sclerosis (MS). According to the Optic Neuritis Treatment Trial, the risk of developing MS at 15 years is 74%. A patient who has optic neuritis and a normal brain MRI has a 23% risk of developing MS by 15 years (A). If brain MRI demonstrates one T2-weighted (or FLAIR) lesion greater than 3 mm in diameter, the 15-year risk increases to 56% (B). With more than six T2-weighted lesions, the risk increases further to 74%.

9. Correct: Obtain complete blood count (CBC), erythrocyte sedimentation rate (ESR), and C-reactive protein (CRP) (B)

The distinction between the ischemic optic neuropathies can sometimes be blurred. Nonarteritic anterior ischemic optic neuropathy (NAION) is generally considered to present as painless vision loss in an older patient with underlying vascular disease, taking antihypertensives at night. The visual field defect is usually an altitudinal defect with segmental optic nerve edema and likely associated hemorrhages. The fellow eye has a small or no cup. The arteritic variety more likely presents with pain and severe vision loss. Patients may have associated systemic signs such as temporal tenderness/headaches, generalized malaise, fatigue, jaw claudication, night sweats, fevers, or unintentional weight loss. The optic nerve tends to be diffusely swollen and chalky white. Some cases can be difficult to tell apart. A patient who seemingly presents with NAION, but has severe vision loss, diffuse optic nerve edema, or any other concerning factors should first have emergent blood work done for CBC, ESR, and CRP. NAION is not known to have a treatment, and can be monitored (**D**), but ruling out temporal arteritis must be a priority. (**A**) and (**C**) are possible treatment options for NAION, although neither has been shown to be effective and is not required.

10. Correct: Obtain carotid Doppler ultrasound (B)

The patient described in this question presents with a classic case of nonarteritic ischemic optic neuropathy (NAION). The figure shows an inferior altitudinal visual field defect. Embolism does not cause NAION. Although caring for underlying cardiovascular disease is important, a carotid Doppler ultrasound is not indicated. While there is currently no known treatment for the current episode, it is imperative to prevent future episodes in the same or fellow eye. Known risk factors are those that cause ischemia to the optic nerve head and include a small, crowded disc and systemic disorders that predispose to hypotension or hypercoagulability. (**A**) Antihypertensives should not be taken at night as nocturnal hypotension may be aggravated. (**C**) Obstructive sleep apnea may also potentiate ischemia of the optic nerve head. At-risk patients should undergo a sleep study and may need treatment with continuous positive airway pressure. (**D**) Diabetic disease also leads to poor perfusion and ischemia and must be controlled.

11. Correct: Ischemic infarction of the posterior orbital optic nerve (A)

The patient's history of severe vision loss after spinal surgery and MRI with (**left**) diffusion-weighted imaging and (**right**) apparent diffusion coefficient confirm ischemia to the posterior orbital optic nerve on the left. Posterior ischemic optic neuropathy is generally due to acute systemic hypotension such as in long spinal surgery with prone positioning or cardiac surgery, severe hemorrhage, hemodialysis, and cardiac arrest. Embolic ophthalmic artery occlusion (**B**) may have a similar presentation but would be expected to show a blonde fundus with cherry-red spot. Early in the process, only a subtle cherry-red spot and mild macular edema may be noted. Retrobulbar hemorrhage (**C**) would be expected to be much more symptomatic with severe pain and proptosis.

12. Correct: Electrocardiogram (D)

The patient's presentation and history are most consistent with Leber's hereditary optic neuropathy (LHON). LHON classically occurs in young males, but it may occur in at any age and gender. Inheritance is mitochondrial with mitochondrial point mutations at positions 11,778, 14,484, and 3,460 being the most common. Patients suspected of having LHON can undergo genetic testing for these common mitochondrial DNA point mutations, with 11,778 being the most common. These patients should be referred for electrocardiogram to rule out possible related cardiac conduction deficits. Choices (**A**), (**B**), and (**C**) are not relevant in evaluation of a patient diagnosed with LHON.

13. Correct: Review medications (C)

Patients presenting with bilateral optic neuropathy may have a number of underlying causes. It is imperative that the physician obtains a complete history to help pinpoint the cause. In the presented patient with a past medical history that includes tuberculosis, it is very important to know all the medications being taken. Ethambutol is commonly used to treat tuberculosis, but is known to sometimes cause a slowly progressive bilateral optic neuropathy. MRI of the orbits and brain (**A**) would evaluate for possible compressive or infiltrative processes. Automated perimetry (**B**) should be performed to evaluate the pattern of vision loss. A decrease in color vision (**D**) may be the first sign of an optic neuropathy. All of these steps should be performed among many other available tests, but a complete history is always the first step.

14. Correct: Flat hyperpigmented skin lesions (A)

The image depicts an MRI with a left optic nerve fusiform mass, consistent with an optic nerve glioma. Optic nerve gliomas tend to occur in children less than 10 years of age. Presentation in adulthood is associated with a worse prognosis. Thirty percent of patients with optic nerve glioma have neurofibromatosis type 1 (NF1). Flat hyperpigmented skin lesions known as café au lait spots are commonly associated with NF1. Hearing loss (**B**) can develop in patients with neurofibromatosis type 2. Hypopigmented skin patches (**C**) known as ash leaf spots are commonly seen in tuberous sclerosis. A facial capillary malformation (**D**) known as a port-wine stain is commonly seen in Sturge–Weber syndrome.

15. Correct: Observation (D)

Imaging is most consistent with an optic nerve sheath meningioma of the right eye. The right lateral cavernous sinus is abnormally thickened and enhances, extending to the optic nerve sheath in the posterior half of the orbital optic nerve with a normal optic nerve, as opposed to the fusiform enlargement seen with optic nerve glioma. The thickened nerve sheath gives a characteristic "railroad" sign. Given the mild visual symptoms, observation would be the best option in managing this patient. Close follow-up with neuro-ophthalmic examinations and Humphrey's visual fields is warranted. Intervention has multiple risks that do not outweigh the benefits in this case. With progression, the patient could undergo radiotherapy (**C**). Surgical resection (**B**) would be a last resort given the high risk of optic nerve damage and vision loss. Biopsy (**A**) can be considered in unusual cases as other processes such as lymphoma may mimic meningioma on imaging.

16. Correct: Reassurance (C)

The color fundus photographs show bilateral irregular optic disc margins with a lumpy appearance. The vessels course normally over the rim. The red-free photographs show bilateral autofluorescence of small bumps of the optic nerve head. These findings are consistent with optic disc drusen. Most patients are asymptomatic throughout life, and reassurance of the benign course can be given. It should be noted in this discussion that some patients can develop transient visual obscurations, visual field loss, and may be at increased risk of nonarteritic anterior ischemic optic neuropathy. QuantiFERON Gold (**A**) is a blood test for tuberculosis, which is not suspected in this case. Orbital MRI (**B**) is not needed, as there is no visual change requiring advanced imaging to rule out optic nerve lesions. CT of the orbits may show the drusen as calcifications at the optic disc. Ultrasound can also show optic nerve head calcifications. Genetic testing (**D**) does not have a role in this case, although optic disc drusen are thought to usually be transmitted in an autosomal dominant fashion.

17. Correct: Endocrine evaluation (D)

The patient has septo-optic dysplasia (de Morsier's syndrome), which includes bilateral optic nerve hypoplasia and midline defects (one or all of absent septum pellucidum, atrophic corpus callosum, pituitary ectopia). The MRI shows absence of the septum pellucidum. Patients with pituitary ectopia may have panhypopituitarism. All patients with septo-optic dysplasia should undergo an endocrine evaluation to prevent any life-threatening complications. Choices (**A**), (**B**), and (**C**) should not be needed in evaluation of septo-optic dysplasia unless indicated by examination.

18. Correct: Corticosteroids (B)

Optic pits may remain asymptomatic but can sometimes lead to the formation of macular serous detachments. Corticosteroids have been used in the past but have not been shown to lead to improvement and are no longer considered an indicated treatment. With observation alone (**A**), about one-third will resolve.

Other treatment options include pars plana vitrectomy (**C**) to relieve vitreous traction and a few rows of photocoagulation (**D**) between the optic disc and the detachment in an attempt to form a barrier of scar tissue.

19. Correct: Anticoagulation (C)

The imaging shows a left transverse sinus filling defect consistent with dural venous sinus thrombosis. The appropriate treatment is anticoagulation. Other treatments aimed at lowering the intracranial pressure may also be needed. Intravenous antibiotics (**A**) and steroids (**B**) are not used to treat thrombosis. Diuresis (**D**) may be needed to lower intracranial pressure, but anticoagulation is the next best treatment.

20. Correct: Diuresis (D)

The patient's presentation and imaging are consistent with idiopathic intracranial hypertension (IIH). The sagittal MRI shows a partially empty sella. The MRV shows stenosis of the transverse sinuses. Depending on symptom severity, treatment will vary from weight loss only to diuresis and headache management to surgical options such as ventriculoperitoneal shunt and optic nerve fenestration. Of the answer choices given, diuresis is the best treatment for this patient. Antibiotics (**A**) and anticoagulation (**C**) are not needed in IIH. Corticosteroids (**B**) are sometimes used in severe optic nerve edema as a possible temporizing measure until a more definitive procedure is performed.

21. Correct: Hemineglect (B)

Balint's syndrome is usually caused by an insult to bilateral parieto-occipital lobes that leads to simultagnosia (**A**), ocular apraxia (**C**), and optic ataxia (**D**). Simultagnosia is when a patient cannot describe an entire scene but is able to describe individual parts of that scene. Ocular apraxia is when a patient cannot fixate on an object that he or she can see in his or her visual field. Optic ataxia is when a patient cannot touch an object that he or she can see. Hemineglect occurs with lesions of the nondominant hemisphere. Patients do not respond to stimuli in the opposite (usually left) visual field and may have a sensorimotor hemiparesis.

22. Correct: The Pulfrich phenomenon (C)

The patient is exhibiting the Pulfrich phenomenon, which is the perception of a pendulum swinging in an elliptical path when it is actually swinging in one plane. This occurs due to the conduction delay of the optic nerves in a unilateral or asymmetric optic neuropathy. Prosopagnosia (**A**) is when patients cannot recognize famous or familiar faces. Ocular apraxia (**B**) is when a patient cannot fixate on an object he or she can see and is seen as part of Balint's syndrome. The Riddoch phenomenon (**D**) occurs when patients have a visual field defect where they cannot see static objects, but can see motion of objects in the blind field.

23. Correct: Anton's syndrome (A)

Anton's syndrome describes a patient who denies vision loss, yet has cerebral blindness. In Charles Bonnet syndrome (**B**), patients with severe vision loss due to anterior disease (such as macular degeneration) experience visual hallucinations due to release of the normal visual cortex without normal anterior pathway input. In visual allesthesia (**C**), patients have brief episodes of seeing a visual stimulus transposed from one hemifield to the other. In metamorphopsia (**D**), patients note a change in size perception.

24. Correct: Left pretectal nucleus (D)

The pupillary light reflex pathway starts with light entering the eye and hitting the retina. Signal from the retinal ganglion cells travels through the optic nerve and to the chiasm, where 55% of fibers cross the contralateral optic tract. Before reaching the lateral geniculate nucleus, pupillary fibers leave the tract via the brachium of the superior colliculus to reach the pretectal nucleus. A lesion of the brachium of the superior colliculus or pretectal nucleus will cause a contralateral relative afferent pupillary defect (RAPD) *without* visual loss. A lesion of the optic tract will cause a contralateral RAPD with a visual field defect. In this patient with no visual defect and a right RAPD, only localization to the contralateral (left) pretectal nucleus is correct.

25. Correct: Intracavernous carotid aneurysm (D)

The patient has a right abduction deficit consistent with a sixth cranial nerve palsy as well as a right-sided Horner's syndrome. The sympathetic fibers run along with the sixth cranial nerve for a short distance in the cavernous sinus. Lesions in this location can demonstrate both a sixth nerve palsy and a Horner syndrome. Third-order lesions will also lack anhidrosis as fibers controlling facial sympathetics split off after the superior cervical ganglion. A carotid aneurysm in the area of the cavernous sinus can cause such a lesion. A demyelinating brainstem lesion (**A**) will cause a first-order Horner's syndrome. An apical lung tumor (**B**) will cause a second-order Horner's syndrome. An internal carotid artery dissection (**C**) will also cause a third-order Horner's syndrome, but a sixth nerve palsy would not be present.

26. Correct: Order an MRI of the brain, orbits, neck, and chest (B)

The child has examination findings consistent with a right Horner syndrome. Without an obvious cause, metastatic neuroblastoma is the major concern and must be ruled out. MRI of the sympathetic chain should

be performed and includes the brain, orbits, neck, and chest. Reassurance would not be a good option (**A**). While an MRI of the abdomen (**C**) would image for a primary neuroblastoma, without clear clinical suspicion, it may be of low yield and requires a separate test with second sedation. MRI of the sympathetic chain would still be required. Urine testing for vanillylmandelic acid and homovanillic acid should also be performed

27. Correct: Pharmacological (A)

The first step in examining anisocoria is to determine if the problem is with the smaller or larger pupil. This is best done by checking the difference in light and dark. With a bigger difference in light, we know the larger pupil is the problem in this case. In pharmacological mydriasis (**A**), the pupil does not react to light or near (accommodation). Nebulized ipratropium bromide is an anticholinergic that can cause mydriasis when it escapes around the mask, as likely occurred in this case. Other anticholinergics include atropine, homatropine, tropicamide, scopolamine, and cyclopentolate. Sympathomimetics such as phenylephrine and adrenaline also cause mydriasis. In Adie's tonic pupil (**B**), light-near dissociation is seen such that the pupil does not or minimally react to light, but reacts to accommodation. This is due to a majority of fibers serving accommodation versus pupilloconstriction. When regeneration after the initial insult causing Adie's tonic pupil occurs, more accommodative fibers may rewire to pupilloconstriction, leading to light-near dissociation. In pupil-involving third nerve palsy (**C**), diplopia is generally noted with decreased adduction, supraduction, and infraduction, as well as ptosis. Traumatic mydriasis (**D**) will have a history of trauma, which is not noted here.

28. Correct: MRI of the brain (C)

From the presentation, it is clear that this patient has a pupil-involving third cranial nerve palsy. The likely causes of the third cranial nerve palsy in this case are pituitary apoplexy or an aneurysm. MRI of the brain should be performed urgently. Pharmacological testing (**A**) is not needed to determine the cause of the anisocoria. Lumbar puncture (**B**) and intravenous corticosteroids (**D**) are not yet indicated.

29. Correct: Right hypertropia worse in left gaze and right head tilt (C)

The three-step test is used to help determine which muscle is not working well in a hyperdeviation. Gaze to the left or right will isolate the appropriate elevators and depressors. In left gaze, the elevators are the right inferior oblique and left superior rectus muscles. The depressors are the right superior oblique and left inferior rectus muscles. In a right hypertropia worse in left gaze, there is either a problem in depressing the right eye or elevating the left eye. Therefore, either the right superior oblique or left superior rectus is not working properly. In right head tilt, the right eye will intort and the left eye will extort. Since the superior oblique is the intorter and the inferior oblique is the extorter, the right superior oblique must be the deficient muscle with worsened right hypertropia. This is why patients with a fourth cranial nerve palsy develop a compensatory head tilt in the opposite direction of the palsied muscle. (**A**), (**B**), and (**D**) do not fit all of these criteria.

30. Correct: Thyroid eye disease (B)

Proptosis has a long differential with many important disorders, but many times it can be easily differentiated. Thyroid eye disease is the most common cause of both unilateral and bilateral proptosis in adults. The MRI shows thickening of the medial rectus muscles bilaterally. Of note, the tendon is spared, which helps differentiate it from inflammatory myositis (**A**), where the muscle and tendon insertion are both inflamed. Orbital cellulitis (**C**), the most common cause of proptosis in children, generally also shows periorbital tissue edema and orbital fat stranding.

31. Correct: Superior oblique (C)

The patient has an acquired Brown syndrome. There is an inflammation of the superior oblique tendon/trochlea. Digital pressure in the area of the trochlea will usually reveal tenderness. Although up and in gaze is in the field of action of the inferior oblique (**D**), it is the restriction of the superior oblique tendon that compromises the ability to look up and in. The superior (**A**) and inferior (**B**) rectus muscles act to elevate and depress the eye, respectively, in lateral gaze.

32. Correct: C-reactive protein (B)

Older patients with transient or constant double vision should undergo evaluation for temporal arteritis. Symptoms of temporal arteritis should be checked on history and examination, and evaluation of platelets for thrombocytosis, erythrocyte sedimentation rate, and C-reactive protein should be ordered urgently. Although myasthenia gravis can cause transient double vision, symptoms usually worsen throughout the day. Myasthenia gravis can be tested with acetylcholine receptor antibodies (**A**) but would not lead to vision loss. Thyroid eye disease can also lead to double vision, but it is usually constant due to muscle restriction. Thyroid-stimulating immunoglobulin (**C**) is a test for thyroid eye disease. Antineutrophil cytoplasmic antibody (**D**) tests for small vessel vasculitides that can lead to vision loss, but it is not the most likely diagnosis in this case.

33. Correct: Atrophy of the maxillary sinus (C)

Causes of enophthalmos include orbital wall fracture, silent sinus syndrome, and metastatic scirrhous breast carcinoma. In silent sinus syndrome, chronic maxillary sinusitis leads to a blockage of the maxillary sinus outlet. This causes negative pressure to develop with collapse of the maxillary sinus and downward bowing of the orbital floor, leading to enophthalmos. Agenesis of the sphenoid wing (**A**) usually occurs in neurofibromatosis type 1. This results in herniation of intracranial contents into the orbit and pulsatile proptosis. Hypertrophy of extraocular muscles (**B**) is seen in thyroid eye disease and myositis. These may lead to proptosis. Orbital fat stranding (**D**) is a common sign in orbital cellulitis, which may show proptosis.

34. Correct: Electrocardiogram (D)

Chronic progressive external ophthalmoplegia (CPEO) presents with ptosis and limitation of extraocular movements over many years. Many patients do not complain of double vision because the eyes are straight in primary gaze. They tend to complain of diplopia with reading. CPEO can be a part of many syndromes. Many of these myopathies are associated with systemic findings, including cardiomyopathy and cardiac conduction deficits. All patient with CPEO must have an electrocardiogram. MRI of the brain and orbits (**A**) may be obtained in these patients but is not as important as the electrocardiogram. CT chest (**B**) and renal ultrasound (**C**) are not indicated in CPEO.

35. Correct: Christmas tree (B)

This patient's presentation is consistent with myotonic dystrophy. It is the most common adult-onset muscular dystrophy. It is autosomal dominant with trinucleotide repeat on chromosome 19. These patients characteristically develop the Christmas tree cataract, which consists of highly reflective, multicolored, crisscrossing needles. Oil droplet (**A**) cataract is associated with galactosemia. Sunflower (**C**) cataract is associated with Wilson's disease. Cerulean (**D**) cataract is associated with Down's syndrome.

36. Correct: Barium swallow (B)

This patient with chronic progressive external ophthalmoplegia (CPEO) and French Canadian ancestry is likely to have oculopharyngeal dystrophy. This is an autosomal dominant disorder with trinucleotide repeat on chromosome 14. Dysphasia is a major part of the disease, and these patients should have evaluation with barium swallow. Choices (**A**), (**C**), and (**D**) are not needed in the evaluation of oculopharyngeal dystrophy.

37. Correct: Acetylcholine receptor antibodies are positive in up to 50% of patients. There is still a chance you have myasthenia gravis (C)

The patient has ptosis with signs and symptoms consistent with ocular myasthenia gravis. Ptosis (and/or double vision) is best upon awakening and worse with time and when tired. The signs exhibited in this patient include an inability to sustain upgaze (the eyelids should not droop back down as upgaze is maintained) and Cogan's lid twitch (downgaze allows the levator palpebrae superioris to fully rest, and when looking straight ahead, the eyelid will overshoot prior to returning to its prior ptotic position). Over 50% of these patients will develop generalized myasthenia gravis. Acetylcholine receptor antibodies are positive in about 50% of patients with ocular myasthenia gravis. They are positive in up to 90% of patients with generalized myasthenia gravis (**A**). Patients with ptosis due to myasthenia gravis should only have surgical intervention as a last resort (**B**). The examiner should be suspicious of negative acetylcholine receptor antibody testing in a patient with signs and symptoms of ocular or generalized myasthenia gravis and should perform other testing (ice test, rest test, edrophonium test, single-fiber electromyography).

38.   Correct: CT chest (A)

About 10% of patients with myasthenia gravis may have a thymoma. Thus, patients diagnosed with myasthenia gravis should have a CT chest to evaluate for this mass. Those with thymoma should undergo thymectomy. Choices (**B**), (**C**), and (**D**) are not required specifically for myasthenia gravis.

39.   Correct: Elevated intracranial pressure (C)

The patient likely has an elevated intracranial pressure causing his left sixth cranial nerve palsy. The sixth cranial nerve nucleus is located in the pons, so a midbrain ischemic lesion (**A**) would not cause a left sixth nerve palsy. The fascicle travels around the seventh nerve nucleus and then travels anteriorly to exit the anterior aspect of the pons. The nerve then enters the subarachnoid space and travels over the edge of the tentorium, where elevated (or low) intracranial pressure may lead to compression of the sixth cranial nerve. Temporal arteritis may cause any cranial nerve palsy, but this patient is not in the appropriate age range, so ESR and CRP (**B**) do not need to be tested. A thickened medial rectus may cause a restrictive strabismus that may initially appear like a sixth nerve palsy. A thickened lateral rectus (**D**) would cause a restrictive pattern (decreased adduction, possibly abduction) and would not affect the vision.

40.   Correct: Difficulty hearing (D)

The patient presents with a bilateral sixth nerve palsy and bilateral seventh nerve palsy. These findings along with the lack of other neurologic findings are consistent with Möbius syndrome. Möbius syndrome is a sporadic congenital agenesis of the sixth and seventh cranial nerve nuclei. The fifth and eighth cranial nerves may also be involved. Patients may have difficulty hearing, facial deformities, endocrine problems, and malformed extremities. Choices (**A**), (**B**), and (**C**) are not associated with this syndrome.

41.   Correct: Miosis during convergence (B)

The patient shows signs of a pseudo–sixth nerve palsy with convergence on attempted left lateral gaze. Most cases in adulthood are functional in nature with an underlying psychiatric disorder or stressor. Noting miosis during convergence on attempted lateral gaze hints toward the nonorganic nature of the gaze restriction. Organic causes of an abduction deficit (sixth nerve palsy, neuromuscular disorders, and restrictive disorders) will not have pupillary involvement on extraocular movements. Miosis occurs normally with convergence, along with accommodation. Concerning signs include convergence-retraction nystagmus (**A**) and limitation of upgaze (**C**), which are signs consistent with dorsal midbrain syndrome. Tonic deviation (**D**) may be found in thalamic hemorrhage. Concern for these two syndromes requires imaging. In this case, in which miosis is noted during convergence without other concerning findings, the patient may be referred for psychological evaluation.

42.   Correct: Exits the midbrain dorsally, crosses contralaterally, and enters the orbit outside the annulus of Zinn (C)

The fourth cranial nerve exits the midbrain dorsally (all other cranial nerves exit ventrally), crosses to the contralateral side, travels in the subarachnoid space (longest intracranial course of all cranial nerves), enters the lateral wall of the cavernous sinus passing below the third cranial nerve and the ophthalmic division of the fifth cranial nerve, and enters the orbit through the superior orbital fissure, outside the annulus of Zinn.

43.   Correct: Right limitation in infraduction and adduction, bilateral ptosis, and supraduction deficit (D)

The patient suffered an ischemic stroke to the right midbrain. Knowledge of the location of the cranial nerve nuclei in the brainstem allows for differentiation between a third and fourth nerve palsy. The third nerve nucleus lies in the midbrain at the level of the superior colliculus. A patient with a fourth nerve palsy would present with a compensatory head tilt in the opposite direction. As the fourth nerve crosses over once it exits the brainstem, an ischemic stroke would cause a hypertropia on the contralateral side (and a compensatory head tilt to the same side as the stroke). Since this is a third nerve nucleus stroke, choices (**A**) and (**B**) are incorrect. Differentiating between (**C**) and (**D**) requires more detailed knowledge of the third nerve subnuclei. Each muscle controlled by the third nerve has its own subnucleus with notable differences: the levator palpebrae superioris has one centrally shared subnucleus and the superior rectus subnucleus controls the contralateral superior rectus. A stroke to the right midbrain would cause a complete ipsilateral third nerve palsy including pupillary dilation. The superior rectus that is controlled by the contralateral midbrain is affected as the exiting fibers cross through the contralateral nucleus (so that bilateral superior recti are affected). Bilateral ptosis also occurs due to the single central levator palpebrae superioris subnucleus.

44. Correct: Either A or C (D)

Most third cranial nerve palsies are ischemic, especially in those over 50 years of age and with ischemic risk factors (diabetes mellitus, heart disease). Ischemic third nerve palsies are generally pupil-sparing, as the parasympathetics are located in the periphery of the nerve, and ischemia mainly affects the center of the nerve. They may be painful. Complete and incomplete palsies in those older than 50 years and with ischemic risk factors should still be imaged (**A**) and followed closely (**C**) to exclude progression to pupillary involvement. Pupil-involving third nerve palsies and any palsy in those under age 50 years without ischemic risk factors should be promptly imaged to rule out a compressive lesion (usually either an aneurysm or sellar mass).

45. Correct: Benedikt's syndrome (B)

The patient has a right third nerve palsy and contralateral tremor, consistent with Benedikt's syndrome. Each of these syndromes occurs due to a brainstem lesion affecting the nerve fascicle. Weber's syndrome (**A**) combines the third nerve palsy with contralateral hemiparesis. Claude's syndrome (**C**) has a contralateral tremor and ataxia. Nothnagel's syndrome (**D**) has ipsilateral ataxia.

46. Correct: Conventional angiography (A)

A pupil-involving third nerve palsy should have a compressive etiology ruled out immediately. MRA may miss small aneurysms. CTA is more sensitive, but may still miss smaller aneurysms. In the face of negative imaging, when clearly indicated, conventional angiography should be obtained to definitively rule out an aneurysm. Temporal arteritis is not likely to cause a third nerve palsy, especially if pupil-involving, thus ESR and CRP (**B**) is not the best test to obtain. Lumbar puncture (**C**) may be helpful in ruling out meningitis or subarachnoid hemorrhage not seen on imaging, but conventional angiography is still the better first test. Acetylcholine receptor antibodies (**D**) for myasthenia gravis are not needed as the extraocular motor deficits will not involve the pupil.

47. Correct: Cavernous sinus (B)

The patient's ophthalmoplegia is most consistent with palsies of the third, fourth, and sixth cranial nerves. The pain is consistent with involvement of V1 and likely V2. As the optic nerve does not pass through the cavernous sinus, the vision is usually not involved in cavernous sinus lesions, while it is involved in orbital apex lesions (**A**). Brainstem lesions (**C**) large enough to involve all of these cranial nerves would show other obvious systemic effects.

48. Correct: Lumbar puncture (D)

Pupil-involving third nerve palsies in children are rarely due to vascular lesions. Most acquired cases are secondary to trauma, posterior fossa tumors, or meningitis. MRI should be obtained to rule out a compressive mass. If MRI is normal, lumbar puncture is the next best step to rule out meningitis. MRA (**A**), CTA (**B**), and angiography (**C**) are generally not needed in children younger than 10 years of age.

49. Correct: Elevated cerebrospinal fluid (CSF) protein (A)

The patient has Miller Fisher syndrome with the classic triad of ataxia, areflexia, and ophthalmoplegia. Facial weakness is common, with normal extremity strength. CSF will show an elevated protein level but is otherwise normal. Serum or CSF antibodies for *Campylobacter jejuni* or anti-GQ1b antibodies may be positive. Miller Fisher syndrome differs from Guillain–Barrè syndrome in that Guillain–Barrè has ascending symmetric limb weakness.

50. Correct: Vitamin B1 (C)

This patient with confusion, ataxia, ophthalmoplegia, and nystagmus is most likely suffering from Wernicke's encephalopathy. MRI with T2 signal hyperintensity in the mammillary bodies helps to confirm this suspicion. T2 signal hyperintensity in the medial thalami, tectal plate, and periaqueductal area may also be seen. The ophthalmoplegia and nystagmus may be of various types. The lateral recti tend to be most affected. Chronic alcoholism and malnutrition are the usual causes. Treatment is with rapid supplementation with vitamin B1, hydration, and nutrition. Choices (**A**), (**B**), and (**D**) are not needed in the treatment of Wernicke's encephalopathy, although vitamin B12 deficiency may also be seen in alcoholics and other malnourished states and should be supplemented.

51. Correct: Left paramedian pontine reticular formation (B)

Horizontal gaze incorporates multiple nuclei and interconnections. The paramedian pontine reticular formation controls ipsilateral horizontal saccades, so a patient would be unable to look quickly at an object to the same side as the lesion. However, smooth pursuit is not affected. The sixth nerve nucleus (**A**) controls movement of the ipsilateral lateral rectus. An interconnection from the sixth nerve nucleus via the medial longitudinal fasciculus (**C**) to the contralateral third nerve medial rectus subnucleus allows co-firing of the contralateral medial rectus. The contralateral third nerve nucleus (**D**) does not control horizontal movement of the other eye. A lesion of the sixth nerve nucleus would inhibit all types of gaze movement to the same side.

52. Correct: Right medial longitudinal fasciculus (D)

A hypertropia that does not map out to a fourth nerve palsy (**B**) according to the three-step test is consistent with skew deviation. In addition, the patient has slowed adduction of the right eye and contralateral nystagmus of the abducting eye. All of these findings describe a right internuclear ophthalmoplegia caused by a lesion of the right media longitudinal fasciculus (MLF). The MLF is the interconnection from the sixth nerve nucleus to the contralateral third nerve medial rectus subnucleus. The MLF runs up the brainstem ipsilateral to the adduction deficit. A left paramedian pontine reticular formation lesion (**C**) will cause a deficit of ipsilateral horizontal saccades. A lesion of the left frontal lobe (frontal eye fields) may cause a gaze deviation to the ipsilateral or contralateral side, depending on if the lesion is destructive or irritative, respectively.

53. Correct: Both A and C (D)

This scenario describes the one-and-a-half syndrome caused by a lesion of the sixth nerve nucleus (**A**) and the medial longitudinal fasciculus (MFL) on the same side (**C**). This causes a complete gaze palsy to the ipsilateral side as the lateral rectus and co-firing contralateral medial rectus are inhibited by the sixth nerve nucleus lesion. The involvement of the ipsilateral MLF also causes a right internuclear ophthalmoplegia with slowed or decreased adduction of the ipsilateral eye and abducting nystagmus of the contralateral eye. A lesion of the right paramedian pontine reticular formation (**B**) would cause a deficit in saccade to the right from both eyes.

54. Correct: Decreased vertical eye movements (C)

The patient is showing symptoms and examination findings of an increased near point of convergence, consistent with convergence insufficiency (CI). In older adults, CI may be secondary to head trauma, Parkinson's disease, or progressive supranuclear palsy (PSP). PSP is a neurodegenerative disease that manifests with loss of balance and difficulty walking, slowing of movement, personality changes, dementia, slurring of speech, and problems with eye movements. Usually vertical eye movements are decreased in addition to developing CI. Treatment is supportive. The patient's examination is not consistent with internuclear ophthalmoplegia (**A**). Patients with Parkinson's disease show, among many other symptoms, a resting tremor that tends to go away with movement, therefore (**B**) is incorrect.

55. Correct: All of the above (D)

Divergence insufficiency, as seen in this case, presents with difficult seeing and double vision at distance. There is a comitant esotropia at distance that is gone or significantly smaller at near. Extraocular motility is full. The cause of divergence insufficiency is generally not known (**A**). The double vision can be treated with prism correction (**B**). MRI of the brain should be ordered as there can sometimes be an underlying lesion (**C**).

56. Left frontal cortex (B)

This patient had an ischemic stroke with left gaze deviation. The deviation is ipsilateral to the ischemia if in the frontal cortex or contralateral if in the brainstem (**C**). A brainstem stroke is much more likely to cause other symptoms, so the left frontal cortex is the most likely site of the lesion. With a supranuclear lesion in the frontal eye fields, patients may be unable to look contralateral to the lesion and develop a gaze preference or tonic deviation ipsilateral to the lesion. As this is supranuclear, doll's head maneuver will elicit full extraocular motility. With brainstem lesions, eye movement to the same side is disrupted, so the eyes may deviate contralaterally (opposite of cerebral lesions). Here the doll's head maneuver will not work. Seizure activity in the frontal lobe will cause a contralateral movement during the ictal phase that may change to ipsilateral during the postictal state.

57. Correct: Bilateral ptosis (C)

A lesion affecting the dorsal midbrain will be preferentially affecting pathways involved in supranuclear control of vertical gaze, especially upgaze. Patients will likely have bilateral eyelid retraction, not ptosis. These patients will also likely exhibit a supranuclear upward gaze palsy (**A**), convergence-retraction nystagmus on attempted upgaze (**B**) (best elicited with a downward rotating optokinetic nystagmus drum), and light-near dissociation (**D**).

58. Correct: Pons (D)

The presented scenario describes locked-in syndrome where large bilateral lesions of the pons lead to quadriplegia, mutism, and absent horizontal eye movements with normal vertical eye movements, blinking, and consciousness. Vertical eye movements are controlled in the midbrain (**C**) by the interstitial nucleus of Cajal and the rostral interstitial nucleus of the medial longitudinal fasciculus. These midbrain nuclei, along with the posterior commissure, input on the third and fourth cranial nerve nuclei. The midbrain is superior to the pons, so vertical eye movements remain intact. Lesions of the thalamus (**B**) and frontal cortex (A) would also not lead to the presented findings.

59. Correct: All of the above (D)

CCF is an abnormal communication between the carotid artery and the cavernous sinus. Direct CCF may be secondary to trauma, aneurysm rupture, or iatrogenic. Indirect CCF is nontraumatic, and generally seen in older women with hypertension, diabetes, collagen vascular disease, or from childbirth. Examination findings include arterialization of the orbital venous system, which may present as "corkscrew" dilated conjunctival vessels (**A**), elevated intraocular pressure (**B**) due to reduced venous outflow and increased episcleral pressure, proptosis (**C**), ophthalmoplegia, a bruit, optic nerve edema, dilated retinal veins, intraretinal hemorrhages, and choroidal thickening/detachment.

60. Correct: Dilated orbital varix on CT during the Valsalva maneuver (C)

The patient has proptosis due to increased pressure from the Valsalva maneuver when picking up packages. A suspicion for an orbital varix should be raised. Obtaining a CT and performing imaging with and without the Valsalva maneuver should reveal a varix that is visible during the Valsalva maneuver and not seen while resting. An audible bruit (**A**) may be noted in patients with carotid-cavernous fistula. Patients with absence of the sphenoid wing, such as in neurofibromatosis type 1, may have a pulsatile proptosis (**B**). CT showing dilation and thrombosis of the cavernous sinus (**D**) would show a constant proptosis, chemosis, and ophthalmoplegia, among other findings not seen in this case.

61. Correct: A normal optokinetic testing response (A)

Congenital nystagmus (CN), or infantile nystagmus, is usually not present at birth, but noted in the first few months. It is almost always horizontal, and may appear as both jerk and pendular. Characteristically, there is reversal of the optokinetic response in which the slow phase is opposite the direction of rotation of the optokinetic drum. Nystagmus is not present during sleep (**B**). CN may be associated with normal or reduced vision (**C**), so a careful evaluation of the visual pathway is warranted and appropriate testing (MRI, electroretinogram, visual evoked potential) performed as needed. There may be a null point and CN is diminished in convergence (**D**).

62. Correct: Check proximal muscle strength (D)

The top panel shows the patient in primary gaze with ptosis of the left eye. The bottom two panels show results of sustained upgaze testing. Supraduction and eyelid position appear normal in the bottom left panel, but with sustained upgaze after 1 minute on the bottom right, the left eye and eyelid are unable to fully maintain their elevated position. These findings are consistent with fatigue in ocular myasthenia gravis. Checking for signs of systemic disease is extremely important, and may be life-saving. Obtaining MRI of the brain and orbits (**A**) and MRA (**C**) are not needed in ptosis

without any other abnormalities. Ptosis in myasthenia gravis is due to a neuromuscular issue, and not levator dehiscence from the tarsal plate (**B**). Surgery should only be used as a last resort.

63. Correct: MRI is recommended for common anterior visual pathway gliomas (A)

While MRI and sometimes electroretinogram are recommended to evaluate for lesions that may cause a spasmus nutans–like nystagmus, spasmus nutans itself is benign and self-limiting (**B**) and not associated with any lesions. The triad of spasmus nutans includes asymmetric rapid pendular eye movements, head nodding, and torticollis (**C D**).

64. Correct: Discontinuation of lithium (A)

Downbeat nystagmus has many causes including medications (lithium, amiodarone, toluene, phenytoin, carbamazepine), nutritional deficiency (alcohol, thiamine and B12 deficiency, low magnesium), trauma, encephalitis, paraneoplastic syndromes, cerebellar degenerations, a Chiari malformation, and other lesions affecting the cervicomedullary junction, foramen magnum, vestibulocerebellum, and medulla. Atenolol (**B**) and midbrain lesions (**C**) are not associated with downbeat nystagmus. Prisms in reading glasses may help to attenuate the nystagmus, but should be placed base-down, not base-up (**D**).

65. Correct: Start baclofen (B)

The patient has periodic alternating nystagmus (PAN), which when acquired tends to be responsive to baclofen. PAN is caused by lesions of the cerebellum, especially involving the nodulus and uvula, and the cervicomedullary junction. Clonazepam (**A**), B12 (**C**), and iron (**D**) supplementation are not used to treat PAN.

66. Correct: Low-frequency, high-amplitude nystagmus in left gaze (B)

The CT shows a left cerebellopontine angle mass (an acoustic neuroma). Mass lesions in this location cause a low-frequency, high-amplitude nystagmus (gaze-paretic) when looking toward the lesion (in this case to the left), and a high-frequency, low-amplitude nystagmus (vestibular) when looking away from the lesion (in this case to the right, making (**A**) incorrect). This is known as Brun's nystagmus. Periodic alternating nystagmus (**C**) is caused by lesions of the nodulus and uvula of the cerebellum and of the cervicomedullary junction. Choice (**D**) describes an internuclear ophthalmoplegia, which is caused by a lesion of the medial longitudinal fasciculus on the side of adduction deficit.

67. Correct: Seesaw nystagmus (C)

Seesaw nystagmus is a pendular nystagmus with elevation and intorsion of one eye, as the other eye depresses and extorts and then reverses back and forth. It is most commonly due to parasellar lesions, such as the pituitary mass presented in this case, craniopharyngiomas, septo-optic dysplasia, and midbrain lesions. Brun's nystagmus (**A**) is associated with masses of the cerebellopontine angle. Periodic alternating nystagmus (**B**) is caused by lesions of the nodulus and uvula of the cerebellum and of the cervicomedullary junction. Dissociated jerk nystagmus (**D**) describes nystagmus that is different in both eyes, such as an internuclear ophthalmoplegia.

68. Correct: Sellar mass (C)

A sellar mass is expected to cause a bitemporal hemianopia as shown in the figure due to compression of bilateral crossing nasal retinal fibers in the optic nerve chiasm. The defect may initially be denser superiorly in pituitary adenoma as the compression comes from below the chiasm. Right homonymous hemianopia would be expected in left optic tract (**A**) or left occipital lobe lesions (**B**). Right superior quadrantanopia would be expected in left temporal lobe (**D**) or inferior bank of the left occipital lobe lesions.

69. Correct: Tremor of the palate (D)

Oculopalatal myoclonus describes the findings of a vertical pendular nystagmus along with a tremor of the palate. Sometimes the facial muscles, larynx, or diaphragm are involved. Symptoms begin a few months after infarction or hemorrhage within the Mollaret triangle. The Mollaret triangle is bounded by the red nucleus superiorly, the inferior olivary nucleus inferiorly, and the dentate nucleus posteriorly. Choices (**A**), (**B**), and (**C**) are not associated with vertical pendular nystagmus.

70. Correct: Intravenous ceftriaxone (C)

Oculomasticatory myorhythmia includes a high-amplitude, low-frequency pendular nystagmus that converges and diverges, a supranuclear vertical gaze palsy, and rhythmic movements of the masticatory muscles. It is pathognomonic for Whipple's disease, a chronic systemic disorder caused by *Tropheryma whippeli*, and is diagnosed with biopsy of involved tissue, for example, the small intestine. Treatment is with appropriate long-term antibiotics. Intravenous corticosteroids (**A**), mannitol (**B**), and heparin (**D**) are not used as primary treatments for Whipple's disease.

71. Correct: Nonorganic vision loss (D)

The Goldmann visual field shows constriction of the visual field, but with crossing of the isopters. Dimmer and smaller test objects should not cross outside of isopter for a brighter and larger test object. This points toward nonorganic visual field loss, which should be supported by normal anatomy of

the visual system. Patients with glaucoma (**A**) may develop a number of different visual field defects such as cecocentral scotomas, inferior and superior arcuate defects, and nasal steps, but peripheral constriction with crossing of the isopters on the Goldmann perimetry should not be seen. Patients with retinitis pigmentosa (**B**) usually develop dense peripheral constriction, but the isopters again do not cross, and multiple examination findings are usually present. Occipital lobe ischemia (**C**) tends to show congruent homonymous quadrantanopia or hemianopia on visual field testing.

72. Correct: Obtain optical coherence tomography (OCT) (A)

The presented patient with blurred vision has fundus examination showing optic nerve edema. Also noted is blunting of the foveal reflex. OCT would be the next best test to evaluate and quantify the macular edema as shown below. B-scan ultrasound (**B**) would be useful when suspecting pseudoedema from optic nerve drusen, but this is not suspected in this case with macular involvement. CT (**C**) and MRI (**D**) of the brain and orbits may be needed if the diagnosis is not clarified, but OCT should be obtained first and may remove the need for further imaging.

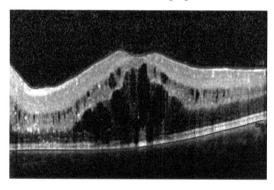

73. Correct: Posterior subcapsular cataracts (D)

The MRI shows meningiomas on each side of the cavernous sinus, with the left side entering the orbit. There is also a vestibular schwannoma. These findings are consistent with neurofibromatosis type 2 (NF2). NF2 is autosomal dominant with the NF2 gene localized to chromosome 22. Bilateral vestibular schwannomas are definitive for NF2, although patients with a unilateral vestibular schwannoma and two or more of either meningiomas, gliomas, schwannomas, or juvenile posterior subcapsular/cortical cataracts likely have NF2, especially with a positive family history. Exposure keratopathy (**A**), anterior uveitis (**B**), and nuclear sclerotic cataracts (**C**) are not associated with increased frequency in NF2.

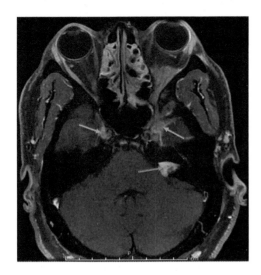

74. Correct: They originate from arachnoid cells (B)

The image shows an MRI with a right sphenoid wing meningioma. These tumors originate from arachnoid meningeal epithelial cell and are generally benign and slow-growing, with proptosis being the most common presentation. Vision loss and extraocular motility deficits can also occur. Incidence is higher in females than males (**A**). They are commonly associated with a loss or change in the NF2 gene on chromosome 22 (**C**). Treatment is either conservative, if no important structure is being impacted, or resection and/or radiation for lesions requiring treatment. Meningiomas are not responsive to steroids. Lymphoma may respond to steroids, but will recur (**D**) and is treated with radiation and/or chemotherapy.

75. Correct: The involved vessel is inferior to the optic nerve (D)

The image shows carotid angiography with an ophthalmic artery aneurysm. The ophthalmic artery runs inferior to the optic nerve, and is a branch of the internal carotid artery (**B**). Aneurysms of the ophthalmic artery are rare (**C**). MRI may show the lesion, but it is best seen with angiographic imaging. A dural tail is associated with meningioma (**A**).

76. Correct: Right homonymous hemianopia sparing the vertical meridian (C)

The calcarine sulcus splits the occipital lobe and its primary visual cortex in the middle. The MRI shows an area of ischemia in the occipital lobe, which is sparing the medial portion, or lip, of the calcarine sulcus. This will lead to a homonymous hemianopia sparing the vertical meridian, as shown in the Humphrey visual field below. Lesions that spare the more lateral base of the calcarine sulcus will spare the horizontal meridian of the visual field (**D**). Lesions that involve the anterior lip of the calcarine fissure will lead to an expected contralateral homonymous field defect along with

an ipsilateral temporal crescent, which is a 30-degree segment of temporal field beginning 60 degrees from fixation. Any lesion of the occipital cortex will lead to a visual field defect (**A**). Central homonymous hemianopia or quadrantanopia is represented by the most posterior portion of the occipital lobe, which is supplied by the middle cerebral artery. Lesions sparing the posterior portion will have macular sparing on the visual field. Larger lesions will lead to complete homonymous hemianopia (**B**).

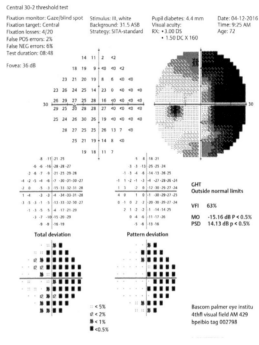

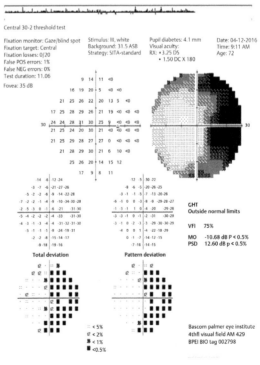

77. Correct: None of the above (D)

The lesion in the image is a mucosa-associated lymphoid tissue (MALT) lymphoma. The only way to truly differentiate MALT lymphoma from meningioma is with biopsy. Lymphoma can mimic multiple different processes and masses. MALT lymphoma will more commonly have an underlying vasogenic edema compared to meningioma, but may be present in either case. Both may have a dural tail (**A**) and will diffusely enhance with gadolinium (**C**). Onset in older populations is similar in both lesions and both have a higher incidence in females (**B**).

78. Correct: Negative for markers CD5 and CD10, but positive for CD23 (B)

The pathological stains show a population of small lymphocytes that are CD20-positive B cells (A). The remaining stains point toward mucosa-associated lymphoid tissue (MALT) lymphoma. MALT lymphoma is negative for CD5, CD10, and CD23. CD23 is positive in small lymphocytic lymphoma. MALT lymphoma is also negative for Cyclin D1, which is positive in mantle cell lymphoma. Primary dural lymphomas, including MALT lymphoma, are associated with immunosuppression (**D**). MALT lymphomas are additionally associated with chronic inflammation from *Helicobacter pylori* and *Chlamydia psittaci* (**C**).

79. Correct: Idiopathic intracranial hypertension (D)

These photographs show left decreased supraduction, infraduction, and adduction, along with ptosis, consistent with a third nerve palsy. Elevated intracranial pressure is most likely to produce sixth nerve palsies due to compression of the nerve, although a pupil-involving third nerve is possible with severe, life-threatening uncal herniation. Ischemia (A) is the most likely cause of a complete third cranial nerve palsy. Aneurysmal compression (**B**) will usually cause a pupil-involving third cranial nerve palsy, but early on may spare the pupil and should remain high on the differential. Myasthenia gravis (**C**) can mimic any cranial neuropathy, as long as the pupil is not involved.

80. Correct: Obtain orbital biopsy (D)

The MRI shows bilateral retro-orbital masses and thickening of the hypophysis. This presentation with central diabetes insipidus and exophthalmos is consistent with Erdheim–Chester disease. Nonetheless, as a suitable biopsy site is available with large orbital masses, a biopsy should be obtained in order to properly tailor treatment as other diseases may mimic this rare disorder. Intravenous corticosteroids (**A**) may be useful as an early temporizing treatment, but a specific diagnosis should be sought after. Infection is unlikely in this case, so intravenous antibiotics are unlikely to help (**B**). Radiation therapy (**C**) may also be a treatment option, but biopsy should be performed first.

81. Correct: More than 50% are positive for the BRAF V600E mutation (C)

Pathological analysis reveals a histiocytosis positive for CD69 and negative for IgG4 and S100, consistent with Erdheim–Chester disease (EDC), a rare non-Langerhans' cell histiocytosis (**D**). The BRAF V600E mutation is detectable in more than 50% of patients, allowing treatment with BRAF V600E inhibitors in resistant cases. First-line therapy is with interferon-α, with many other treatment options available. Rarely does surgical debulking help in this disease (**A**). EDC does not have a cure and has a variable prognosis with central nervous system and orbital and cardiac involvement being poor prognostic factors (**B**).

82. Correct: Order MRI or MRA (C)

The patient has aberrant regeneration after third nerve palsy, which is a concerning sign of compression. MRI and MRA (or CTA) should be performed to evaluate aneurysm or mass. Trauma can also cause aberrant regeneration but would be noted on history. Myasthenia gravis (**B**) and ischemic causes (**A**) and (**D**) do not cause aberrant regeneration.

83. Correct: Imaging (A)

The case describes hemifacial spasm, which is often idiopathic, but includes a broad differential: seventh nerve intermittent vascular compression by vascular loop, seventh nerve compression from a mass, inflammation, and infection. Imaging (MRI/MRA) should be obtained to rule out any of these causes. Often, there is a history of a previous or nonresolved seventh nerve palsy from a variety of causes. Chemodenervation (**B**) is generally the treatment of choice, unless other treatable cause is found. Imaging is the more important step (although chemodenervation can be performed immediately for patient relief). Hemifacial spasm is generally nonresolving (**C**).

84. Correct: Sudden-onset headache after exercise (D)

Severe, sudden headaches that are different than a normal migraine should alert a patient and provider to seek emergent imaging for a possible life-threatening cause. Migraine headaches are debilitating headaches that may or may not have a visual aura or other prodrome. The aura, if present, typically lasts 5 to 60 minutes, followed by a severe unilateral headache that lasts 4 to 72 hours (can alternate between episodes) and may be associated with nausea, vomiting (**A**), photophobia (**B**), phonophobia, and other neurologic symptoms such as cranial nerve palsies, Horner's syndrome (**C**), and limb weakness.

85. Correct: Anticoagulation (B)

The patient presents with right-sided neck pain and right Horner's syndrome, raising concern for carotid dissection. The CTA in the figure reveals a right internal carotid dissection, which can be seen as the hyperintense vessels on the right, with the dissection appearing enlarged within a separate lumen, compared to the adjacent and contralateral normal vessels. The patient should be started on anticoagulation if cleared of intracerebral hemorrhage, and then evaluated for possible endovascular or surgical treatment, if needed. There is no mass to resect (**A**). Intravenous corticosteroids (**C**) and observation (**D**) would not be appropriate in a dissection.

86. Correct: Sixth cranial nerve palsy (D)

The MRI shows a lesion in the left pons on both diffusion-weighted imaging (*left panel*) and T2-weighted imaging (*right panel*). The lesion is affecting the seventh nerve nucleus. Additionally, the sixth nerve fascicle wraps around the seventh nerve nucleus, and is involved in the ischemic lesion. Exposure keratopathy (**A**) will not cause binocular diplopia. Focal ischemic pontine lesions affecting the seventh cranial nerve will not affect the third cranial nerve (**B**) in the midbrain or cause an internuclear ophthalmoplegia (**C**), which is located more anteriorly and travels from the pons to the midbrain.

87. Correct: No known treatment will improve your vision. We will observe (C)

The prognosis of vision after traumatic optic neuropathy is difficult to predict. Some patients experience significant recovery with or without intervention, while others have no visual improvement. The International Optic Nerve Trauma Study compared surgical optic canal decompression (**A**), high-dose systemic corticosteroids (**B**), and observation. Results showed a visual acuity improvement of three lines or more in 32% of the decompression group, 52% of the corticosteroid group, and 57% of the observation group. The study did have multiple weaknesses, including being nonrandomized and limited in power with small sample size in the observation group. Nonetheless, results were not convincing that surgery or steroids lead to significant improvement compared to observation. The options should still be reviewed with the patient on a case-by-case basis, with risks and benefits of each option (if indicated as an option) explained. Of note, patients with traumatic optic neuropathy likely also have traumatic brain injury (TBI). Corticosteroids are considered contraindicated in TBI as they have been correlated with an increased risk of death when used in treating TBI.

88. Correct: Orbitotomy for mass excision (A)

Surgical orbital procedures should be avoided when the disease is not vision-threatening, and other nonsurgical options are available. The patient has an orbital mass with IgG4-positive staining on histology, consistent with IgG4-related orbital disease.

IgG4 is an autoimmune disorder of unknown etiology. Pathology shows a fibroinflammatory reaction seen as tumefactive lesions with dense lymphoplasmacytic infiltration, and IgG4 staining of more than 50 cells per high-power field. Serum IgG4 levels may be normal but can be helpful to monitor treatment when elevated. Treatment is aimed at decreasing inflammation, which corticosteroids (**B**), corticosteroid-sparing agents such as rituximab (**C**), and radiation therapy (**D**) treat.

89. Correct: Oral prednisone dosed at 1 mg/kg (A)

Patients with optic neuritis should not be treated with oral prednisone dosed at 1 mg/kg, as the Optic Neuritis Treatment Trial showed that oral steroids had about two times higher risk of development of multiple sclerosis compared to intravenous steroids (**B**) in the first 3 years (and about the same risk as placebo). The protective effect of intravenous steroids was not seen in the past 3 years. Rituximab (**C**) and intravenous immunoglobulin (**D**) are sometimes used to treat optic neuritis resistant to steroids.

90. Correct: Start steroids and antivirals (D)

The presented patient has varicella-zoster virus (VZV) infection around the right ear causing a vesicular rash and facial nerve palsy, also known as Ramsay Hunt syndrome. Some patients may experience hearing loss, tinnitus, or vertigo. Steroids and antivirals should be started. Antibiotics could be useful if a coexistent cellulitis is suspected (**B**). MRI (**A**) is not needed for this clinical diagnosis but can be obtained in cases that are not straightforward to rule out compression. Lumbar puncture (**C**) is sometimes obtained in difficult cases concerning for meningitis or encephalitis.

91. Correct: Large fusion amplitudes (B)

Normal vertical fusion amplitudes are 3 to 5 PD. In congenital fourth nerve palsy, they are over 10 PD. The most common cause of acquired fourth nerve palsy is trauma; however, trauma can cause a congenital fourth nerve palsy to become symptomatic. Other causes include hypertension and diabetes (**A**), a mass that may cause headaches (**C**), and inflammatory causes such as multiple sclerosis. Patients with congenital fourth nerve palsy usually have a head tilt, which may be noted in old photographs (**D**).

92. Correct: Lumbar puncture for opening pressure (C)

The patient in the photograph has restriction in upgaze of the left eye. Lumbar puncture for opening pressure will not help in this case. High or low intracranial pressure will most likely cause a sixth cranial nerve palsy with difficulty abducting one or both eyes. CT of the orbits (**A**) can help to rule out muscle entrapment in a fracture, myositis, enlarged muscles

133

in thyroid disease, or lesions inhibiting muscle movement. Acetylcholine receptor antibody (**B**) test for myasthenia gravis can cause a variety of extraocular motility deficits. Thyroid-stimulating immunoglobulins (**D**) can help test for thyroid eye disease.

93. Correct: Orbital surgery (D)

CT shows entrapment of the left inferior rectus muscle, which is causing upgaze restriction. This occurs in orbital floor fractures, especially in younger patients with more flexible bone, where the fracture opens and then snaps back as it traps the muscle underneath it. It should be repaired urgently to relieve oculocardiac reflex and to prevent muscle ischemia. Corticosteroids (**A**) can be used to treat restriction caused by myositis and myasthenia gravis. Thyroidectomy (**B**) is performed to treat thyroid disease but will not improve the muscle restriction. Pyridostigmine (**C**) is used to improve the double vision and other symptoms of myasthenia gravis.

94. Correct: Refer for carotid endarterectomy (B)

The patient presents with right ocular ischemic syndrome. Carotid disease, especially when asymmetric, can cause ocular ischemic syndrome. According to the North American Symptomatic Carotid Endarterectomy Trial, symptomatic patients with 70 to 100% blockage should undergo carotid endarterectomy. Symptomatic patients with 50 to 69% blockage may also benefit from carotid endarterectomy. As this patient does not have any symptoms of giant cell arteritis with normal ESR and CRP, intravenous corticosteroids (**A**) are not appropriate. MRI of the orbits (**B**) may be helpful to rule out compression but will likely be unrevealing without any other orbital signs. Any systemic issue that causes ischemia such as diabetes mellitus can lead to ocular ischemia, although it is usually bilateral.

95. Correct: Prognosis for final visual acuity ranges from 20/200 to 20/400 (A)

The patient has dominant optic atrophy. Visual acuity is usually moderate, ranging from 20/50 to 20/70, although visual acuity loss to 20/200 does occur. Examination will show bilateral optic atrophy, either a temporal segment or diffuse (**B**). It is inherited in an autosomal dominant (**C**) fashion and usually presents within the first decade of life (**D**). There is no known treatment although maximizing mitochondrial function may be attempted.

96. Correct: About 10% of patients have sensorineural hearing loss (B)

The patient has Wolfram's syndrome, or DIDMOAD (diabetes insipidus, diabetes mellitus, optic atrophy, deafness). About 50% of patients exhibit sensorineural hearing loss. Patients usually first manifest diabetes mellitus, followed by optic atrophy. The age of onset varies, but most patients begin to show symptoms in adolescence. About 50% of patients develop diabetes insipidus (**A**). Wolfram's syndrome is inherited in an autosomal recessive (**C**) manner and is caused by a mutation in *WFS1* or *WFS2* (**D**).

97. Correct: Cerebellar atrophy (C)

Ataxia–telangiectasia is an autosomal recessive disorder with progressive cerebellar ataxia, oculocutaneous telangiectasia, and immunodeficiency with recurrent sinopulmonary infections. MRI of the brain would show cerebellar atrophy as the cause of the ataxia. Serum IgA is reduced in most cases. Midbrain (**A**) and optic nerve (**C**) atrophy are not part of this disorder.

98. Correct: Astrocytic hamartomas are the only ocular involvement (C)

Tuberous sclerosis complex involves multiple organ systems. Ocular changes include astrocytic hamartomas (pale retinal lesions, which are sometimes calcified), coloboma, and papilledema secondary to hydrocephalus. Almost 50% of patients have learning disabilities (**A**). Angiomyolipomas of the kidneys may develop and often lead to hematuria (**B**). Rarely, these may lead to life-threatening hemorrhage even with mild trauma. Inheritance is autosomal dominant (**D**). Many may start as a sporadic mutation that can then be passed down. The currently known genetic loci are in *TSC1* and *TSC2*.

99. Correct: Skin biopsy (B)

von Hippel–Lindau syndrome is a systemic disorder featuring multiple visceral cysts and tumors that may have malignant potential. Skin changes are rare, though some patients may have café-au-lait spots. Skin biopsy is generally not needed in these patients. Retinal and central nervous system hemangioblastomas are common. They may also develop in the spine (**D**). Renal cell carcinoma is the leading cause of death, so abdominal ultrasound (**A**) or other imaging is necessary. Imaging or urinary catecholamine metabolite (**C**) testing is also needed to monitor for pheochromocytomas.

100. Correct: Trauma is the underlying mechanism (A)

This patient has Parry–Romberg syndrome, which is characterized by a progressive hemiatrophy of the face. Trauma is not associated with Parry–Romberg syndrome. Patients may develop a depressed facial scar called the "coup de sabre" given its appearance of trauma from a blow by a sabre. The scar may begin with a scleroderma patch with hair loss that then extends down through the midface. The disorder is considered to be autoimmune, and likely a variant of scleroderma (**B**) given the indistinguishable scleroderma lesion. Patients may have neurologic effects such as trigeminal neuralgia (as in the presented patient), seizures, and Horner's syndrome (**C**) (underlying sympathectomy has been considered part of the pathogenesis). Patients may develop ipsilateral hemiatrophy (**D**).

Chapter 5

Oculofacial, Plastics, and Orbit

Anne Barmettler, Ashley A. Campbell, Larissa Kadar Ghadiali, Peter MacIntosh, Lora R. Dagi Glass

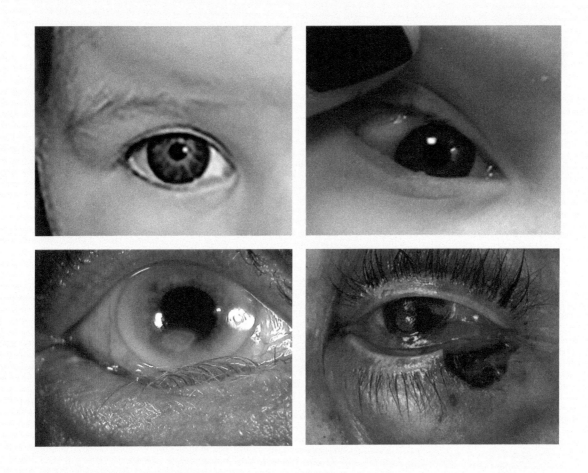

5.1 Questions

Easy	Medium	Hard

1. An 87-year-old man presents after slipping on his grandson's firetruck and falling. Upon presentation, he is noted to have significant periocular edema and ecchymosis. A CT of the orbits is ordered as part of his work-up. Which of the following were most likely impacted by his injury?

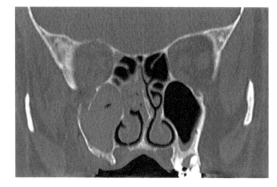

A. Frontal and sphenoid bones

B. Zygomatic and sphenoid bones

C. Ethmoid, lacrimal, maxillary, and sphenoid bones

D. Zygomatic, maxillary, and palatine bones

2. A 64-year-old woman presents with chronic, constant epiphora OS for the past year. Irrigation of the nasolacrimal system reveals a complete nasolacrimal duct obstruction, and the patient is consented for a dacryocystorhinostomy with nasolacrimal intubation. As you explain the procedure to her, you demonstrate the anatomic location of nasolacrimal duct outflow, as well as the location in which a new bony ostium is created. Where was the original, and where will the new one most likely be?

A. Inferior meatus (beneath the inferior turbinate), and in the region anterior to the middle turbinate

B. Middle meatus (beneath the middle turbinate), and in the middle turbinate

C. Inferior meatus (beneath the inferior turbinate), and between the middle turbinate and the superior turbinate

D. Middle meatus (beneath the middle turbinate), and in the region underneath or anterior to the superior turbinate

3. Which of the following complications could occur secondary to surgical disruption of the medial orbital wall above the frontoethmoidal suture?

A. Optic neuropathy

B. Disruption of the cribriform plate

C. Orbital tissue necrosis

D. Disruption of innervation to the inferior oblique muscle

4. A patient needs an incisional lacrimal gland biopsy to rule out lymphoma. Which of the following techniques would be preferred?

A. Lid crease approach with palpebral lobe biopsy

B. Conjunctival approach with palpebral lobe biopsy

C. Lid crease approach with orbital lobe biopsy

D. Conjunctival approach with orbital lobe biopsy

5. A patient presents with unilateral contractions of her eyelids, cheek, and mouth. Imaging shows no pathology. You discuss treatment, and your patient asks you to "give her a little extra" along her forehead and laugh lines on the uninvolved side—"after all, you have a deal going on, my insurance is paying for it!" What should you do?

A. Inject botulinum toxin type A along regions impacted by the seventh nerve unilaterally, and then perform the cosmetic injection; submit the insurance claim for the total quantity injected and wasted.

B. Inject botulinum toxin type A along regions impacted by the third nerve unilaterally, and perform the cosmetic injection; submit the insurance claim for the quantity injected and wasted for the functional purposes alone, and bill the patient separately for the cosmetic injection.

C. Inject botulinum toxin type A along regions impacted by the seventh nerve unilaterally, and then perform the cosmetic injection; submit the insurance claim for the quantity injected and wasted for the functional purposes alone, and bill the patient separately for the cosmetic injection.

D. Inject botulinum toxin type A along regions impacted by the third nerve unilaterally, and then perform the cosmetic injection; submit the insurance claim for the total quantity injected and wasted.

6. Interventional radiology wants your help accessing a carotid-cavernous sinus fistula by exposing a large vein. Which of the following is your vein of choice?

A. Superior ophthalmic vein

B. Inferior ophthalmic vein

C. Angular vein

D. Facial vein

7. A mother brings in her toddler, as she has noticed a swelling of the right brow area. It doesn't appear to bother her toddler, and isn't tender, but it has been slowly increasing in size since birth. You discuss options and decide to perform a lesion excision. What is the pathology most likely to show?

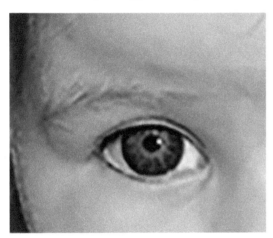

A. Endothelium-lined capillary channels in a lobular configuration

B. Keratinized epithelial lining, hair follicles, and sebaceous glands

C. Keratin-filled cyst

D. Spindle cells with occasional cross-striations

8. A pediatrician urgently refers a male infant for evaluation of an orbital mass. The child was the product of a normal pregnancy and delivery. He looks comfortable. After seeing the following on examination, what do you advise the parents to do?

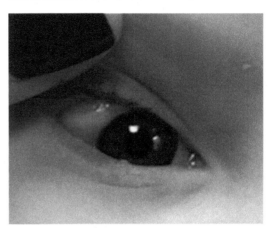

A. Perform an excisional biopsy.

B. Perform a partial excision if irritating.

C. Perform an incisional biopsy.

D. Never biopsy or excise.

9. A 6-month-old male infant with known Crouzon's syndrome presents for ophthalmic examination. Which of the following is incorrect?

A. He will never be able to interact meaningfully with his environment.

B. He should be managed in a multidisciplinary manner with services including neurosurgery, ENT, and ophthalmology.

C. He will need routine, chronic monitoring for evidence of exposure keratopathy, and elevated intracranial pressure.

D. He should be carefully refracted to help prevent refractive amblyopia.

10. You receive a call from the Newborn Nursery regarding a 1-day-old who appears to be missing an eye. After examining the newborn, you diagnose microphthalmia of the left eye; the right eye is normal. What is the next best step?

A. Patch therapy OD.

B. Enucleation OS with placement of gradually larger conformers.

C. Retain microphthalmic eye OS and use gradually increasing conformers with possible dermis-fat graft in the future.

D. Perform an immediate dermis-fat graft.

11. A 61-year-old woman presents with diplopia of 2 month's duration. She has no past medical history. Examination shows limited supraduction OS and retraction of the left upper eyelid. Which of the following studies would be most helpful in diagnosing the underlying etiology of her diplopia?

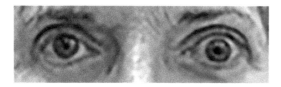

A. Complete blood count with differential

B. Thyroid-stimulating immunoglobulin

C. Acetylcholine receptor binding, blocking, and modulating antibodies

D. Erythrocyte sedimentation rate

12. A 24-year-old patient with recent diagnosis of hyperthyroidism presents with acute proptosis OD. History is also notable for a deep ache OD. Further examination reveals chemosis OD, mild bilateral upper eyelid retraction, and left upper lid lateral flare. A CT scan of the orbits is performed. What is the most likely finding?

A. Tendon-sparing enlargement of the superior oblique muscle

B. Diffuse enlargement of the medial rectus muscle

C. Cavernous hemangioma

D. Fatty proliferation

13. A 68-year-old woman with thyroid eye disease (TED) is very distressed by her right upper eyelid retraction. She would like you to "make things right" as quickly as possible. Her examination is otherwise notable mild chemosis OD, rare punctate keratopathy OU, and new resolution of a mild supraduction deficit. What is your treatment plan for this patient?

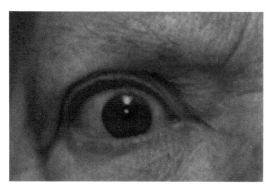

A. IV methylprednisolone infusions for the next 12 weeks

B. Surgical right upper eyelid recession

C. Artificial tears four times a day OU

D. Orbital radiotherapy

14. A 44-year-old woman presents with an enlarged lacrimal gland. After serum laboratory work shows elevated immunoglobulin G4 (IgG4) levels, you maintain a high suspicion for IgG4-related orbital disease and decide to biopsy the lacrimal gland. Which of the following is unlikely to be present upon histopathologic review of the biopsy specimen?

A. Cribriform appearance

B. Storiform fibrosis

C. Obliterative phlebitis

D. Elevated IgG4/IgG ratio

15. A 49-year-old man presents with scleritis and swelling of the superomedial eyelid. He reports a history of glomerulonephritis. Imaging is consistent with a bone-destructive process of the sinuses. Which of the following is incorrect?

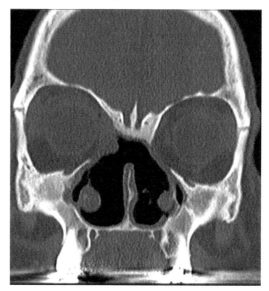

A. Histopathologic examination of the affected tissue would show vasculitis, granulomatous inflammation, and necrosis.

B. Treatment with cyclophosphamide should be initiated.

C. This disease process can be fatal.

D. Serum cytoplasmic antineutrophil cytoplasmic antibody (c-ANCA) is specific for this disease process; if it is negative, this process can be ruled out.

16. A previously healthy 7-year-old patient presents with bilateral dacryoadenitis, abdominal pain, and vomiting. Which of the following is true?

A. There is no need to rule out systemic infection.

B. Treatment with steroids should begin immediately.

C. In adults, this condition is typically unilateral and without systemic symptoms.

D. Imaging is likely to show tendon-sparing enlargement of the extraocular muscles.

17. A 5-year-old, otherwise healthy girl presents with acute periocular edema and proptosis OD in the setting of sinus congestion. She has no relative afferent pupillary defect and her vision remains intact, though her adduction and abduction are painful and restricted. You obtain her CT scan. Which of the following is the best next step?

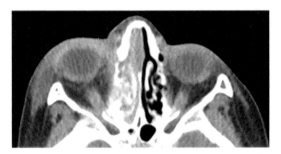

A. Anterior orbitotomy with drainage
B. Initiation of IV antibiotic therapy
C. Initiation of oral antibiotic therapy
D. Functional endoscopic sinus surgery

18. A 29-year-old woman presents with acute-onset, progressive periocular edema and erythema OS. Her history is notable for a recent scratch near her left eye. Which of the following is the most important bacteria to cover for when treating?

A. *Haemophilus influenzae*
B. *Staphylococcus aureus*
C. *Klebsiella pneumoniae*
D. *Actinomyces israelii*

19. A 39-year-old poorly controlled diabetic presents with rapidly progressive discoloration of his right periocular tissue after recently hitting a cabinet corner; the eyelid is swollen and painful, and the color has turned from rose to blue-gray. The emergency room attending sends him home with oral antibiotics. Which of the following is most likely to be accurate?

A. He must be monitored for shock and has a high mortality risk.
B. Histopathologic review would show a thrombosing vasculitis involving nonseptate hyphae.
C. Amphotericin B should be administered systemically.
D. Surgical debridement will not be necessary.

20. A 45-year-old Black woman presents with dacryoadenitis and skin nodules. A skin biopsy reveals the following. Which of the following is helpful in the diagnosis of cases such as this?

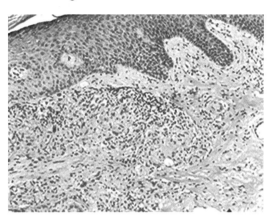

A. Conjunctival biopsy
B. PPD testing
C. Chest X-ray
D. Bone marrow biopsy

21. A 74-year-old man presents with at least 4 months of foreign body sensation in both eyes. The most common type of this eyelid malposition in the lower lid is _____, while the most common type of this eyelid malposition in the upper lid is _____.

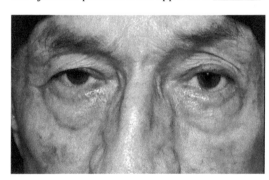

A. cicatricial, spastic
B. involutional, cicatricial
C. involutional, congenital
D. spastic, congenital

22. A 60-year-old woman with a history of pernicious anemia and Graves' disease complains of droopy upper lids, left worse than right. She notes that it seems to be worse when she is tired, when she has had a few glasses of wine, and at the end of each day. The medical student and the resident get into an argument over the margin to reflex distance 1 (MRD1) measurement only to be disappointed when neither of their measurements match the attending's. What is the next best step?

A. Ptosis repair at the ambulatory surgical center after cardiac clearance

B. Laboratory work-up of acetylcholine receptor antibodies

C. MRI of the brain or spine with aquaporin-4 antibodies

D. MRI or MRA of the internal auditory canal

23. A patient presents complaining of droopy upper lids. Examination reveals a high upper eyelid crease and normal levator function. What is the most likely type of ptosis?

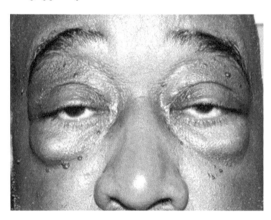

A. Aponeurotic
B. Neurogenic
C. Myogenic
D. Mechanical

24. A 4-month-old male infant is referred for evaluation of tearing in both eyes. His mom reports that he hates direct sunlight and constantly has tears rolling down his cheeks. What is the most likely etiology?

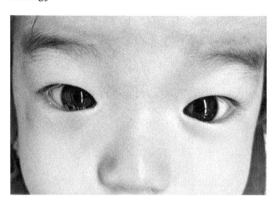

A. Epiblepharon
B. Euryblepharon
C. Entropion
D. Congenital glaucoma

25. What are the three anatomic issues that must be addressed in the surgical treatment of involutional entropion?

A. Scarring of the posterior lamella, horizontal laxity, and trichiasis

B. Horizontal laxity, capsulopalpebral fascia dehiscence, and trichiasis

C. Capsulopalpebral fascia dehiscence, overriding orbicularis, and horizontal laxity

D. Overriding orbicularis, scarring of the posterior lamella, and capsulopalpebral fascia dehiscence

26. A patient presents complaining of droopy upper lids. Examination is significant for decreased levator function, eyelid lag on downgaze, and lagophthalmos. What is the most likely type of ptosis?

A. Aponeurotic
B. Neurogenic
C. Myogenic
D. Mechanical

27. A 67-year-old patient with a history of diabetes type 2, hypertension, and hyperlipidemia comes in complaining of binocular diplopia, worse in left gaze, starting after a lower lid blepharoplasty by an outside surgeon. What is the most likely cause?

A. Iatrogenic left cranial nerve VI palsy
B. Damage to the left lateral rectus muscle
C. Damage to the left inferior oblique muscle
D. Damage to the right inferior oblique muscle

28. A 23-year-old female model presents with left upper lid ptosis (margin to reflex distance 1 [MRD1]: right 4.5 and left 3) and a levator function of 14. Her ptosis resolves with instillation of phenylephrine. What is the best option for surgical repair?

A. Levator advancement

B. Conjunctivomullerectomy

C. Frontalis sling

D. Bick's procedure

29. A patient presents with stable eyelid changes. He is tired of getting funny looks and is requesting treatment. Examination is normal except for the following appearance. What is the next step?

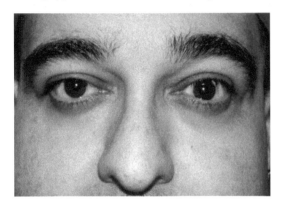

A. Ptosis repair of the right upper lid

B. Retraction repair of the left upper lid

C. Radioactive iodine

D. Check free T_4, TSH, and thyroid antibodies

30. A 50-year-old woman presents with droopy upper lids. She complains that they are getting in her way, worsening over the last few years, and she has to lift her lids with her hands to see. She says this runs in her family (her dad and her paternal grandmother have the same problems). Her examination is significant for margin to reflex distance 1 (MRD1) of 1 OU and a levator function of 12 OU. Her examination is otherwise normal. Which of the following would be most consistent with this presentation?

A. Red ragged fibers on muscle biopsy.

B. Delayed swallow study and genetic mutations of *PABPN1*.

C. Ptosis improves with opening of the jaw.

D. After looking down and then back in primary gaze, the upper eyelid will overshoot and appear to open briefly before returning to its normal position.

31. A 58-year-old woman complains of spasms that have worsened to the point where she has difficulty opening her eyes. She reports that it has gotten so bad that she is scared of leaving the house. Which of the following is true?

A. The medication she should receive takes about 2 to 3 days to work, peaks in effect 7 to 10 days later, and lasts about 3 to 4 months.

B. The medication she should receive inhibits acetylcholine binding in the postsynaptic neuron.

C. She should get an MRI to rule out pathology of the pons.

D. The most common cause of this disorder is vascular compression of the facial nerve at the brainstem.

32. A 58-year-old woman complains of spasms around her right eye. On examination, you note that her lower face on the right also twitches. Which of the following is true?

A. Neurosurgical decompression of the facial nerve should be recommended.

B. The spasms likely occur at nighttime, when she is asleep.

C. She may have a history of ipsilateral facial nerve palsy, and this represents unilateral aberrant synkinetic facial movements.

D. B and C.

33. A 67-year-old man complains of droopy upper lids. Examination reveals heaviness in the upper eyelid area, especially temporally. The amount of skin between the eyelid margin and the inferior aspect of the brow measures 20 mm. Palpation reveals the brow position to be below the superior orbital rim. The margin to reflex distance 1 (MRD1) is 4 in both eyes. What is the best surgical option?

A. Upper eyelid blepharoplasty

B. Upper eyelid fractional CO_2 laser

C. Levator advancement

D. Brow lift

34. A 67-year-old man complains of redness and copious tearing in both eyes. He reports he recently went on long trip abroad and got a great deal on a surgery to make him look younger. Which of the following are possible solutions?

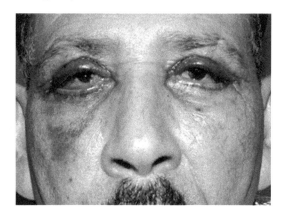

A. Artificial tears and ointment
B. Full-thickness skin graft
C. Midface lifting
D. All of the above

35. A budding oculoplastic surgeon approaches you for advice on how to surgically approach an ectropion. There is no cicatricial component. Which of the following is your recommendation?

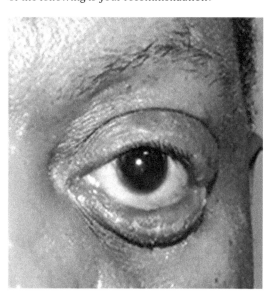

A. Lateral tarsal strip
B. Lateral tarsal strip with medial spindle procedure
C. Weiss procedure
D. Quickert suture

36. A 44-year-old man with a past medical history of diabetes mellitus (DM), hypertension (HTN), hyperlipidemia (HL), and morbid obesity complains of red eyes associated with discharge. Which of the following disorders are associated with this entity?

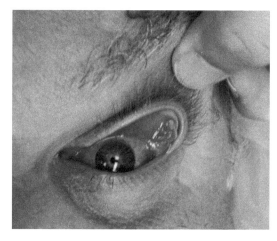

A. Keratoconus
B. Obstructive sleep apnea
C. Obesity
D. All of the above

37. In addition to an ectropion of the right lower lid, which other right-sided eyelid malpositions are associated with the etiology of this right lower lid ectropion?

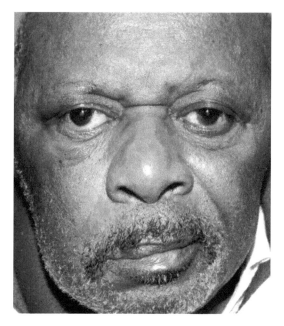

A. Dermatochalasis
B. Blepharoptosis
C. Blepharochalasis
D. Lagophthalmos

38. The following examination finding is discovered on a work-up for ptosis of the right upper lid. What is the best explanation for the changes that occur in this figure?

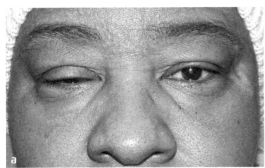

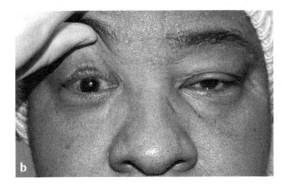

A. Hering's law
B. Sherrington's law
C. Cogan's lid twitch
D. Harada–Ito sign

39. A 48-year-old eye makeup model presents with foreign body sensation of the right eye for several years. On examination, she is noted to have trichiasis. For which of the following situations would radiofrequency epilation be the best solution?

A. She is White and not Black.
B. She has just three trichiatic lashes scattered throughout both upper and lower eyelids.
C. She has a 4-mm segment on the right lower lid that is completely trichiatic.
D. She has many trichiatic lashes on the lower lid, they are scattered diffusely, and the eyelid margin appears rounded.

40. A 37-year-old Irish woman comes in complaining of aging changes in her lower face. She notices fine lines throughout, especially around her lips. She admits to being a heavy smoker until last year, when she quit to pursue a vegan/yoga lifestyle. What are some possible nonsurgical options for her?

A. Hyaluronic acid fillers to the fine perioral lines
B. Fractionated CO_2 laser throughout the lower face (with option for adding upper face)
C. Botox injection to the fine perioral lines
D. A and B

41. A 9-month-old female infant has group E retinoblastoma of the left eye. What is the best surgical option for this eye?

A. Exenteration
B. Evisceration with 18-mm silicone implant
C. Enucleation with dermis-fat graft
D. Enucleation with 18-mm silicone implant

42. A patient presents with a remote history of left eye enucleation with implant placement. What can be done to correct her secondary eyelid problem?

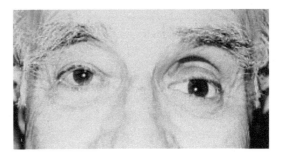

A. Subperiosteal orbital floor implant OS
B. Brow lift OD
C. External levator advancement OS
D. Blepharoplasty OD

43. One week after an enucleation for a blind, painful right eye, the tarsorrhaphy is removed. One week later, the conformer falls out while the patient was showering and is lost down the drain. The patient calls to let you know, and also states that there is no pain, discharge, or bleeding. He is very happy with the results so far. What should you do?

A. Confirm his follow-up with the ocularist at postoperative week 6.
B. Ask him to come urgently to clinic.
C. Schedule surgery to replace the conformer.
D. Recommend lubrication with antibiotic ointment and see him as scheduled in 2 weeks.

44. A 59-year-old man comes for routine eye examination. He has a prosthesis in the left eye related to an enucleation for a severe chemical eye injury many years ago with "some tissue taken from his mouth." What complication might he have suffered from his injury?

A. Anophthalmic ptosis
B. Fornix contracture
C. Deep superior fornix
D. Implant exposure

45. A 65-year-old patient has a blind painful eye from neovascular glaucoma. You recommend removing the eye, but she is concerned about motility postoperatively. What is the best option for this patient?

A. Enucleation with acrylic sphere

B. Evisceration with acrylic sphere

C. Enucleation with acrylic sphere wrapped in sclera with muscles attached to it

D. Enucleation with dermis-fat graft

46. A 79-year-old woman walks in to see you 6 months after enucleation for a blind, painful eye. She had removed her prosthesis to clean it, and a translucent sphere "popped out." On examination, you notice a deflation of her anophthalmic socket and disruption of her conjunctiva. Which of the following factors is least likely to contribute to this scenario?

A. Oversized implant

B. Suturing the extraocular muscles to each other over the anterior surface of the implant

C. Improper Tenon's closure

D. Improper conjunctival closure

47. A 45-year-old patient is referred to you for removal of his blind, painful eye. You present the options of enucleation and evisceration to him. What do you describe as an advantage of enucleation over evisceration?

A. Better motility

B. Treatment of endophthalmitis

C. Less disruption of orbital anatomy

D. Reduced risk of sympathetic ophthalmia

48. Which of the following is true regarding the lacrimal drainage system?

A. By the 10th week of gestation, the nasolacrimal groove forms as a furrow lying between the nasal and maxillary prominence.

B. The canalicular system is an outgrowth of the lacrimal gland.

C. Caudally, the developing nasolacrimal duct exits in the middle meatus.

D. Canalization of the nasolacrimal duct is usually complete around the time of birth.

49. Referring to the four images below, examining from images a to d in sequence, which description is the most accurate?

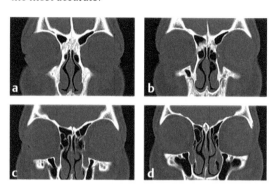

A. Normal lacrimal sac, scrolling anterior to posterior

B. Post dacryocystorhinostomy surgery, scrolling anterior to posterior

C. Normal lacrimal sac, scrolling posterior to anterior

D. Post dacryocystorhinostomy surgery, scrolling posterior to anterior

50. The parents of a 3-month-old male infant note that he has been tearing excessively since birth, with occasional crusting of his eyelashes. There is no evidence of erythema, edema, or purulent discharge on examination. Which statement is true?

A. The obstruction is presumed to be an imperforate valve of Rosenmuller.

B. A dacryocystorhinostomy is the initial procedure of choice.

C. This condition can rarely be associated with life-threatening respiratory compromise.

D. Approximately 50% of symptomatic congenital nasolacrimal duct obstructions resolve in the first year of life.

51. A 66-year-old woman comes in complaining of tearing bilaterally. You decide to perform testing in order to better understand the nature of her tearing. Which of the following tests are considered "physiologic?"

1. Jones I

2. Jones II

3. Dacryoscintigraphy

4. Dacryocystogram

A. 1 and 2

B. 3 and 4

C. 2 and 4

D. 1 and 3

52. What are the correct locations and names of the valves in the tear drainage system?

A. Middle meatus Hasner, upper canaliculus Rosenmuller

B. Superior meatus Rosenmuller, lower canaliculus Hasner

C. Inferior meatus Hasner, common canaliculus Rosenmuller

D. Middle meatus Hasner, lower lacrimal sac Rosenmuller

53. A medical student scrubs in on your dacryocystorhinostomy case. In an attempt to explain the procedure, which bones do you tell her you are planning to remove?

A. Lacrimal and ethmoid

B. Ethmoid and maxillary

C. Maxillary and lacrimal

D. Maxillary, lacrimal, and ethmoid

54. What is the least urgent step in management of this patient?

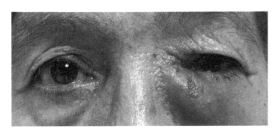

A. Incision and drainage

B. Full eye examination

C. Oral antibiotics

D. Complete blood count

55. A 34-year-old man presents with epiphora. Irrigation testing reveals a left nasolacrimal duct obstruction. Which is the best next step in management?

A. CT orbits with contrast

B. External dacryocystorhinostomy (DCR)

C. Endoscopic DCR

D. Contrast dacryocystography

56. A 50-year-old man presents with painful and progressive proptosis and hypoglobus of the left eye for the last 6 months. Visual acuity is normal. Imaging reveals a well-circumscribed tumor in the left lacrimal gland. What is the best management for this condition?

A. Tumor excision without biopsy

B. Biopsy, tumor excision, and adjuvant proton therapy

C. Neoadjuvant radiation, tumor excision, and chemotherapy without biopsy

D. Biopsy, exenteration, and chemotherapy

57. You perform probing and irrigation on a 57-year-old woman due to epiphora in the right eye. The puncta appear normal in size. She has prolonged dye disappearance test in the right eye. You encounter a "hard stop" when probing the upper and lower canaliculi. On irrigation testing of both canaliculi, there is no reflux and the patient senses fluid in the nasopharynx. What procedure would you recommend?

A. None

B. Balloon dacryoplasty

C. Dacryocystorhinostomy

D. Conjunctivodacryocystorhinostomy

58. An otherwise normal 2-year-old child presents with epiphora. What is the best additional information to confirm the location of the blockage in this patient?

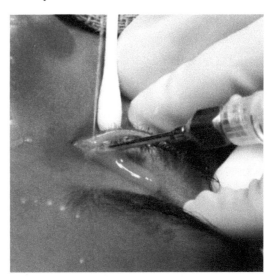

A. None

B. Duration of symptoms

C. Results of canalicular probing

D. MRI maxillofacial

59. A 63-year-old man presents with an erythematous, hot medial lower lid. When placing pressure over the medial lid, purulent discharge is expressed from the punctum. You decide to perform a curative procedure in the office, and note several concretions are able to be removed. What is the most common cause of this finding?

A. Trauma

B. Actinomyces israelii

C. Candida

D. Idiopathic

60. A 15-year-old adolescent boy presents with acute right upper lid swelling and pain. You notice an S shape to the lid, and he is tender to palpation superolaterally. Upon lifting his lid, you note purulent discharge from the lacrimal gland. What is the most common infectious cause of this condition?

A. Gram-positive bacteria

B. Epstein–Barr virus

C. Tuberculosis

D. Adenovirus

61. An 87-year-old man presents for consultation for a right optic nerve lesion. On examination, his vision is 20/50 in the right eye; there is an afferent pupillary defect; there is inferior depression on his visual field; and he has 5 mm of proptosis. Below is his MRI scan (T1-weighted pre-gadolinium and post-gadolinium, respectively). Based on this appearance, which is the most likely diagnosis?

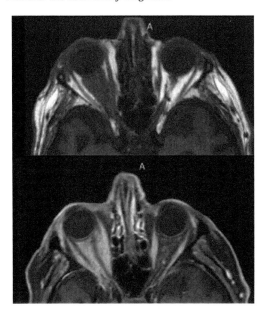

A. Optic nerve glioma

B. Optic nerve meningioma

C. Cavernous hemangioma

D. Solitary fibrous tumor

62. A 6-year-old boy presents with no light perception vision and an optic nerve lesion as seen in the MRI and corresponding pathology. What genetic disorder is most often associated with this abnormality?

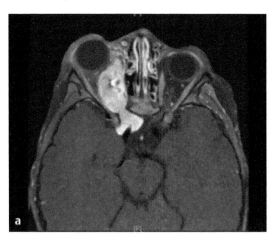

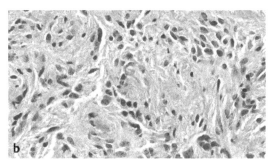

A. Neurofibromatosis 1 (NF1)

B. von Hippel–Lindau disease

C. Neurofibromatosis 2 (NF2)

D. Sturge–Weber syndrome

63. A 72-year-old man presents with proptosis and downward displacement of the left eye with a scan showing a well-circumscribed, expansile sinus mass with bony erosion extending into the orbit. Which of the following is true of this lesion?

A. Most commonly results from chronic noninvasive fungal sinusitis from the ethmoid sinus.

B. Usually presents in children.

C. MRI is the best imaging modality.

D. The frontal sinus is the most common place for mucocele development to occur.

64. A 6-year-old girl falls and hits her head while playing with her brother. On examination, her vision is intact, intraocular pressure (IOP) is within normal limits, and the motility in the right eye is severely limited in upgaze with associated double vision. Coronal and sagittal cut of her CT is shown below. What is the best next step in her management?

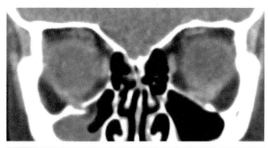

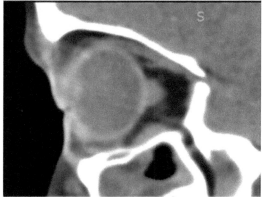

A. Proceed to the OR immediately for exploration and management of the entrapped fracture.

B. Reassure the parents that this will resolve over time on its own.

C. Perform an emergent lateral canthotomy and cantholysis.

D. Send the patient home and advise her to return to the clinic in a week for reevaluation.

65. A 37-year-old man presents with an eyelid laceration after a neighbor's pit bull bit him. Which of the following is not necessary when planning and performing a repair of a canalicular laceration?

A. A complete ophthalmic examination, including a dilated examination, is recommended.

B. Repair should be performed under general anesthesia.

C. A stent should be left in place temporarily.

D. The repair can be done within 24 to 72 hours after the injury.

66. A 70-year old man presents to the emergency room after sustaining a fall while at home with a bicanalicular laceration and medial canthal tendon avulsion. Reattachment of the medial canthal tendon to which of the following structures is necessary for reconstruction of the normal eyelid anatomy?

A. Anterior process of the maxilla

B. Anterior lacrimal crest

C. Lacrimal sac fossa

D. Posterior lacrimal crest

67. A 32-year-old man presents to the emergency room after getting punched in the right eye during a bar fight. Which of the following are indications for an emergent lateral canthotomy and cantholysis?

A. Elevated IOP, limitation in upgaze

B. Elevated IOP, decreased vision

C. Limitation in upgaze, diplopia

D. Diplopia, decreased vision

68. A 65-year-old man trips on the sidewalk while walking his dog and falls onto his face sustaining an orbital floor fracture. What is not an indication to repair the fracture?

A. Enophthalmos that exceeds 2 mm

B. Diplopia in primary gaze with limitation in upgaze that persists for 2 weeks

C. Hypoesthesia in the V2 distribution

D. Fractures involving approximately 50% of the orbital floor

69. A 25-year-old woman presents after getting assaulted with a large orbital floor fracture of the right eye, −1 limitation in upgaze, and 3 mm of enophthalmos. Which of the following is considered to be the optimal timing for repair of this fracture?

A. Within 6 weeks following the injury

B. Within 2 weeks following the injury

C. Within 1 to 3 days following the injury

D. Within 24 hours of injury

70. A patient presents concerned after an MRI performed for headaches reveals the following (see figure). Which of the following is true regarding lesions such as this?

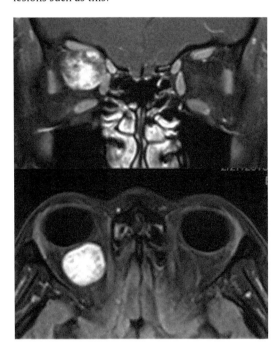

A. Pathology is characterized by "staghorn" vascular sinusoids.

B. Usually presents with significant pain that improves with steroids.

C. May be treated with propranolol.

D. Represents the most common benign orbital tumor in adults.

71. This is an 8-year-old girl who presented with significant proptosis and hypoglobus in the right eye. Which of the following subtype is associated with the worst prognosis?

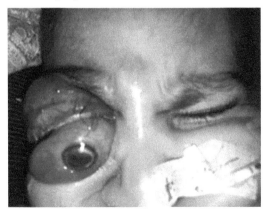

A. Botryoid

B. Embryonal

C. Alveolar

D. Pleomorphic

72. Which of the following statements is true about the most likely entity shown in the figure below?

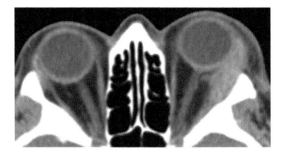

A. Most commonly B-cell-associated.

B. Most commonly T-cell-associated.

C. About 90% is associated with systemic disease.

D. About 80% presents in the lacrimal fossa.

73. If planning a biopsy of the above lesion, what is the most appropriate way to submit the tissue to pathology?

A. Formalin-fixed

B. Fresh

C. Frozen

D. Alcohol-fixed

74. An 8-month-old female infant presented with a bruise around her eye, abnormal eye movements, and a mass in her adrenal gland. Her scan is shown below. Which of the following statements about her condition is true?

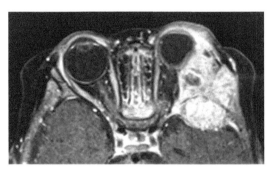

A. Almost 90% survival when present in patients younger than 1 year.

B. Debulking of the orbital mass should be performed.

C. Associated with ocular apraxia.

D. Should obtain serum catecholamine levels.

75. A 60-year-old woman presents with sudden proptosis of the left eye and periorbital ecchymosis around the eye. She recently recovered from an upper respiratory infection. Imaging shows lesions with fluid levels. Which of the following is not an appropriate treatment option?

A. Refer to interventional radiology for sclerotherapy.

B. Observe with or without steroidal therapy.

C. Perform an orbitotomy with debulking of the lesion.

D. Refer for orbital radiotherapy.

76. A 35-year-old woman presents with 3 months of boring pain around the right eye. CT imaging demonstrates a poorly circumscribed lesion in the lacrimal fossa with bone destruction. Which is the most likely diagnosis?

A. Pleomorphic adenoma

B. Adenoid cystic carcinoma of the lacrimal gland

C. Adenocarcinoma of the lacrimal gland

D. Nonspecific orbital inflammation

77. A 23-year-old man gets hit in the face with a softball while playing second base during a recreational game. Imaging demonstrates a right-sided small orbital floor fracture extending to the orbital rim and ipsilateral disruption of the zygoma. All of the following except which one can be associated with this type of fracture?

A. Trismus

B. V2 hypoesthesia

C. Epiphora

D. Lateral canthal dystopia

78. A 65-year-old woman presents with a metastatic mass of the left orbit. What is the most likely site of origin?

A. Lung

B. Colon

C. Breast

D. Melanoma

79. A 44-year-old woman presents with a slowly progressive distortion of the globe such that it appears to be pushed inferomedially. You palpate a firm mass in the superolateral quadrant of the orbit. Which of the following is most likely false about this mass?

A. Most common benign epithelial neoplasm of the lacrimal gland.

B. Excision should be performed to avoid rupture of tumor's pseudocapsule.

C. Characterized by gradual progressive proptosis with no associated pain.

D. Has the potential of transforming into adenoid cystic carcinoma.

80. Which of the following scenarios involving an orbital foreign body requires urgent exploration?

A. History of tripping over a bush and falling on eye while running from police with evidence of air pockets in the orbit on CT scan

B. BB pellet in the posterior orbit with otherwise normal examination

C. Shards of shrapnel in the orbit with associated sclopetaria after a bomb explosion

D. History of being ejected from the windshield after a car accident

81. A 90-year-old woman comes to you with tearing, worse in the wind and cold. She notes that her tears well up laterally and run down her face. Her lower lids are well opposed to the globe with no signs of trichiasis or in-turning of the eyelid. You note a snap test of 10 seconds and a distraction test of 10 mm. A trial of taping the lower lid laterally results in complete resolution of her symptoms. What condition does this woman likely suffer from?

A. Functional nasolacrimal duct obstruction

B. Cicatricial ectropion

C. Involutional ectropion

D. Involutional entropion

82. You are asked to see a 97-year-old woman patient whose "lower lids are hanging." On examination, you note bilateral outward-turning lids with significant horizontal eyelid laxity. There are no associated cicatricial changes or skin lesions. Which of the following conditions can be corrected by horizontal eyelid shortening alone?

A. Cicatricial ectropion

B. Involutional ectropion

C. Spastic entropion

D. Mechanical ectropion

83. Which of the following is not a feature of this condition?

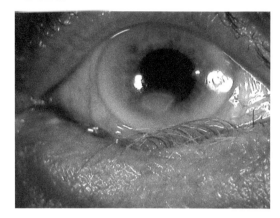

A. Horizontal eyelid laxity
B. Posterior lamellar scaring
C. Overriding by the preseptal orbicularis
D. Disinsertion of the lower eyelid retractors

84. A 70-year-old man comes to you with pain, photophobia, and tearing of the right eye. On examination, you note in-turning of the right lower eyelid. You also note significant horizontal eyelid laxity and inferior corneal staining. Which of the following procedures could not temporarily improve his signs and symptoms?

A. chemodenervation of the lower lid orbicularis
B. Quickert's sutures
C. Eyelid taping
D. Medial spindle procedure

85. A young child presents to you for a routine eye examination after his pediatrician noticed atypical-appearing eyelids. His parents are nonplussed (see figure). Which type of epicanthus is correctly paired with its description?

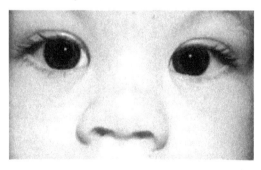

A. Epicanthus tarsalis—the fold is most prominent in the lower eyelid.
B. Epicanthus tarsalis—the fold is most prominent in the upper eyelid.
C. Epicanthus palpebralis—the fold is most prominent in the lower eyelid.
D. Epicanthus palpebralis—the fold is most prominent in the upper eyelid.

86. A 3-year-old child presents with vertically positioned lower eyelashes. The lower eyelid lashes are noted to be touching the inferior cornea when the child looks down. There is no staining of the cornea, and the parents have not noted any eye redness or apparent discomfort. Which of the following is the most appropriate treatment option?

A. A skin and muscle flap should be excised in the area of the misdirected lashes in order to prevent corneal decompensation.
B. The child should be observed and followed carefully for any signs of corneal decompensation.
C. The lashes should be epilated to prevent corneal decompensation.
D. A lateral tarsal strip with reinsertion of the lower eyelid retractors should be performed.

87. A 56-year-old man with a history of obesity presents to clinic complaining of mucous discharge and eye irritation. You note easy eversion of the upper eyelids and a chronic papillary conjunctivitis of the upper eyelid. Which of the following conditions is not associated with his ocular problem?

A. Obstructive sleep apnea
B. Christmas tree cataract
C. Keratoconus
D. Obesity

88. A 14-year-old adolescent girl comes to you for routine eye examination. Her mother mentions that she is an honor roll student and currently applying college. On examination, you note areas of madarosis and lashes in different stages of regrowth. Her eyelid skin appears normal and she has no past medical history. What is the most likely diagnosis?

A. Sebaceous cell carcinoma
B. Thyroid eye disease
C. Trichotillomania
D. Merkel cell carcinoma

89. You see a 9-year-old boy demonstrated in the figure below. His father has similar eyelid features. What is the inheritance pattern of this condition?

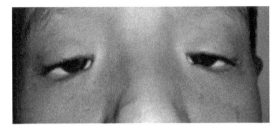

A. Autosomal recessive

B. Autosomal dominant

C. X-linked

D. X-linked recessive

90. A 35-year-old woman with rosy cheeks complains of a "bump" of her right upper eyelid for approximately 6 months. On examination, you note meibomian gland inspissation in both eyelids and a red firm elevated lesion that appears to be internal to the tarsus. She has been using warm compresses with a warming facial mask and lid massage for the past 3 months without improvement. Which of the following would you recommend?

A. Oral trimethoprim–sulfamethoxazole

B. Incision and curettage

C. Ofloxacin eyedrops

D. Artificial tears

91. A 93-year-old woman with no history of skin cancer presents to you for routine eye examination. You note a 1 × 1 mm pigmented lesion of her left lower lid. The lesion is uniform in color, non-ulcerating, and does not distort the eyelid margin. You note multiple lashes growing through the lesion. Which of the following is not a clinical sign suggesting eyelid malignancy?

A. Swelling

B. Ulceration

C. Madarosis

D. Distorted margin architecture

92. A 67-year-old Irish runner presents with the eyelid lesion depicted. She notes the lesion occurred gradually over the past several months. What is the most appropriate treatment?

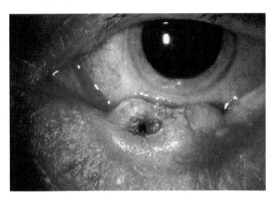

A. External photographs and observation

B. Warm compresses and lid massage

C. Incisional biopsy for diagnosis

D. Intralesional steroid injection

93. An 80-year-old woman is referred to you for a second opinion regarding a chalazion of her right upper lid. The referring physician has drained the lesion three times, but the lesion has not resolved and continues to grow. You send an excisional biopsy of the lesion, and the pathology comes back consistent with adenocarcinoma. Which of the following statements regarding adenocarcinoma is incorrect?

A. Wide surgical excision with map biopsies of the conjunctiva should be performed.

B. Orbital exenteration may be considered.

C. Sentinel lymph node biopsy may be considered.

D. Excisional biopsy is frequently all that is required.

94. You have diagnosed a 70-year-old man with melanoma of the upper eyelid by excisional biopsy. Your wide margins are clear, and there are no signs of vascular or lymphatic invasion on pathology. Your patient is happy with your periocular reconstruction and asks you more about malignant melanoma in the periocular region. Which of the following statements is incorrect?

A. Primary cutaneous melanoma of the eyelid is relatively common, accounting for approximately half of eyelid malignancies.

B. Primary cutaneous melanoma of the eyelid is rare, accounting for less than 0.1% of eyelid malignancies.

C. Lentigo maligna melanoma, nodular melanoma, superficial spreading melanoma, and acral lentiginous melanoma are the four types of cutaneous melanoma that may affect the eyelid.

D. Thin lesions (< 0.75 mm) have a high 5-year survival rate (98%).

95. You are examining a patient in the emergency room who sustained a penetrating injury to the lower eyelid during a motor vehicle collision. A CT of the orbits reveals no foreign body or orbital fractures. On your examination, you note normal visual acuity, pupils, extraocular motility, slit lamp examination, and dilated fundus examination findings. You note a central lower eyelid laceration 10 mm in length, which does not involve the eyelid margin or canalicular system. A small amount of orbital fat is visible through the wound. Which of the following statements is correct regarding your repair?

A. The presence of orbital fat indicates that the orbital septum has been violated, and the patient requires surgical exploration and repair of the lower eyelid focusing on meticulous closure of the orbital septum.

B. The presence of orbital fat in the wound is of no clinical significance, and the orbital septum has not necessarily been violated.

C. The presence of orbital fat in the wound indicates the orbital septum has been violated, and the wound should be carefully explored for signs of foreign bodies and copiously irrigated. The orbital septum should not be sutured, but the overlying orbicularis and skin should be closed.

D. The laceration is relatively small, and therefore, the wound should be left to heal by secondary intension.

96. You are examining a 24-year-old man in the emergency room who has sustained a full-thickness eyelid laceration involving the upper lid margin from a dog bite. The laceration is in the center of the eyelid. Which of the following statements is correct regarding your treatment?

A. The patient should immediately receive systemic antibiotics and tetanus vaccine; the eyelid lesion should be copiously irrigated and repaired.

B. During the repair, full-thickness tarsal bites should be taken above the eyelid margin to ensure adequate closure.

C. Permanent marginal sutures should always be used to repair the eyelid margin.

D. The patient should immediately receive systemic antibiotics, tetanus vaccine, and copious irrigation. However, repair of the laceration should be delayed several days to ensure that there are no signs of infection.

97. A 79-year-old woman presents to you for lower eyelid reconstruction following Mohs' surgery for a basal cell carcinoma. The canalicular system and canthal tissues are uninvolved. Which of the following is unlikely to be a viable surgical option for this patient?

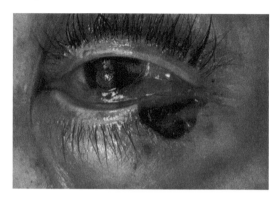

A. A tarsoconjunctival flap from the upper eyelid is used to reconstruct the posterior lamella of the lower eyelid, and a skin graft is used to reconstruct the anterior lamella of the upper eyelid.

B. A tarsoconjunctival flap from the upper eyelid is used to reconstruct the posterior lamella of the lower eyelid, and a skin advancement flap is used to reconstruct the anterior lamella of the upper eyelid.

C. A free tarsoconjunctival graft from the opposite upper eyelid is used to reconstruct the posterior lamella of the lower eyelid, and a skin graft is used to reconstruct the anterior lamella of the upper eyelid.

D. A free tarsoconjunctival graft from the opposite upper eyelid is used to reconstruct the posterior lamella of the lower eyelid and a skin-muscle flap is used to reconstruct the anterior lamella of the upper eyelid.

98. A 68-year-old man presents to you for upper eyelid reconstruction following Mohs' surgery for a squamous cell carcinoma. You note that the upper eyelid defect is small, involving approximately 30% of the upper eyelid. The canalicular system and canthal tissues are uninvolved. Which of the following is likely the best surgical option for this patient?

A. Full-thickness lower eyelid advancement flap (Cutler–Beard procedure)

B. Free tarsoconjunctival skin graft from the opposite upper eyelid and free postauricular skin graft

C. Primary closure of the defect with superior crus lateral cantholysis if necessary

D. Tarsoconjunctival flap from the lower lid with a free postauricular skin graft

99. A 76-year-old farmer presents to you for reconstruction following excision of an advanced basal cell carcinoma of the medial canthus. The defect is large and extends onto the lateral nasal side wall. There is no involvement of the canalicular system. Which of the following is the most viable surgical option for him?

A. Healing by secondary intension

B. Free skin graft

C. Undermining with direct closure

D. Forehead or glabellar flap

100. You see a young man in the emergency room after a physical altercation with a friend. The patient believes his friend's finger pulled off his lower eyelid. You are suspicious for lower eyelid medial canthal avulsion. His vision, pupils, pressure, extraocular motility, slit lamp examination, and dilated fundus examination are all normal. He has no orbital fractures on CT can. Which of the following is not a critical next step in your examination?

A. Dilation and probing of puncta with irrigation

B. Looking for signs of medial canthal rounding

C. Gonioscopy

D. Grasping the lid with toothed forceps and gently tugging away from the injury while palpating the insertion of the tendon

5.2 Answers and Explanations

Easy	Medium	Hard

1. Correct: Zygomatic, maxillary, and palatine bones (D)

This image demonstrates a fracture of the right orbital floor in the setting of a mechanical fall. The orbital floor is comprised of the zygomatic, maxillary, and palatine bones. (**A**) The orbital roof is comprised of the frontal and lesser wing of the sphenoid bones. (**B**) The lateral wall of the orbit is comprised of the zygomatic and greater wing of the sphenoid bones. (**C**) The medial wall of the orbit is comprised of the ethmoid, lacrimal, maxillary, and lesser wing of the sphenoid bones.

2. Correct: Inferior meatus (beneath the inferior turbinate), and in the region underneath the middle turbinate (A)

Tears ultimately drain through the inferior meatus, an opening beneath the inferior turbinate; in a dacryocystorhinostomy, a new ostium is typically created anterior to the middle turbinate. (**B**) The maxillary, frontal, and some ethmoidal sinuses drain into the middle meatus; the middle turbinate itself is not the site of a new bony ostium during dacryocystorhinostomy. (**C**) The new ostium does not sit superior to the middle turbinate; in fact, the superior attachment of the middle turbinate marks the region of the cribriform plate, and this is a high-risk zone for surgery. (**D**) The new ostium is not created in the region of the superior turbinate.

3. Correct: Disruption of the cribriform plate (B)

The frontoethmoidal suture marks the entrance of the anterior and posterior ethmoidal arteries and the general level of the cribriform plate or the floor of the anterior cranial fossa; it therefore also marks the roof of the ethmoid sinuses. (**A**) The optic nerve traverses the optic canal, which is seated in the lesser wing of the sphenoid. While the lesser wing of the sphenoid bone is one of the bones comprising the medial wall of the orbit, the optic canal is lateral to the frontoethmoidal suture. (**C**) Since the anterior and posterior ethmoidal arteries enter through the region of the suture, disruption of the suture or a region just superior to it could cause hemorrhage, rather than necrosis. (**D**) The inferior oblique muscle is innervated by the inferior division of the third cranial nerve, which enters the orbit through the superior orbital fissure and inside the annulus of Zinn. The branch innervating the inferior oblique muscle travels along the lateral aspect of the inferior rectus and pierces the inferior oblique posteriorly.

4. Correct: Lid crease approach with orbital lobe biopsy (C)

An anterior orbitotomy allows for a surgical approach of the orbital lobe of the lacrimal gland. The lacrimal gland, which sits in the lacrimal fossa, is divided into two lobes—orbital and palpebral—by the lateral horn of the levator aponeurosis. The ducts of the orbital lobe travel through the palpebral lobe prior to exiting. (**A, B**) Since all lacrimal gland ducts exit via the palpebral lobe, it is unwise to perform an incisional biopsy of the palpebral lobe from any approach. (**D**) The visible lobe of the lacrimal gland in the superotemporal fornix is palpebral. The aptly named orbital lobe is deeper in the orbit.

5. Correct: Inject botulinum toxin type A along regions impacted by the seventh nerve unilaterally, and then perform the cosmetic injection; submit the insurance claim for the quantity injected and wasted for the functional purposes alone, and bill the patient separately for the cosmetic injection (C)

It is unethical and fraudulent to bill insurance for cosmetic injections and procedures. Botulinum toxin type A can be injected for both functional and cosmetic reasons. For example, insurance will typically cover injections for hemifacial spasm or blepharospasm. However, injections for cosmetic paralysis of mobile rhytids, such as forehead lines or crow's feet, are considered noncovered entities. In this case, the patient is presenting with hemifacial spasm, involving muscle innervated by the seventh cranial nerve. The patient's insurance should be billed for the functional injection alone; the patient is fully responsible for any fees covering the cost of cosmetic botulinum injection and time. (**A and D**) Insurance should not be billed for cosmetic botulinum toxin use; only the quantity injected for functional purposes should be recorded for an insurance claim. (**B and D**) The patient presented with complaints consistent with hemifacial spasm, involving muscles of facial expression innervated by the seventh cranial nerve or the facial nerve. The third cranial nerve, or oculomotor nerve, innervates the inferior rectus, inferior oblique, superior rectus, medial rectus, and levator palpebrae superioris muscles.

6. Correct: Superior ophthalmic vein (A)

The superior ophthalmic vein drains most of the orbit, originating superonasally and traveling diagonally before entering the superior orbital fissure and draining into the cavernous sinus. (**B**) The inferior ophthalmic vein splits into two sites of drainage: (1) the pterygoid plexus and (2) the cavernous sinus, commonly by entering with the superior ophthalmic vein. It is therefore less ideal for direct cavernous sinus access. (**C and D**) The angular vein, which is a superior continuation of the facial vein, connects with the inferior and superior ophthalmic veins; therefore, neither the facial nor the angular veins are direct conduits to the cavernous sinus.

7. Correct: Keratinized epithelial lining, hair follicles, and sebaceous glands (B)

Dermoid cysts are one of the most common congenital orbital tumors; they tend to slowly, progressively enlarge and, if superficial enough, can be noted in early or late childhood. Deeper orbital cysts may not present until adulthood. Histopathology demonstrates a keratinized lining with dermal components, such as hair or sebaceous glands. The lateral eyebrow is the most common site of dermoid cyst occurrence, typically adjacent to the frontozygomatic suture line. They can be mobile, adherent to periosteum, or even continuous with an inner orbital cyst in a dumbbell pattern. They are well defined on imaging, with enhancing walls and a lumen that is nonenhancing (lacking in blood vessels internally), hypointense compared to orbital fat on T1, and hyperintense compared to orbital fat on T2. (**A**) Capillary hemangiomas are commonly noted in eyelids; they are present at birth or, more typically, soon thereafter, progressively grow for months, and involute over the course of years. Typically, involution occurs by school age. Histopathology demonstrates endothelium-lined capillary channels in a lobular configuration, though

they may be more cellular with nests of endothelial cells in early stages, and fibrosis and hyalinization with luminal occlusion once involuted. Treatment is aimed at prevention of amblyopia if in the eyelid region, and can include occlusion therapy, steroid, beta blockers, excision if well defined (rare), and laser of the skin if superficial. (**C**) Another frequent congenital hamartoma is an epidermoid cyst, which is an epithelium-lined cyst containing keratin. The lack of dermal appendages differentiates an epidermoid from a dermoid cyst. (**D**) Rhabdomyosarcoma is the most common primary orbital malignancy of childhood and typically presents acutely with rapid proptosis. There are three subtypes of which embryonal is the most common; pleomorphic has the best prognosis; and alveolar has the worst prognosis. Embryonal rhabdomyosarcoma shows spindle cells with occasional cross-striations upon biopsy. Emergent biopsy with histopathologic diagnosis is key for prompt, multidisciplinary treatment.

8. Correct: Perform a partial excision if irritating (B)

This lesion is a classic dermolipoma; it has both pink and yellow hues and is in the superolateral quadrant. The finding of several fine hairs overlying it is an excellent indication. Dermolipomas are benign, solid tumors over the lateral aspect of the globe; while they appear superficial and anterior, they extend posteriorly and can involve the levator aponeurosis, lacrimal gland region, and extraocular muscles. (**A, C, and D**) For this reason, they are typically left alone unless physically irritating or cosmetically concerning to the patient. If surgery is needed, it is typically an incomplete removal of only the visible portion, and attempts are made to spare the conjunctiva.

9. Correct: He will never be able to interact meaningfully with his environment (A)

Patients with craniosynostosis typically demonstrate normal IQ if their intracranial pressure is monitored and appropriately managed. (**B**) It is crucial to work in a multidisciplinary fashion to allow for management of elevated intracranial pressure, as well as to attempt to improve functional and cosmetic concerns. Surgical treatment is typically performed over multiple stages. (**C and D**) From an ophthalmic perspective, there is risk of proptosis with exposure keratopathy, ptosis, hypertelorism, nasolacrimal duct obstruction, strabismus, significant refractive error, and optic neuropathy. For this reason, in addition to lubrication as needed, bony orbital manipulation may be performed in concert with other services; eyelid, nasolacrimal, and strabismus surgery are frequently necessary; careful refraction is crucial; and optic nerve function and appearance should be routinely monitored.

10. Correct: Retain microphthalmic eye OS and use gradually increasing conformers with possible dermis-fat graft in the future (C)

Microphthalmia is on a spectrum with anophthalmia and coloboma; cases may be unilateral or bilateral and can include any combination of the spectrum. A range of chromosomal and single gene mutations have been identified as linked to the spectrum, and patients may suffer from a variety of associated syndromes. Ophthalmologically speaking, in cases of anophthalmia and microphthalmia, focus must be placed on expansion of the otherwise retarded bony socket. (**A**) Microphthalmic eyes typically have no visual potential, so bone expansion is initiated as soon as possible after birth, rather than focusing on visual potential. (**B**) Any microphthalmic globe can help with volume-induced expansion of the orbit, and so the anomalous globe is kept; conformers and prostheses can generally be fit as needed around it, with the potential exception of microphthalmia with orbital cyst—though a cyst can be very helpful in bone expansion; at times it can grow too large and require removal for prosthesis fitting. (**C**) In general, conformers or implants of increasing size are placed in the socket to allow for expansion, at times followed by a dermis-fat graft that can grow with the child once the minimum space for this is available, with the ultimate expectation of prosthesis placement.

11. Correct: Thyroid-stimulating immunoglobulin (B)

Thyroid eye disease (TED) is the most common cause of upper eyelid retraction in adults. TED can also cause retraction of the lower eyelid, proptosis, and limited extraocular muscle movement. Though both orbits are often affected, it can present asymmetrically. Severe TED can cause a compressive optic neuropathy. Laboratory work evaluation should include thyroid studies (thyroid-stimulating hormone, free T_4, T_3), and the following antibodies: thyroid peroxidase antibody, thyroid-stimulating hormone receptor antibody, thyroid-stimulating immunoglobulin, and thyrotropin-binding inhibitory immunoglobulin. (**A**) Infections might be demonstrated with an elevated white blood cell count but would typically present with significantly more erythema and injection, as well as a more acute pattern of onset. (**C**) Myasthenia gravis is associated with TED but is far less common. It can cause variable extraocular muscle and eyelid movement. Acetylcholine receptor antibodies can be positive in the setting of myasthenia gravis. (**D**) Temporal arteritis can cause elevated erythrocyte sedimentation rate and platelet count but would cause a cranial nerve palsy rather than restricted eye movement and retraction.

12. Correct: Fatty proliferation (D)

Orbital fibroblasts play a significant role in thyroid eye disease (TED). They carry the same CD40 surface receptor as B cells, and when engaged by proinflammatory T cells, they increase hyaluronan and glycosaminoglycan synthesis. Orbital fibroblasts are also capable of differentiating into adipocytes, which can secondarily cause fatty hypertrophy of the affected orbit. Fatty proliferation is more typical of younger TED patients, as opposed to those older than 40 years. (**A**) The oblique muscles are rarely a prominent feature of muscle enlargement in TED. (**B**) The inferior and medial recti are frequently involved; the superior rectus/levator muscle complex and lateral rectus can also be involved, though less frequently. Typically, the muscle enlargement is tendon-sparing. (**C**) In this patient with known Graves' disease and bilateral, asymmetric signs of TED, it would be unlikely to find a secondary orbital process. Of note, TED is the most common cause of unilateral or bilateral proptosis in general.

13. Correct: Artificial tears four times a day OU (C)

TED has both active and stable phases and can be classified according to severity. In this patient, her findings are consistent with actively improving TED. Additionally, her upper eyelid retraction is not causing significant exposure keratopathy. For this reason, management can be conservative, with head elevation, ocular surface lubrication, and continued control of euthyroid state. Selenium supplementation may also have a role in this example of mild TED. (**A, D**) Intravenous methylprednisolone infusion is reserved for more severe TED; if optic nerve compression is present, there is also indication for urgent orbital decompression. It is of note that orbital radiotherapy is without consensus. Though some advocate its use in severe TED, it can cause retinopathy and should not be used in diabetics or other patients who may already have risk of retinopathy. (**B**) Surgical right upper eyelid recession is an excellent way to improve cosmesis and decrease exposure keratopathy, but should be reserved until the patient is in a stable TED state, without evidence of changing disease (improvement or progression) for at least 6 months. It should typically be performed after any planned decompression or strabismus surgery.

14. Correct: Cribriform appearance (A)

Adenoid cystic carcinoma can demonstrate multiple histologic patterns, but cribriform changes (Swiss cheese) are the most common. Adenoid cystic carcinoma of the lacrimal gland is a destructive, invasive, and typically painful (due to nerve invasion) malignancy. (**B–D**) IgG4 disease can cause mass lesions throughout the body, potentially impacting multiple organ systems. In IgG4-related ophthalmic disease, the lacrimal glands are most commonly affected. Bilateral lacrimal gland involvement portends a high risk of systemic disease. Serum IgG4 levels are commonly, but not definitionally, elevated. Histopathologic review of an IgG4-related biopsy classically demonstrates lymphoplasmacytic infiltrate with a high number of IgG4+ plasma cells, a high IgG4/IgG ratio, storiform fibrosis, and obliterative phlebitis. In conjunction with rheumatology, systemic imaging and laboratory work should be performed to search for other impacted organs; treatment is frequently initiated with steroids, though steroid-sparing agents can also be used.

15. Correct: Serum cytoplasmic antineutrophil cytoplasmic antibody (c-ANCA) is specific for this disease process; if it is negative, this process can be ruled out (D)

This patient presents with classic signs of granulomatosis with polyangiitis (GPA, formerly Wegener's granulomatosis). c-ANCA is specific for GPA but can be negative in the early stages, particularly when involvement is more local in nature. (**A**) Histopathologic examination of affected tissue typically demonstrates a necrotizing granulomatous process with vasculitis. GPA can involve multiple systems, including the upper and lower respiratory tract, the kidneys, and any small vessels. (**B, C**) For this reason, vasculitic changes can cause multiorgan damage, and the disease can be fatal. Though systemic steroids can be used acutely, cyclophosphamide is the treatment of choice and leads to lower mortality rates than steroid use alone. This is a disease process that benefits from multiteam management.

16. Correct: In adults, this condition is typically unilateral and without systemic symptoms (C)

A child presenting with bilateral signs of orbital inflammation, headache, fever, nausea/vomiting, and lethargy may ultimately be demonstrated to have nonspecific orbital inflammation (NSOI). Approximately two-thirds of childhood NSOI cases, and typical adult forms of NSOI, are unilateral; adults do not tend to present with systemic symptoms, whereas half of pediatric cases do. (**A**) NSOI is a diagnosis of exclusion. Systemic infections could cause similar findings (i.e., Epstein–Barr virus and mumps), as could lymphoproliferative neoplasms or systemic inflammatory conditions, such as the immunoglobulin G4 disease spectrum. For this reason, it is best to perform laboratory work and, if infection is not found, a biopsy is performed to better understand the condition and classify it as accurately as possible. Biopsied tissue classically demonstrates pleomorphic inflammatory cellular infiltrate, including eosinophils, and progressive fibrosis. For this reason, steroids are more helpful in early stages. (**B**), (**D**)

NSOI can affect extraocular muscles, the lacrimal gland, and other orbital tissue to varying degrees (i.e., apical inflammation). When myositis occurs, it is typically not tendon-sparing, as opposed to thyroid eye disease. NSOI can also present as scleritis/uveitis. Laboratory work-up may show elevated inflammatory markers and eosinophilia.

17. Correct: Initiation of IV antibiotic therapy (B)

Pediatric and adult orbital cellulitis with abscess tend to differ significantly in terms of treatment needs. Though both can present with orbital and systemic signs, and are frequently related to sinusitis, pediatric cases tend to be single gram-positive organisms, and adult cases tend to be due to multiple organisms, including anaerobes. Adults typically need drainage, whereas children younger than 9 years are typically able to be treated with IV antibiotic therapy alone as long as the abscess is solely medial, small or medium in size, without gas on CT (anaerobic sign), without evidence of optic neuropathy, without evidence of chronic sinusitis, without dental involvement (anaerobic risk), and non-recurrent. (**A**) In children 9 years and older and adults, or in those children at significant risk (i.e. optic neuropathy), anterior orbitotomy with drainage may be urgently indicated or at least very likely, even after an initial cool-down with IV antibiotic therapy. (**C**) Oral antibiotic therapy is not indicated when initiating abscess treatment, though it may be warranted after IV antibiotic treatment (and orbitotomy as needed) to continue a complete antibiotic course once the orbit has significantly improved. (**D**) Functional endoscopic sinus surgery is potentially very important in sinusitis-related orbital cellulitis. However, it is not indicated as the next step alone.

18. Correct: *Staphylococcus aureus* (B)

Staphylococcus aureus is a common cause of preseptal cellulitis in the setting of trauma. It is important to note that the incidence of methicillin-resistant *S. aureus* (MRSA) is increasing in the community. Community-acquired MRSA is particularly aggressive compared to methicillin-sensitive *S. aureus* but is treatable with oral antibiotics (i.e., TMP-SMX, clindamycin). MRSA often presents with an abscess, which should be drained. Should any infection prove resistant to oral antibiotics, intravenous therapy may be necessary. (**A**) *Haemophilus influenzae* is a known cause of preseptal cellulitis. Prior to the introduction of the vaccine, *H. influenzae* was a common cause of preseptal cellulitis, meningitis, and bacteremia; it is now rarer. (**C**) *Klebsiella pneumoniae* can cause preseptal cellulitis, as can a wide range of bacteria. Preseptal cellulitis may be secondary to sinusitis, especially in children, as well as dacryocystitis or any skin trauma (such as a bite or scratch). In pediatric populations, *Streptococcus* species are common. In third world regions, tuberculosis and anthrax can be culprits as well. (**D**) *Actinomyces israelii* is the most common cause of canaliculitis.

19. Correct: He must be monitored for shock and has a high mortality risk (A)

Necrotizing fasciitis is a rapidly progressive bacterial infection of the subcutaneous soft tissue and often tracks along avascular planes; the infection can cause toxic shock with rapid deterioration and a mortality rate as high as 30%. It is typically due to group A β–hemolytic *Streptococcus*, though other organisms can also be causative. Though immunocompetent patients can present with necrotizing fasciitis, it is more common in immunocompromised patients. Patients may present with numbness or pain; skin color changes from rose to blue-gray and ultimately can show evidence of necrosis. Admission for IV antibiotics and intensive systemic monitoring is crucial, as is team-based care; missing this potential diagnosis can result in death. (**D**) Surgical debridement is typically necessary and should be performed early in the course of necrotizing fasciitis treatment. (**B, C**) Mucormycosis (aka zygomycosis, phycomycosis) is a fungal, destructive process that typically starts in a sinus before invading the orbit. As with all fungal disease, immunocompromised status is a predisposing risk factor. Surgical debridement and IV antifungal therapy are usually combined. IV amphotericin B is typically used. Histopathologic review would show nonseptate hyphae causing a thrombosing vasculitis, in contrast to aspergillosis, which shows septate branching hyphae.

20. Correct: Chest X-Ray (C)

This figure demonstrates a noncaseating granuloma pattern consistent with sarcoidosis. Sarcoidosis can cause granulomatous inflammation in multiple organs and sites, including orbital tissue. The lacrimal gland is the most commonly affected orbital tissue, but the lungs are the most commonly affected site in general. Chest X-ray or CT can demonstrate hilar adenopathy or infiltrates, and sometimes bronchoscopy can be used to demonstrate granulomas in washings or lung biopsies. Demonstration of involvement in other sites, including the lungs, changes monitoring and treatment needs; this work-up can be performed in conjunction with a rheumatologist. Serum blood work may demonstrate elevated angiotensin-converting enzyme, lysozyme, and calcium. (**A**) Conjunctival biopsy of a discrete lesion may be helpful but random conjunctival biopsies are not. In this case, without a particular conjunctival lesion to biopsy, random conjunctival biopsy would neither contribute to the diagnosis nor tailor the treatment plan. (**B**) Tuberculosis causes caseating granulomas. (**D**) Bone marrow biopsy would be useful in situations concerning for lymphoproliferative neoplasm.

21. Correct: involutional, cicatricial (B)

This image demonstrates a lower lid entropion. There are four types of entropion: involutional, congenital, spastic, and cicatricial. Involutional entropion is the most common type of entropion involving the lower lids and typically is due to horizontal laxity, capsulopalpebral fascia disinsertion, and orbicularis override. Cicatricial entropion is a rotation of the eyelid margin due to scarring from disorders, such as ocular cicatricial pemphigoid, Stevens–Johnson syndrome, trachoma, prior surgeries, and long-standing topical glaucoma drop use. Cicatricial entropion is the most common cause of upper eyelid entropion. Therefore, answer choice (**B**) is correct. Answer choices (**A**), (**C**), and (**D**) are incorrect, because spastic and congenital entropion are not the most common types of entropion. Spastic entropion is typically due to a combination of eyelid laxity and ocular surface irritation. Congenital entropion is rare and represents an eyelid margin that has rotated inward. This should be differentiated from congenital epiblepharon, where the eyelid margin is in the correct position, but the eyelashes are rotated toward the cornea by a fold of skin.

22. Correct: Laboratory work-up of acetylcholine receptor antibodies (B)

(**A**) Ptosis with variability/fatiguability should be worked up for myasthenia gravis (MG) *prior* to surgical intervention. (**B**) MG is an autoimmune disorder, which can be diagnosed with acetylcholine receptor antibodies. Ocular MG may present with negative antibodies in up to 50% of patients, so edrophonium challenge, electromyography, and other tests, like a CT scan to rule out thymus gland tumor, can be indicated in cases of high suspicion. Ptosis due to MG not only has diurnal variation but also varies in severity and sometimes can respond to systemic medications and treatments, such as pyridostigmine (Mestinon), intravenous immunoglobulin (IVIg), and the monoclonal antibody rituximab (Rituxan). (**C**) Aquaporin-4 is a water channel protein, for which the antibody is a serum marker for neuromyelitis optica, an autoimmune disorder that affects both the optic nerve and spinal cord. In neuromyelitis optica, vision would be affected, not the eyelid. (**D**) MRI/MRA with attention to the internal auditory canal (mirroring the path of cranial nerve VII) is typically done in patients with hemifacial spasm to rule out vascular contact with the facial nerve root exit zone. Hemifacial spasm would not cause a bilateral upper lid ptosis with variability/fatiguability.

23. Correct: Aponeurotic (A)

Aponeurotic ptosis is caused by dehiscence of the levator palpebrae superioris muscle. The attachments of the levator muscle to the overlying skin create a lid crease. In cases of levator dehiscence,

157

the muscle still works well, so the levator function remains normal (above 11 mm); since the muscle is stretched (dehisced), the lid crease typically moves superiorly. (**B**) A neurogenic ptosis, like a complete cranial nerve III palsy, would have a severely reduced levator function, if any. (**C**) Myogenic ptosis, which is the most common cause of congenital ptosis, is a congenital defect in the levator palpebrae superioris muscle. This typically translates to decreased levator function and a poorly visible lid crease. (**D**) Mechanical ptosis is due to excess weight on the upper lid, causing the eyelid to fall. This can be due to a tumor, edema, or infection.

24. Correct: Epiblepharon (A)

Epiblepharon is a congenital condition, more typically affecting children of Asian descent. Although the eyelid margin is in the correct position, the eyelashes are pushed inward toward the eye by the skin and the overriding orbicularis oculi muscle. As the facial bones grow, this typically resolves spontaneously. Cases in which the cornea is being damaged or there is significant discomfort, removal of skin and orbicularis can be considered. During skin closure, incorporating the capsulopalpebral fascia can ensure that there will no longer be orbicularis override. (**C**) In contrast, a congenital entropion has an abnormal eyelid margin position and is rare. (**B**) Euryblepharon is due to a congenital horizontal enlargement, which can be seen in blepharophimosis syndrome or independently. If causing symptoms, a lateral tarsal strip can be performed. (**D**) Finally, congenital glaucoma can cause tearing and light sensitivity. However, the typical clinical triad also includes blepharospasm. Additionally, there may also be corneal clouding or buphthalmos (ocular enlargement, due to the immature cornea and sclera stretching in response to the increased intraocular pressure). In this case, there is no corneal clouding, history of blepharospasm, and the corneal diameter appears within normal limits (normal horizontal diameter in newborns is 9.5–10.5 mm and increases to 10–11.5 mm by 1 year of age). Diameter greater than 1 mm above the normal range should be of concern. In cases in which the etiology is unclear, an intraocular pressure check is critical.

25. Correct: Capsulopalpebral fascia dehiscence, overriding orbicularis, and horizontal laxity (C)

Surgical management of involutional entropion requires reattachment of the capsulopalpebral fascia to address the dehiscence, suturing the infraciliary skin closure sutures to incorporate the underlying capsulopalpebral fascia or removing a strip of orbicularis muscle to prevent orbicularis override, and a lateral tarsal strip to address the horizontal laxity. Answer choices (**A**) and (**D**) are incorrect, because scarring of the posterior lamella would be a

different kind of entropion—cicatricial, which typically requires a surgery like a Weiss procedure. (**A, B**) Additionally, trichiasis is defined as correct eyelid position with incorrect eyelash orientation. Trichiasis is treated depending on the distribution and number of misguided lashes. For example, if there are only one or two aberrant lashes, radiofrequency epilation is effective, although this typically requires several treatments. If there is one area of trichiatic lashes, removal of that area of the eyelid via pentagonal wedge excision can be considered. Diffuse trichiasis involving the entire lid should be reexamined as many cases are actually misdiagnosed entropion.

26. Correct: Myogenic (C)

Myogenic ptosis most commonly is congenital in onset and is a muscle disorder causing ptosis. In this case, the muscle doesn't work well, so the eyelid struggles to move superiorly (poor levator function) and inferiorly (eyelid lag on downgaze, lagophthalmos). (**A**) Aponeurotic ptosis is due to a dehiscence of the levator palpebrae superioris muscle, but the muscle itself is not affected, so levator function is normal and eyelid closure should also be complete. Because of the dehisced (stretched) levator muscle, the lid tends to be even more ptotic on downgaze. (**B**) Neurogenic ptosis (due to a cranial nerve III disorder) would have poor levator function but would not have lagophthalmos, as this would require a concurrent cranial nerve VII palsy. (**D**) Mechanical ptosis is due to a weight on the upper lid, causing droopiness. This would most likely still have complete eyelid closure (no lagophthalmos) and would not have eyelid lag on downgaze.

27. Correct: Damage to the right inferior oblique muscle (D)

The inferior oblique muscle passes between the medial and middle orbital fat pads in the lower eyelid. This is why careful dissection should be done to identify the muscle prior to orbital fat removal in lower lid blepharoplasties. With this knowledge, answer choices involving the lateral rectus (**A and B**) can be ruled out. Left cranial nerve VI or lateral rectus muscle damage would cause diplopia worse in left gaze, but these structures do not pass in the lower lid blepharoplasty surgical field. In primary gaze, the inferior oblique muscle extorts, elevates, and abducts the eye. On looking toward the nose, the torsional action is minimized, and the inferior oblique's ability to elevate is more easily assessed. In left gaze, the left superior rectus and right inferior oblique elevate, while the left inferior rectus and right superior oblique depress. So, if a patient is having diplopia worse in left gaze, this represents damage to the right inferior oblique muscle. (**C**) Left inferior oblique muscle damage would have diplopia worse in right gaze.

28. Correct: Conjunctivomullerectomy (B)

With good levator function, surgical options for ptosis repair are levator advancement or conjunctivomullerectomy. (**A**) In this case, where the patient is young and is a model, a conjunctivomullerectomy is ideal, as the patient does not have extra skin to remove (which could be done concurrently in a levator advancement), and there will be no visible scar. Conjunctivomullerectomy is typically ideal for repair of minimal ptosis (< 2 mm), so the asymmetry here fits this soft criterion. (**C**) Frontalis sling would be done for a levator function of less than 4 mm, and the levator function is reported to be good here. (**D**) A Bick procedure is removal of a full-thickness lower lid wedge, described for senile entropion and ectropion.

29. Correct: Check free T$_4$, TSH, and thyroid antibodies (D)

The most common cause of eyelid retraction is thyroid eye disease. (**A**) Retraction of one eyelid can cause the contralateral eyelid to look ptotic, but surgical correction of the ptosis will not address the true problem, which is the thyroid eye disease and retraction of the left upper lid. The correct next step is to confirm the diagnosis of thyroid eye disease. Thyroid eye disease requires two of the following to be positive: (1) clinical changes such as eyelid retraction with temporal flare, new proptosis, chemosis, caruncular erythema/edema, compressive optic neuropathy, and restrictive strabismus, (2) autoimmune thyroiditis (Graves', Hashimoto's, or euthyroid with thyroid antibodies), (3) radiographic changes (fusiform enlargement of one or more of the extraocular muscles). (**B**) Retraction repair would be the correct surgical solution here, but diagnosis with establishment of 6 months of stability would be desirable first. (**C**) Once Graves' hyperthyroidism is confirmed, one possible option for treatment is radioactive iodine, but risk for worsening the thyroid ophthalmopathy should be considered.

30. Correct: Delayed swallow study and genetic mutations of *PABPN1* (B)

This question is describing a patient with oculopharyngeal dystrophy. This autosomal dominant disorder tends to have an onset in the late 40s to early 50s with ptosis preceding dysphagia by a few years. Diagnosis is established via the presence of disease in two or more generations, swallow studies, and ptosis. Genetic studies showing mutations of *PABPN1* can be done for confirmation. (**A**) Muscle biopsy showing ragged red fibers would be consistent with a mitochondrial disease, such as chronic progressive external ophthalmoplegia

(CPEO). However, in CPEO, the patient would also have decreased extraocular motility and a flat effect (see figure). Mitochondrial disorders are also only passed down maternally (mitochondrial DNA is only passed from the egg), so her father would not have been able to pass CPEO to her. (**C**) Marcus Gunn jaw wink, an abnormal connection between the levator muscle and the pterygoid muscles, can be congenital or acquired. However, this condition is typically sporadic and certainly not autosomal dominant, as described in this question step, where three generations are affected. (**D**) An overshooting upper eyelid on downgaze followed by primary gaze describes Cogan's lid twitch, which has a 99% specificity and 75% sensitivity for myasthenia gravis.

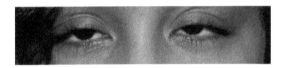

31. Correct: The medication she should receive takes about 2 to 3 days to work, peaks in effect 7 to 10 days later, and lasts about 3 to 4 months (A)

Bilateral periocular spasms most likely represent benign essential blepharospasm (BEB). As the name describes, this is a benign process, but it can be so disabling that patients cannot leave their house or pursue normal daily activities, because they are not sure if they will be able to open their eyes. In cases with underlying dry eye syndrome, dryness should be treated. For those without dry eye or who have maximized dry eye therapy, periocular botulinum toxin type A injections addresses this problem in the majority of patients and the onset, peak effect, and duration as described above for the commonly used Botox (onabotulinum) brand. (**B**) The mechanism of action is inhibiting acetylcholine *release* from the *presynaptic* neuron, not binding at the postsynaptic neuron. Other possible treatment options include surgical orbicularis oculi myectomy (but this is reserved for those poorly responsive to botulinum therapy), surgical ablation of the facial nerve (but there is a risk of recurrence and paralysis often results), and medical therapy (but this is rarely effective and the side effect profile is high). (**C**) MRI is not indicated for BEB, but it is indicated for hemifacial spasm (which is a spasm that affects only one side of the face, as its name describes) to rule out pons pathology. (**D**) The cause for BEB is posited to be a disorder of the basal ganglia, but this is not proven. The most common cause of hemifacial spasm is a vascular irritation of cranial nerve VII at its exit at the brainstem, and MRI with attention to the pathway of cranial nerve VII can confirm this.

32. Correct: B and C (D)

The question stem is describing hemifacial spasm—right-sided periocular spasms with right lower face spasms. The most common cause of hemifacial spasm is a vascular irritation of the facial nerve at the brainstem, and MRI is indicated to rule out pons or cranial VII pathology. (**A**) Neurosurgical decompression can be considered, but onabotulinum (botulinum toxin type A) injections are much less invasive and typically have excellent results, so should be considered first. (**B**) Hemifacial spasms (unlike benign essential blepharospasm) can occur during sleep. (**C**) History of facial nerve injury (Bell's palsy, trauma, etc.) is not uncommon in hemifacial spasm, which then represents a form of synkinesis.

33. Correct: Brow lift (D)

A brow that is below the superior orbital rim is considered ptotic. In women, the brow tends to be higher and more arched, so it may appear ptotic before it is below the superior orbital rim. Brow lift is the best surgical option here to address the true underlying problem of brow ptosis. Options include a direct brow approach (incision is directly superior to the brow and thus conspicuous), endoscopic brow lift (incisions are hidden posterior to the hairline), and pretrichial brow lift (incisions are at the hairline, so it is best for patients with bangs). Typically, 20 mm of skin between the eyelid and inferior aspect of the brow is a conservative amount of skin for this area. (**A, B**) For example, when a blepharoplasty is done, a safe amount to leave behind is 20 mm of skin (which is the amount of skin this patient has currently), so additional skin removal should be considered with great caution, as the risk of postoperative lagophthalmos increases with less skin. Also, aggressive blepharoplasty will result in further depression of the brow. Thus, upper eyelid blepharoplasty or CO_2 laser (which tightens skin) would be less desirable, as both decrease the amount of skin between the brow and lid margin. (**C**) There is no indication of blepharoptosis in this patient, as the MRD1 is symmetric and at a normal height of 4 mm, so levator advancement would not be indicated.

34. Correct: All of the above (D)

The patient underwent aggressive lower eyelid blepharoplasty with resulting lower eyelid retraction, right worse than left, as well as lagophthalmos. The lid margin is everted and retracted inferiorly with resulting conjunctival injection. (**A–C**) All of the solutions proposed are reasonable options, depending on the severity of the symptoms and signs. Additionally, there can be a role for a posterior lamellar spacer graft, conventionally a hard palate or ear cartilage graft, and more recently an acellular dermal matrix (such as Alloderm, Surgimend, Enduragen). Other lower lid blepharoplasty complications include retrobulbar hemorrhage with visual loss and diplopia from oblique muscle damage.

35. Correct: Lateral tarsal strip with medial spindle procedure (B)

The figure shows a patient with left lower lid ectropion—specifically, a tarsal ectropion. In cases where the entire lower lid tarsus everts and the etiology is involutional, a medial spindle procedure will help rotate the lid back inward. (**A**) There is typically also horizontal laxity, which should be addressed with a lateral tarsal strip, but this alone will likely be insufficient. (**C, D**) The other two answer choices are entropion repair procedures with a Quickert suture being a fast but usually temporizing measure to reinsert the retractors and a Weiss procedure being an eyelid margin rotation surgery.

36. Correct: All of the above (D)

A morbidly obese patient with eyelids that easily stretch off the globe with gentle traction, causing conjunctival injection and discharge, represents a case of floppy eyelid syndrome. (**A–C**) Floppy eyelid syndrome is associated with obesity, obstructive sleep apnea, and keratoconus, along with other issues (like Down's syndrome, HTN, DM, HL, and hyperglycemia). Treatment of the obstructive sleep apnea with continuous positive airway pressure can result in resolution of sleep apnea symptoms. Conservative management involves taping the eyelids and lubrication. Surgical treatment involves tightening the eyelids by removing excess tissue, for example, via lateral tarsal strip.

37. Correct: Lagophthalmos (D)

The patient in this figure has a right-sided cranial nerve VII palsy. This can be deduced from the following: asymmetric left-sided frontalis rhytids with absence of right frontalis rhytids, right-sided brow ptosis, right lower lid ectropion, right-sided loss of the nasolabial fold, and a right-sided ptosis of the oral commissure. Facial nerve palsies tend to present with a paralytic ectropion and concomitant lagophthalmos (incomplete closure of the eyelids). Treatment depends on severity and expected duration of paralysis. Conservative measures include lubrication, moisture chambers, and taping of the temporal lower lid. Other surgical options include tarsorrhaphy, canthoplasty, grafts to elevate the lower lid, suspension of the lower lid, horizontal tightening of the lower lid, and lid weights to the upper lid. (**A, B**) Dermatochalasis and blepharoptosis are not associated with facial nerve palsy. In fact, a facial nerve palsy can cause a relative upper eyelid retraction due to poor orbicularis muscle function. Both can be seen with normal aging; blepharoptosis has many other causes besides age-related aponeurotic ptosis such as myogenic (typically congenital, but also muscular dystrophy, chronic progressive external ophthalmoplegia, oculopharyngeal dystrophy), neurogenic (cranial nerve III palsy, Horner's syndrome, Marcus Gunn jaw winking), mechanical, and traumatic. (**C**) Blepharochalasis is not an age-related change; it is a rare familial type of angioneurotic edema. This is more typically seen in younger patients with a female preponderance and is characterized by intermittent episodes of eyelid edema, which causes the skin to stretch and then become wrinkly when the edema resolves. The eyelid edema also causes blepharoptosis, herniated lacrimal glands, orbital fat pad atrophy, and prominent eyelid vascularity. This is difficult to resolve surgically as the intermittent episodes typically continue.

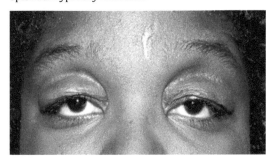

38. Correct: Hering's law (A)

Hering's law is also known as overcompensation for a contralateral ptosis. In the figure panel A, the patient has a ptosis of the eyelids, worse on the right than the left. The margin to reflex distance on the right is −2 (the pupillary reflex is not even visible). The margin to reflex distance on the left is 1.5 mm. In the figure panel B, the right upper eyelid is manually lifted and the left upper lid drops with the margin to reflex distance of −1. This occurs because the brain sends the same amount of innervation to each eye, so when one eyelid is droopier than the other, the brain sends out as much innervation as possible to each side to attempt to lift the more ptotic side. Once the more ptotic side is elevated (manually or surgically), the brain will no longer send out as much innervation to lift each eyelid, so the nonsurgical side may drop. (**B**) Sherrington's law is the law of reciprocal innervation, which means that when one muscle contracts, the opposite muscle will relax. For example, when the right medial rectus contracts, the right lateral rectus muscle relaxes. (**C**) Cogan's lid twitch is an overshooting upper eyelid on downgaze followed by primary gaze, which is highly specific for myasthenia gravis. (**D**) Finally, Harada–Ito is not a sign, but a procedure, done for a cranial nerve IV palsy. The superior oblique

is split, and the anterior fibers, which are responsible for incyclotorsion, are moved anteriorly and laterally to improve excyclotorsion.

39. Correct: She has just three trichiatic lashes scattered throughout both upper and lower eyelids (B)

In cases of sparse scattered trichiasis, radiofrequency is ideal because of its high success rate with multiple sessions and minimal collateral damage (unlike electrolysis or argon laser). (**A**) Having lighter skin pigmentation impacts cryotherapy choice, not radiofrequency epilation. The side effects of cryotherapy include edema, eyelid notching, and skin hypopigmentation (which is why you would avoid cryotherapy in a darker-skinned or appearance-conscious patient such as this). (**C**) A 4-mm segment of trichiasis is considered segmental trichiasis, which would not be a reason to choose radiofrequency epilation. In this scenario, cryotherapy via the double freeze–thaw technique or surgical resection with pentagonal resection could be considered. Radiofrequency could still be considered, but she is only in the country for a month and radiofrequency epilation typically requires multiple treatments, spaced by at least about 1 month. (**D**) Trichiasis that is diffusely through an eyelid should be reexamined to rule out entropion. This can be easy to miss; clues for diagnosis include a rounded eyelid margin (instead of the normal rectangular shape) and anterior migration of the mucocutaneous junction. If marginal entropion is the cause, tarsal fracture surgery can be considered. Otherwise, if eyelid position is normal, radiofrequency epilation, cryotherapy, or argon laser can also be considered.

40. Correct: A and B (D)

There are many options for fine facial lines, depending on their location, etiology, and skin type. (**A**) For example, hyaluronic acid is a naturally occurring substance that can be used to fill in wrinkles but should be used with caution in areas near vasculature due to a risk of vascular compromise/obstruction. These fillers are a temporary volumizer, which can last on average 6 months to a year, depending on the specific type of filler. Different fillers also have different properties in terms of firmness (known as G'), molecule size, and cross-linking with each of these having an effect on the ideal filler type for a location and purpose. Fillers for fine lines and wrinkles of the lower face would be one possible option for the patient in this question stem. (**B**) While fillers can be used on all skin types, CO_2 lasers are associated with a higher risk of hyperpigmentation in patients with a Fitzpatrick skin type of 3 and above (1 is very fair, always burns, can't tan; 2 is fair, usually burns, sometimes tans; 3 is sometimes burns, usually tans; 4 is olive, rarely burns, always tans; 5 brown/black, never burns, always tans). In an Irish patient, likely a Fitzpatrick 1 skin type, CO_2 laser would be a great option. (**C**) On the other hand, botulinum toxin works by preventing muscles from contracting, so use in the perioral fine wrinkles (smoker's lines) would likely result in the patient being unable to move her lips properly, possibly biting them, and drooling! Botulinum toxin can be used in the perioral area to improve a gummy smile or downturned oral commissures, but this should only be done very carefully.

41. Correct: Enucleation with 18-mm silicone implant (D)

There are two concerns in this patient. First, in a pediatric patient, enucleation may lead to underdevelopment of the surrounding bony orbit with secondary facial and eyelid asymmetry. Orbital soft-tissue volume is critical for orbital bone growth. The surgeon must select the technique that will replace the most orbital volume without undue tension on the wounds. The autogenous dermis-fat graft has been shown to grow and expand the orbit more symmetrically with the contralateral side. However, the second issue is that in the case of retinoblastoma, the dermis-fat graft (**C**) may mask a recurrence of tumor in the orbit, and for this reason it should be avoided. The next best option is thus to enucleate and place the largest synthetic sphere that can fit. (**A**) Without the description of extension through the sclera, exenteration is not indicated. (**B**) Evisceration is never indicated in retinoblastoma, as it disrupts the sclera and risks seeding the orbit with tumor.

42. Correct: Subperiosteal orbital floor implant OS (A)

This patient has a deep right superior sulcus after an enucleation and an implant that provided inadequate volume replacement. The surgeon can correct the deformity by increasing the orbital volume through placement of a subperiosteal secondary implant on the orbital floor to lift the spherical implant and orbital fat to better fill out the superior sulcus. Other options include replacing the original spherical implant with a larger one or with a dermis-fat graft or implanting fat into the upper eyelid. (**B**) The right upper brow may appear ptotic, but it is an illusion due to the deep superior sulcus. (**C**) The patient has the illusion of a high right superior eyelid skin fold, but it is secondary to the deep superior sulcus and the margin to reflex distance 1 is similar between the two eyes, so there is no blepharoptosis. (**D**) The left upper eyelid has a fuller appearance than the right, but the left eyelid is normal, and the real problem is the hollow right superior sulcus.

43. Correct: Ask him to come urgently to clinic (B)

After an enucleation, patients are typically sent for prosthesis fitting around postoperative week 6. It is critical that the conformer remain in place until the final prosthesis is made to avoid adhesion formation and contraction of the fornix. If the conformer falls out early, it should be reinserted expeditiously. Many patients can reinsert it themselves if they still have it; otherwise the surgeon should have the patient come in the same or next day to reinsert it for them if they don't feel comfortable or to replace it if it is lost. (**A**) While an appointment with the ocularist is appropriate at postoperative week 6, the conformer must be replaced immediately. (**C**) If the conformer stayed in place for a week after the tarsorrhaphy was removed, it is likely appropriately sized and just needs to be replaced. No surgery is needed for this procedure. (**D**) The conformer must be replaced right away. Lubrication alone is inadequate to prevent adhesions and contracture and waiting 2 more weeks is too long.

44. Correct: Fornix contracture (B)

The history of enucleation after a chemical injury raises concern for secondary socket contracture. After surgically opening the contracted tissue, an oral mucous membrane graft may be placed in the defect to expand the socket to accommodate a prosthesis. (**A**) Anophthalmic ptosis would be addressed with an external levator advancement or Muller's conjunctival resection surgery. (**C**) Deep superior fornix syndrome is treated with an orbital floor implant or orbital fat placed in the defect. (**D**) Although small implant exposures may be managed conservatively, when surgical correction is needed, it typically requires a tough tissue such as sclera, hard palate, or temporalis fascia. The implant may extrude again through the delicate oral mucous membrane.

45. Correct: Evisceration with acrylic sphere (B)

Evisceration will give the best motility since the extraocular muscles are left attached to the sclera, and there is less dissection within the orbit. (**A**) Enucleation with simple acrylic sphere will not achieve very good motility, since the muscles have been cut and not attached to the sphere or conjunctiva. (**C**) Enucleation with acrylic sphere wrapped in sclera and muscles attached will give good motility, but not as good as evisceration, since there is still disruption to the extraocular muscles and significant orbital dissection. (**D**) Enucleation separates the extraocular muscles from the globe, and although they can be sutured to the dermis-fat graft, the resulting motility will be less than is achievable with evisceration.

46. Correct: Improper conjunctival closure (D)

Conjunctival closure is important to create a completely mucosalized socket, and a meticulous conjunctival closure is important to avoid cyst formation. However, Tenon's closure (**C**) is more important for preventing implant extrusion. (**A**) An oversized implant is more likely to be pushed anteriorly and extrude. (**B**) While suturing the extraocular muscles over the implant, it may at first hold the implant back, if the muscles slip posteriorly, they may actually cause anterior migration of the implant. Alternatively, the muscles may be sutured to the implant itself or to sclera wrapped around the implant to prevent extrusion and provide better motility.

47. Correct: Reduced risk of sympathetic ophthalmia (D)

Theoretically, the risk of sympathetic ophthalmia is less with enucleation than evisceration since the globe is not disrupted in the former. (**A**) Evisceration leaves the muscles attached to the sclera, offering better motility than enucleation. (**B**) Evisceration is preferred by some surgeons for endophthalmitis, because extirpation and drainage of the ocular contents can occur without invasion of the orbit, reducing the risk of orbital cellulitis and intracranial spread of infection. (**C**) Evisceration does not sever the extraocular muscles, nerves, or fat. The relationship between the muscles, globe, eyelids, and fornices remains undisturbed.

48. Correct: Canalization of the nasolacrimal duct is usually complete around the time of birth (D)

Congenital nasolacrimal duct obstruction is clinically evident in only 2 to 6% of newborns around 1 month of age. (**A**) The nasolacrimal groove forms by the fifth week of gestation. (**B**) The canalicular system is an outgrowth of the lacrimal sac. (**C**) Caudally, the developing nasolacrimal duct exits in the inferior meatus. The middle meatus is the location of the osteotomy for a dacryocystorhinostomy surgery.

49. Correct: Normal lacrimal sac, scrolling anterior to posterior (A)

You should recognize the most commonly used imaging modalities and their important ocular structures. This is a coronal orbital CT scan in bone window. The bone window allows us to better examine the bony walls of the orbit than does the soft-tissue window. In this case, we can determine that the bony lacrimal sac fossa is intact (image a). (**B, D**) Post dacryocystorhinostomy, the coronal CT would show a bony defect in the middle meatus (image b). There is

no evidence of a dacryocystorhinostomy procedure. (**C**) The normal duct travels inferiorly, laterally, and posteriorly. Scrolling anteriorly from the lacrimal sac would scroll away from the duct and place it out of view. As you follow through the images, you will see in image a, the lacrimal sac, and in images b to d, sequentially more inferior segments of the lacrimal duct. Thus, we must be scrolling posteriorly, since each successive image shows a more inferior and lateral segment of the duct.

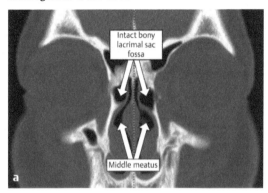

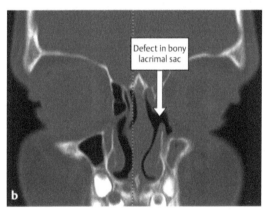

50. Correct: This condition can rarely be associated with life-threatening respiratory compromise (C)

Nasal extension of an enlarged lacrimal sac or dacryocystitis may secondarily obstruct the airway, particularly in infants who are obligate nose breathers in the first few months of life. This situation may necessitate urgent or even emergent surgery if the patient is in respiratory distress. (**A**) The obstruction is presumed to be at the level of the valve of Hasner. (**B**) Many of these cases will resolve with conservative measures including observation, lacrimal sac massage, and/or antibiotic eyedrops, while the others will require probing and possibly stenting. Dacryocystorhinostomy surgery is rarely required. (**D**) The vast majority of congenital nasolacrimal duct obstructions will resolve within the first year of life. The number often quoted is 90%.

51. Correct: 1 and 3 (D)

Jones I testing is considered physiologic. It is also called the primary dye test. The examiner instills fluorescein into the conjunctival fornices and recovers it in the inferior nasal meatus with a cotton-tipped applicator passed into the nose at 2 and 5 minutes. Dacryoscintigraphy is also considered physiologic. In this test, radionucleotide eyedrops are instilled in the fornix, and the natural flow of the drops in the lacrimal system is evaluated using a scintigram. (**A–C**) Jones II testing is considered nonphysiologic, as it determines the presence or absence of fluorescein in irrigating solution retrieved from the nose. The act of irrigating makes this nonphysiologic, since it may overcome a functional block and falsely suggest patency. The dacryocystogram is performed by irrigating dye into the lacrimal sac, and so again is nonphysiologic. After injection, the patient is scanned to evaluate the anatomy of the lacrimal drainage system.

52. Correct: Inferior meatus Hasner, common canaliculus Rosenmuller (C)

The upper and lower canaliculi originate at their respective puncta and travel vertically superiorly and inferiorly, respectively, for 2 mm, before turning 90 degrees to travel horizontally for 8 to 10 mm into the common canaliculus and then the lacrimal sac via the valve of Rosenmuller. The lacrimal sac measures 12 to 15 mm, emptying into the 12-to-18-mm-long nasolacrimal duct, which empties via the valve of Hasner into the inferior meatus.

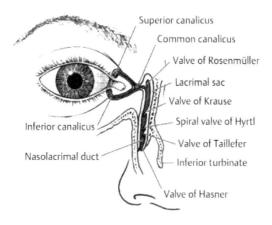

53. Correct: Maxillary and lacrimal (C)

The maxillary and lacrimal bones make up the lacrimal sac fossa, and these are the bones removed in dacryocystorhinostomy surgery. In the special circumstance of an agger nasi ethmoid air cell, a portion of the ethmoid may also be removed. As a reminder, the medial orbital wall is comprised of the ethmoid, lacrimal, maxillary, and lesser wing of the sphenoid bones.

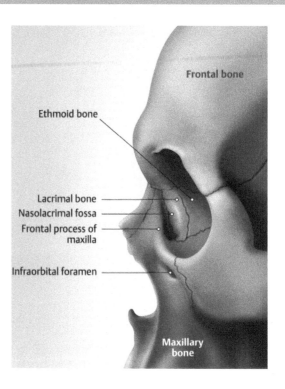

54. Correct: Incision and drainage (A)

Localized abscess of the lacrimal sac may require incision and drainage but usually only after failing more conservative measures such as oral antibiotics (**C**). However, full eye examination (**B**) and white cell count (**D**) are important to rule out orbital cellulitis that will require more aggressive antibiotic coverage and often inpatient admission.

55. Correct: CT orbits with contrast (A)

A 34-year-old man is an atypical demographic for acquired nasolacrimal duct obstruction. Tumor should be ruled out, and CT or MRI should be the next step. (**B**) An external DCR might be appropriate eventually but not before imaging to evaluate for tumor. (**C**) Although an endoscopic DCR can provide tissue for biopsy, the external DCR provides better exposure when there is concern for tumor. Regardless, no type of DCR should be performed before imaging in this case. (**D**) Contrast dacryocystography has fallen by the wayside since simple probing and irrigation provide similar information, and CT provides better information.

56. Correct: Biopsy, tumor excision, and adjuvant proton therapy (B)

This presentation is concerning for adenoid cystic carcinoma (ACC). The correct surgical first step is incisional biopsy to confirm the diagnosis of ACC histologically. Exenteration has failed to produce improvement in long-term survival rates, so the trend is now to perform globe-sparing surgery followed by high-dose radiation, such as proton therapy. (**A**) Pleomorphic adenoma (PA), on the other hand, is a benign tumor of the lacrimal gland that should not undergo incisional biopsy due to the risk of malignant transformation from that procedure. PA should be managed with excisional biopsy. ACC and PA are usually distinguishable based on the presence of pain in ACC but lack thereof in PA and duration of symptoms is less than 1 year for ACC but more than 1 year for PA. If there is diagnostic confusion between ACC and PA, then excisional biopsy should be considered. (**C**) Tissue confirmation should be obtained first, and the proton therapy is performed after the tumor is resected (adjuvant therapy) rather than before (neoadjuvant therapy). (**D**) The trend is toward globe-sparing surgery, since exenteration has not demonstrated improved survival. Adjuvant therapy should include high-dose radiation.

The patient's symptoms of right epiphora along with the abnormal right eye dye disappearance test (DDT) but normal irrigation test suggest a partially stenosed right lacrimal duct. This problem can be addressed with a balloon dacryoplasty, which dilates the stenosed nasolacrimal duct, followed by surgical intubation to keep it patent. (**A**) The patient is symptomatic and has an abnormal DDT, so she should be treated. (**C**) There is a functional blockage in this patient, and we know this since the physiologic DDT is abnormal, but the nonphysiologic irrigation test was normal. These test results suggest there is a functional blockage that can be overcome by the force of manual irrigation but not by the weaker physiologic tear pump mechanism. A dacryocystorhinostomy will not be needed at this time, since the nasolacrimal duct is not completely occluded. (**D**) The description of "reaching a hard stop" suggests the canaliculi are patent. The conjunctivodacryocystorhinostomy is intended to bypass obstructed canaliculi, which manifest with a soft stop on irrigation, so this procedure is not indicated.

The results of canalicular probing will reveal either a soft or a hard stop. A hard stop suggests no canalicular obstruction, making the blockage distal in the nasolacrimal duct. A soft stop suggests canalicular obstruction, and if irrigating fluid flushes from the contralateral punctum, then it is the common canaliculus that is obstructed. (**A**) Without additional information, you cannot tell exactly where the blockage is, as described above. (**B**) Although symptoms present since birth suggest an imperforate valve of Hasner, there are other possible causes, and so the duration of symptoms will not definitively indicate the location of the blockage. (**D**) While an MRI might be helpful in identifying a tumor in the duct, it may require sedation, and the probing test is a simpler and faster way to provide additional information.

This patient presents with canaliculitis; the definitive treatment of canaliculitis is a canaliculotomy; medical treatment alone is not typically curative. In most cases, no inciting event or abnormality is identified as the cause of dacryoliths, or concretions. (**B, C**) They may form less likely from infections with *Actinomyces israelii* or *Candida*. (**A**) Trauma may cause an obstruction that can predispose to dacryoliths, but this is rare.

This patient is presenting with signs and symptoms of infectious dacryoadenitis. Although acute noninfectious inflammation is the most common cause of dacryoadenitis, bacterial etiology is the most common cause of infectious dacryoadenitis; this is typically a gram-positive infection, though gram-negative infection is possible. (**B**) Epstein–Barr virus is the most common cause of viral dacryoadenitis, but overall it is less common than bacterial causes. (**C**) Tuberculous dacryoadenitis is rare. (**D**) There are rare case reports of adenoviral dacryoadenitis. Although not listed as an option, mumps is another common viral cause of dacryoadenitis.

This T1-weighted pre- and post-gadolinium MRI can demonstrate an optic nerve meningioma. The image characteristic of an optic nerve meningioma is a mass that appears within the optic nerve that is isointense to gray matter on T1- and T2-weighted imaging with enhancement that differs with the nonenhancing optic nerve. This gives rise to the "tram-track" sign, as seen here. Optic nerve gliomas are characterized on MRI by an enlarged optic nerve showing low T1 and high central T2 signal with variable enhancement (**A**). Cavernous hemangiomas can be located anywhere in the orbit yet are typically in the intraconal compartment. These are usually well-circumscribed with an oval shape. These are isointense to muscle on T1 and hyperintense compared with muscle on T2 with low-intensity septations (**C**). Orbital lymphoma typically presents in the superior lateral quadrant near the lacrimal gland. Given its highly cellular nature, the imaging characteristics are iso- to hypointense to muscle on T1 and iso- to hyperintense to muscle on T2. There is increased signal intensity on diffusion-weighted imaging with restricted diffusion (**D**).

The MRI shown in the figure is most consistent with an optic nerve glioma extending through the optic canal and abutting the chiasm. Pathology shows characteristic pleomorphic neoplastic astrocytes with Rosenthal fibers. These tumors usually present

165

in children and often occur in the setting of NF1, as known as von Recklinghausen disease. Other manifestations include café-au-lait spots, neurofibromas, iris hamartomas, and sphenoid wing dysplasia. von Hippel–Lindau disease is characterized by central nervous system and retinal hemangioblastomas, pheochromocytomas, increased risk of renal cell carcinoma, and pancreatic cysts (**B**). NF2 is characterized by vestibular schwannomas and spinal schwannomas, meningiomas, and ependymomas (**C**). Sturge–Weber syndrome is characterized by facial port-wine stains usually in the V1 distribution and pial angiomas. One-third of patients have choroidal or scleral angiomatous involvement (**D**).

63. Correct: The frontal sinus is the most common place for mucocele development to occur (D)

Approximately two-thirds of paranasal sinus mucoceles originate from the frontal sinus. They usually occur as a result of an obstruction of the ostium of a sinus due to trauma, inflammation, etc. with ensuing accumulation of mucus and expansion of the sinus. While chronic noninvasive fungal sinusitis has been associated with formation of mucoceles, the frontal sinus is most commonly affected with the ethmoid sinus being the second most common. The maxillary and sphenoid sinuses are rarely involved (**A**). It usually presents in adults, not children (**B**). CT imaging tends to be favored over MRI, as it allows for better bone visualization and identification of whether there has been bony resorption (**C**).

64. Correct: Proceed to the OR immediately for exploration and management of the entrapped fracture (A)

This vignette describes an entrapped or "trapdoor" orbital floor fracture. The oculocardiac reflex does not have to be present in order to diagnose an entrapped fracture. Further, a fracture is not always visible on CT scan. Therefore, one must have a high level of suspicion in a child with limited motility after trauma. When one is suspicious of an entrapped fracture, it is necessary to proceed to the OR as soon as possible for exploration and release of the entrapped fracture. It is not appropriate to anticipate that this will resolve on its own (**B**). A lateral canthotomy and cantholysis is not indicated in the absence of a retrobulbar hemorrhage with elevated IOP (**C**). The patient should not be sent home for reevaluation at a later date. Failure to release the entrapment in a time-sensitive manner can result in permanent ischemic injury to the inferior rectus muscle (**D**).

65. Correct: Repair should be performed under general anesthesia (B)

Repair of canalicular lacerations does not need to be performed under general anesthesia. Depending on patient cooperation and degree of the trauma, some canalicular lacerations can be performed in a minor procedure room with placement of a Mini Monoka stent. A complete ophthalmic examination, including a dilated examination is mandatory prior to any periocular repair to rule out any more serious trauma to the eye, such as an open globe, traumatic optic neuropathy, or intraocular hemorrhage (**A**). A stent should be left in place temporarily, typically anywhere from 2 to 6 months (**C**). While it is an optimal patient experience to repair the laceration as soon as possible, it remains possible to fix a canalicular laceration for several days (**D**).

66. Correct: Posterior lacrimal crest (D)

The medial canthal tendon supports the medial aspect of the eyelids and the canalicular system. In cases of medial canthal avulsion, it is most important to reattach the tendon to the posterior lacrimal crest where the posterior crura of the medial canthal tendon attaches. Reattachment to the anterior process of the maxilla, the anterior lacrimal crest (where the anterior crura of the medial canthal tendon attaches), and the lacrimal sac fossa (which exists between the anterior and posterior lacrimal crests and contains the lacrimal sac) is not indicated (**A–C**).

67. Correct: Elevated IOP, decreased vision (B)

In a patient presenting with a retrobulbar hemorrhage after trauma, the main indication for performing a lateral canthotomy and cantholysis is a markedly elevated intraocular pressure (IOP) with associated decrease in vision via compression of the optic nerve that impedes arterial perfusion. Limitations in upgaze and diplopia are not indications (**A, C, D**).

68. Correct: Hypoesthesia in the V2 distribution (C)

Although indications for repair of an orbital floor fracture are controversial, commonly followed guidelines include enophthalmos that exceeds 2 mm (**A**), diplopia in primary gaze with limitation in upgaze that persists for 2 weeks (**B**), and large fractures involving approximately 50% of the orbital floor (**D**). While hypoesthesia in the V2 distribution is common given that the infraorbital canal is often disrupted, it is not an indication for surgery. This hypoesthesia usually resolves in 3 to 6 months after the initial injury.

69. Correct: Within 2 weeks following the injury (B)

With the exception of an entrapped orbital floor fracture, most orbital floor fractures are repaired within 2 weeks of the initial trauma. This allows for enough time for the initial swelling to subside, yet before any scarring and fibrosis occur which would make surgery more difficult. By 6 weeks, there is some scarring of the prolapsed tissue which makes fracture repair more difficult, though still possible

(**A**). There is still swelling to content with at 1 to 3 days following injury (**C**). Repair within 24 hours is reserved for entrapped orbital floor fractures (**D**).

70. Correct: Represents the most common benign orbital tumor in adults (D)

Cavernous hemangiomas are the most common benign tumor in adults. Women are affected far more than men. Imaging via MRI usually shows a well-circumscribed round mass that contains small vascular channels. Pathology shows dilated vascular spaces lined by endothelial cells that are filled with blood and separated by connective tissue stroma. "Staghorn" vascular sinusoids are most consistent with a hemangiopericytoma (**A**). Cavernous hemangiomas typically present with slowly progressive proptosis, not significant pain that improves with steroids (**B**). Treatment consists of surgical excision if there is optic nerve compression. Capillary hemangiomas are sometimes treated with propranolol (**C**).

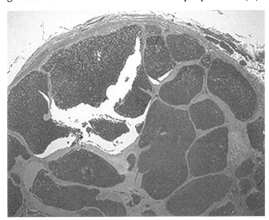

71. Correct: Alveolar (C)

This is a photograph of a patient with rhabdomyosarcoma, the most common primary orbital malignancy of childhood. Typically, children present with sudden onset and rapid progression of unilateral proptosis. Of the four subtypes, alveolar is the most malignant form with a 10-year survival rate of 10%. Botryoid is rare and typically presents primarily from the paranasal sinuses (**A**). Embryonal is the most common type, representing 80% of all cases. They are associated with an excellent survival rate (94%) (**B**). Pleomorphic is the least common and associated with the best prognosis (97%) (**D**).

72. Correct: Most commonly B-cell-associated (A)

The most common type of lymphoma in the orbit is non-Hodgkin's B-cell lymphoma, which accounts for 90% of orbital lymphoproliferative disease. T-cell lymphomas are rare and associated with a worse prognosis (**B**). There is a 20 to 30% chance of periocular lymphoproliferative lesions having a history of prior or concurrent systemic disease, with an additional 30% developing it over 5 years. Conjunctival lesions have the lowest risk of systemic involvement, orbital lesions have slightly higher risk, and eyelid lesions have the highest risk (**C**). Bilateral involvement increases the risk of systemic disease. About 50% of lymphoproliferative disease in the orbit resides in the lacrimal fossa (**D**).

73. Correct: Fresh (B)

If lymphoproliferative disease is on the differential, a portion of the biopsy should be sent fresh to allow for possible flow cytometry and polymerase chain reaction analysis (**B**). While formalin-fixed is appropriate for most diseases, it would not allow for molecular diagnostics in the case of lymphoproliferative disease, which helps more specific characterization (**A**). Frozen tissue may be sent intraoperatively to aid in diagnosis and management but should also be sent for fresh (**C**). Alcohol-fixed is not appropriate in this case.

74. Correct: Almost 90% survival when present in patients younger than 1 year (A)

This vignette is most consistent with a diagnosis of neuroblastoma. This usually presents with abrupt ecchymotic proptosis. On imaging, there can be evidence of bone destruction, especially in the lateral orbital wall or sphenoid marrow. The primary tumor is usually in the abdomen, mediastinum, or neck. When a patient presents younger than 1 year of age, the prognosis is significantly better than when he or she presents older than 1 year of age. It can be associated with opsoclonus–myoclonus, not ocular apraxia (**C**). Urine catecholamines (vanillylmandelic acid and homovanillic acid can aid in diagnosis (**D**). Treatment may include chemotherapy, immunotherapy, radiation, stem cell transplantation, and surgery. The goal of orbital surgery (typically performed after neoadjuvant medical therapy) is tumor excision, rather than debulking (**B**).

75. Correct: Refer for orbital radiotherapy (D)

This vignette is intended to describe a case of a lymphatic malformation, or lymphangioma. These lesions usually contain both venous and lymphatic components and may enlarge during upper respiratory tract infections. Spontaneous hemorrhage within the lesion can cause sudden proptosis and pain. Treatment is not straightforward, and may involve a few strategies. These include sclerotherapy with interventional radiology (**A**), observation with steroid therapy (**B**), and surgical debulking (**C**). Orbital radiotherapy is not considered a therapy (**D**).

76. Correct: Adenoid cystic carcinoma of the lacrimal gland (B)

A patient presenting with pain and a lacrimal fossa lesion with CT scan showing a poorly circumscribed lesion with bone destruction is most consistent

167

with adenoid cystic carcinoma, the most common malignant tumor of the lacrimal gland. Usually, this tumor presents rather rapidly, typically less than a year. Pain is a key feature of the presentation, differentiating it from pleomorphic adenoma. Pleomorphic adenoma presents as a progressive and painless lesion causing downward displacement of the globe. On imaging, the lesion looks well circumscribed with enlargement or expansion of the lacrimal fossa (**A**). Adenocarcinoma is a rare lacrimal gland neoplasm (**C**).Nonspecific orbital inflammation can present with pain but is rare to have bony destruction (**D**).

77. Correct: Epiphora (C)

Zygomaticomaxillary complex (ZMC) fractures, or tripod fractures, involve fracture of the zygoma at four of its sutures—the lateral orbital rim, the inferior orbital rim, the zygomatic arch, and the zygomaticomaxillary buttress. The lacrimal system is unaffected, therefore epiphora is not a common sequela of these fractures. ZMC fractures can be associated with trismus (limitation of mandibular opening) if the fractures impinge the coronoid process of the mandible (**A**). V2 hypoesthesia can develop, especially if the fracture involves the orbital floor (**B**). Significant lateral canthal dystopia is a reason for repair and can occur if there is significant displacement of the zygoma (**D**).

78. Correct: Breast (C)

The most common source of a primary tumor metastatic to the orbit in women is breast. Typically, orbital metastasis presents with pain, proptosis, inflammation, bone destruction, and early ophthalmoplegia. In 75% of cases, there is a positive history of known primary tumor. In 25% of cases, the primary tumor is unknown. The most common origin of orbital metastasis in men is the lung (**A**). Colon and melanoma are less common primary sources (**B, D**).

79. Correct: Has the potential of transforming into adenoid cystic carcinoma (D)

Pleomorphic adenoma, or benign mixed tumor, has the potential of transforming into a malignant mixed tumor over many years if the initial lesion was not completely excised or if there is violation of the pseudocapsule. It does not transform into adenoid cystic carcinoma. It is the most common benign epithelial neoplasm of the lacrimal gland (comprises 50% of epithelial tumors) (**A**). Excision should be performed to avoid rupture of the tumor's pseudocapsule so as to avoid future malignant transformation (**B**). It presents as gradual progressive proptosis with no associated pain (**C**).

80. Correct: History of tripping over a bush and falling on eye while running from police with evidence of air pockets in the orbit on CT scan (A)

A history of tripping over a bush and falling on the eye with air pockets visible on CT scan is suspicious for vegetative matter in the orbit. Vegetative matter poses a significant risk of infection in the orbit, and therefore exploration of the orbit should be performed as soon as possible. Vegetable matter is usually radiopaque, and therefore can be hard to detect on CT imaging. BB pellets are common intraorbital foreign bodies and are usually best left in place, unless they are easily accessible in the anterior orbit (**B**). Shards of shrapnel in the orbit can also be observed, especially if there are numerous fragments making complete removal difficult (**C**). A history of being ejected from the windshield after a car accident is suggestive of glass in the orbit. This can also be left in place as long as the rest of the examination is normal (**D**).

81. Correct: Involutional ectropion (C)

This patient has significant involutional eyelid changes that are likely contributing to her epiphora (**C**). Involutional ectropion occurs due to horizontal eyelid laxity. Patients frequently note epiphora, which is worse in the wind and cold. Tears often well up laterally (as opposed to medially as in nasolacrimal duct obstruction). An abnormal snap test (> 2 seconds) and distraction test (> 2mm) aid in diagnosis. Functional nasolacrimal duct obstruction is used to describe patients with tearing who have no apparent signs of nasolacrimal duct obstruction or eyelid malposition (**A**). Cicatricial ectropion (**B**) occurs due to shortening of the anterior lamella in the upper or lower eyelid following burns, trauma, chronic sun exposure, or from dermatologic conditions. In this case, the lower eyelid is well opposed to the globe, making ectropion unlikely. Involutional entropion (**D**) occurs due to horizontal eyelid laxity, overriding orbicularis muscle, and disinsertion of the lower eyelid retractors. In involutional entropion, the lid is noted to turn inward, which may cause abrasion of the corneal surface via the keratinized surface of the skin or eyelashes.

82. Correct: Involutional ectropion (B)

Involutional ectropion results from horizontal eyelid laxity and can therefore be repaired by horizontal eyelid shortening alone in the form of a lateral tarsal strip. In this procedure, the lateral canthal tendon is disinserted and a strip of tarsus fashioned and reattached at the lateral orbital tubercle (Whitnall's tubercle). The lateral orbital tubercle is the site of attachment for the lateral canthal tendon, the check ligament of the lateral rectus muscle, the suspensory ligament of Lockwood, and the levator palpebrae muscle (**B**). Cicatricial ectropion (**A**) occurs due to shortening of the anterior lamella in the upper or lower eyelid following burns, trauma, chronic sun exposure, or from dermatologic conditions. Cicatricial ectropion is generally treated by releasing the cicatrix, lengthening the anterior lamella with a skin graft or midface lift, and tightening the lid horizontally via a lateral tarsal strip procedure. Spastic entropion (**C**) occurs as a result of orbicularis contraction due to ocular irritation. It is treated by treating the underlying cause of the ocular irritation. Temporary treatment options include Quickert's suture placement, chemodenervation of the lower eyelid orbicularis muscle (botulinum toxin), and taping of the eyelid. Definitive surgical management includes reinsertion of the lower lid retractors, stripping of the overriding orbicularis, and horizontal tightening via a lateral tarsal strip. Mechanical ectropion (**D**) is frequently repaired via excision of the eyelid lesion.

83. Correct: Posterior lamellar scaring (B)

Involutional entropion generally occurs in the lower eyelid and is believed to occur due to a combination of horizontal eyelid laxity (**A**), overriding by the preseptal orbicularis (**C**), and disinsertion of the lower eyelid retractors (**D**). Cicatricial entropion is caused by posterior lamellar scaring (**B**).

84. Correct: Medial spindle procedure (D)

Involutional entropion is thought to result from a combination of horizontal eyelid laxity, overriding by the preseptal orbicularis, and disinsertion of the lower eyelid retractors. Permanent surgical correction of this condition generally addresses these three conditions via horizontal eyelid tightening, reinsertion of the lower eyelid retractors, and stripping of the overriding orbicularis. Temporary treatment options are indicated in cases of corneal decompensation until definitive surgery can be performed. Some temporary treatment options include (**A**) chemodenervation of the lower lid orbicularis, (**B**) Quickert's sutures, and (**C**) eyelid taping. The medial spindle procedure is used in cases of ectropion with punctal eversion.

85. Correct: Epicanthus tarsalis—the fold is most prominent in the upper eyelid (B)

Epicanthus is a term used to describe a congenital anomaly in which the medial canthal fold is present. Four types of epicanthus are described: (1) epicanthus tarsalis in which the medial canthal fold is more prominent in the upper eyelid, (2) epicanthus inversus in which the medial canthal fold is more prominent in the lower eyelid, (3) epicanthus palpebralis in which the medial canthal fold is equally distributed in the upper and lower eyelid, and (4) epicanthus supraciliaris in which the fold arises from the eyebrow region running to the lacrimal sac.

86. Correct: The child should be observed and followed carefully for any signs of corneal decompensation (B)

In epiblepharon, the lower lid lashes are verticalized due to the lower eyelid pretarsal muscle overriding the lower eyelid margin. (**A**) A skin and muscle flap should be excised in the area of the misdirected lashes in order to prevent corneal decompensation in rare cases in which epiblepharon results in corneal decompensation. In the majority of cases, the lashes do not touch the cornea except in downgaze, and there is no corneal staining. In these cases (**B**), the child should be observed and followed carefully for any signs of corneal breakdown. Lash epilation (**C**) is not a viable long-term option, as lashes will regrow, and when short, it may cause worsened keratopathy. (**D**) Lateral tarsal strip with reinsertion of the lower eyelid retractors should be performed in cases of involutional ectropion to correct horizontal and vertical laxity.

87. Correct: Christmas tree cataract (B)

Floppy eyelid syndrome is a condition in which the upper lids are loose and easily everted. Other findings include chronic papillary conjunctivitis of the upper lid and a rubbery appearance of the tarsus. Patients may complain of eye irritation and mucous discharge. Obstructive sleep apnea (**A**), keratoconus (**C**), and obesity (**D**) are associated with floppy eyelid syndrome. A Christmas tree cataract is a highly reflective, often multicolored, needle-shaped cataract, which may be idiopathic or associated with myotonic dystrophy.

88. Correct: Trichotillomania (C)

(**A**) Sebaceous cell carcinoma is a highly malignant tumor that arises from sebaceous cells (meibomian glands, glands of Zeis, sebaceous glands of caruncle). Loss of lashes may be seen, but the disease occurs more frequently in patients over the age of 50. The eyelid skin would not appear normal in sebaceous cell carcinoma. (**B**) Thyroid eye disease is an autoimmune disease, which is characterized by eyelid retraction, lid lag, proptosis, restrictive strabismus, and compressive optic neuropathy. While more frequently associated with Graves' disease and hyperthyroidism, it may also occur in Hashimoto's thyroiditis and hypothyroidism. Hypothyroidism has been associated with hair thinning and lash loss, but in this young girl with other psychological symptoms and lashes in different stages of regrowth, trichotillomania is the more likely diagnosis. (**C**) Trichotillomania is frequently seen in young girls and is considered an impulse control disorder characterized by the inability to refrain from pulling out hairs. Eyebrow hairs and eyelashes of different lengths may be seen. Treatment options include psychotherapy and psychotropic medication. (**D**) Merkel cell carcinoma is a rare and highly malignant eyelid lesion that presents as a painless, erythematous nodule with overlying telangiectatic blood vessels. While it may be associated with madarosis, it is most frequently seen in White people aged 60 to 80.

89. Correct: Autosomal dominant (B)

Blepharophimosis syndrome is an autosomal dominant (**B**) eyelid syndrome characterized by telecanthus, epicanthus inversus, and ptosis. The condition is associated with premature ovarian failure. Therefore, females with blepharophimosis syndrome should be referred to endocrinology.

90. Correct: Incision and curettage (B)

A chalazion is a result of focal inflammation due to obstruction of a meibomian gland. Chalazia are more common in patients with acne rosacea. In the acute phase, warm compresses and eyelid hygiene are indicated. Use of oral trimethoprim–sulfamethoxazole (**A**) is not indicated, as the cause of this condition is thought to be inflammatory rather than infectious. Doxycycline or tetracycline may be used in the long-term treatment of meibomian gland dysfunction for its anti-inflammatory benefits. A chronic chalazion may require surgical incision and curettage in order to clear the inflammation when conservative management has failed. As chalazia are due to chronic inflammation and are not infectious in origin, (**C**) topical antibiotic drops are unlikely to be curative. While acne rosacea and any other blepharitis are associated with dry eye syndrome due to poor meibomian gland dysfunction, a chalazion is unlikely to resolve with artificial tears (**D**).

91. Correct: Swelling (A)

Eyelid swelling is a nonspecific sign and may be associated with infection, inflammation, or orbital processes. Ulcerating eyelid lesions (**B**), madarosis (**C**), and destruction of normal eyelid margin architecture (**D**) are some clinical signs suggesting eyelid malignancy.

92. Correct: Incisional biopsy for diagnosis (C)

This lesion likely represents a basal cell carcinoma (BCC). BCC is the most common eyelid malignancy. Patients with fair skin, sun exposure, and smoking history are at higher risk of developing BCC. Diagnosis

is made via incisional biopsy. BCC originates from the stratum basale of the epidermis. On histopathology, the nodular form demonstrates nests of basal cells and may show peripheral palisading (see figure below). The morpheaform type appears as thin chords with proliferation of connective tissue. Once the diagnosis is confirmed via incisional biopsy, treatment is with excisional biopsy (often by a Mohs surgeon) and reconstruction of the lid (often by an oculoplastic surgeon). Observation (**A**), warm compresses and lid massage (**B**), and intralesional steroid injection (**D**) are not appropriate, as this is a malignant lesion that requires definitive surgical treatment.

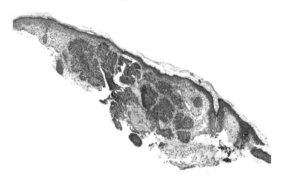

93. Correct: Excisional biopsy is frequently all that is required (D)

Sebaceous adenocarcinoma is a highly malignant and aggressive neoplasm arising from the meibomian glands, glands of Zeiss, or sebaceous glands of the caruncle, or oil glands of the face. It is most frequently seen in the upper eyelid and occurs more commonly in the Asian Indian population. This tumor may be mistaken for a chalazion or blepharitis and occurs more frequently in women and in the upper lid. Intraepidermal growth in the lid and conjunctiva and skip areas make complete excision difficult. Wide surgical excision with map biopsies of the conjunctiva should be performed, as there are frequently skip areas and pagetoid spread. Special stains, such as oil red o, are used to stain for lipids. (**A**) Cryotherapy may be employed in cases of local invasion, and orbital exenteration may be considered in cases of orbital extension (**B**) Metastasis is frequently to regional lymph nodes, so sentinel lymph node biopsy is considered for patients with eyelid sebaceous cell adenocarcinoma (**C**) Lymph node biopsy provides information regarding prognosis and need for further systemic treatment. Because of its tendency for skip areas and pagetoid spread, excisional biopsy (**D**) is frequently insufficient.

94. Correct: Primary cutaneous melanoma of the eyelid is relatively common, accounting for approximately half of eyelid malignancies (A)

While cutaneous melanoma accounts for approximately 5% of cutaneous malignancies, primary cutaneous melanoma of the eyelid is rare, accounting for less than 0.1% of eyelid malignancies (**B**). Lentigo maligna melanoma, nodular melanoma, superficial spreading melanoma, and acral lentiginous melanoma are the four types of cutaneous melanoma (**C**). Thin lesions (< 0.75 mm in depth) have a high 5-year survival rate (98%) (**D**), while the survival rate for lesions greater than 4 mm in depth with ulceration is less than 50%. Unlike conjunctival melanomas, in which excisional rather than incisional biopsy should be performed in order to prevent tumor seeding, incisional biopsy of eyelid lesions does not increase the risk of metastasis. Incisional biopsy should be performed through the center of the lesion in order to determine an accurate depth. In melanomatous lesions greater than 1.5 mm, a metastatic work-up is indicated. Regional lymph node biopsy is suggested in lesions that show lymphatic or vascular invasion, or thickness greater than 1 mm.

---

95. Correct: The presence of orbital fat in the wound indicates the orbital septum has been violated, and the wound should be carefully explored for signs of foreign bodies and copiously irrigated. The orbital septum should not be sutured, but the overlying orbicularis and skin should be closed (C)

Eyelid lacerations that do not involve the margin or canalicular system should be carefully explored for signs of foreign bodies, irrigated, and repaired. The presence of orbital fat indicates that the septum has been violated (**B**). The orbital septum should not be repaired surgically, as this may lead to eyelid retraction (**A**). The overlying orbicularis and eyelid skin should be repaired meticulously. Long lacerations, as in this case, should be repaired and not be left to heal by secondary intension (**D**).

---

96. Correct: The patient should immediately receive systemic antibiotics and tetanus vaccine; the eyelid vaccine should be copiously irrigated and repaired (A)

In dog and human bites, the patient should immediately receive systemic antibiotics, tetanus vaccine, copious irrigation, and repair of the eyelid laceration. Surgical repair should not be delayed (**D**). The eyelid margin is repaired with at least two marginal vertical mattress sutures, one through the gray line and one through the meibomian gland orifice line (tarsal plate), with attention to eversion of the eyelid margin. An additional interrupted stitch is placed through the lash line. These sutures may be permanent (example: silk) or absorbable (example: Vicryl). Absorbable sutures should be used in children or in adults in whom poor follow-up is expected (**C**). Partial-thickness tarsal bites should be taken below the margin to prevent corneal decompensation by sutures rubbing on the cornea (**B**).

---

97. Correct: A free tarsoconjunctival graft from the opposite upper eyelid is used to reconstruct the posterior lamella of the lower eyelid, and a skin graft is used to reconstruct the anterior lamella of the upper eyelid (C)

In general, two free grafts can be placed next to each other, but not layered on top of the other, as there is significant probability of necrosis. In eyelid reconstruction, either the anterior or the posterior lamella may be reconstructed with a free graft (but not both). Therefore, in a large lower eyelid defect involving more than 50% of the lower eyelid, a tarsoconjunctival flap with either a free skin graft (**A**) or a skin (or skin-muscle) flap (**B**) are viable options. Alternatively, a free tarsoconjunctival graft from the opposite upper eyelid may be used, however, this graft must be combined with an advancement flap (**D**), rather than a free skin graft (**C**).

---

98. Correct: Primary closure of the defect with superior crus lateral cantholysis if necessary (C)

Small defects of the upper eyelid (< 33% of the upper eyelid) can usually be repaired via direct closure. If there is excessive tension with direct closure, a superior crus lateral cantholysis can be combined with this procedure (**C**). A full-thickness lower eyelid advancement flap (Cutler–Beard procedure) is employed in large upper eyelid defects (> 50% of the upper eyelid) (**A**). A smaller defect such as this would not typically require free grafts. Other important concepts regarding surgical options B and D are as follows: in eyelid reconstruction, either the anterior or the posterior lamella can be reconstructed with a free graft (but not both) (**B**). A tarsoconjunctival flap from the upper lid with a free postauricular skin graft can be used to reconstruct a lower eyelid defect. However, a tarsoconjunctival flap cannot be fashioned from a lower eyelid as the lower eyelid tarsus measures only 4 mm in vertical height, as opposed to 10 to 12 mm of vertical height in the upper eyelid, and therefore there is insufficient lower lid tarsal tissue for a tarsoconjunctival flap (**D**).

---

99. Correct: Forehead or glabellar flap (D)

The medial canthal region may be a challenging area to reconstruct. If the defect is small, healing by secondary intention (**A**) and undermining with direct closure (**C**) are viable options. Free skin grafts can be used in small- or medium-sized defects without significant depth (**B**). However, large defects extending onto the nasal bridge often require the use of a forehead or glabellar flap. These flaps tend to be cosmetically inferior due to their thickness. A second-stage procedure is required in a forehead flap. Additionally, the thickness of the flap makes early recurrence of tumor difficult to detect.

100. Correct: Gonioscopy (C)

The medial canthal tendon splits into two crura, which envelope the lacrimal sac. The anterior crus originates at the frontal process of the maxillary bone, and the posterior crus originates at the lacrimal bone. In cases of suspected medial canthal evulsion, it is important to assess the canalicular system via dilation and probing of puncta with irrigation (**A**). Medial canthal rounding is frequently seen with medial canthal avulsion (**B**). Careful assessment of the medial canthal tendon integrity can be performed by grasping the lid with toothed forceps and tugging away from the injury while palpating the insertion of the tendon (**D**). In this case, the patient's intraocular pressure and anterior eye examination are normal, therefore, gonioscopy is not critical at this time.

Chapter 6

Pediatric Ophthalmology and Strabismus

Sylvia H. Yoo, Allison R. Loh, Catherine S. Choi, Michelle Trager Cabrera, Maanasa Indaram, Euna B. Koo

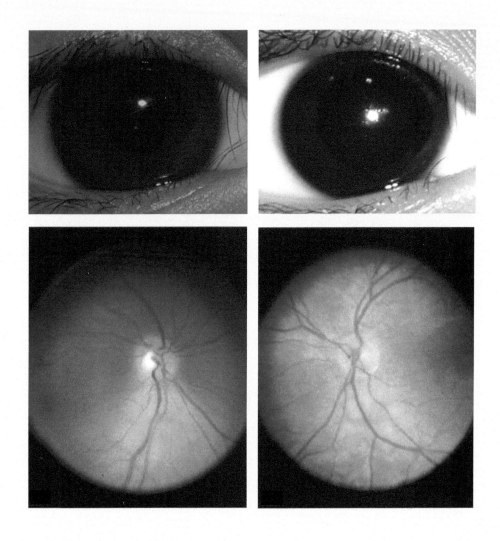

6.1 Questions

Easy	Medium	Hard

1. A 2-year-old girl presents for strabismus evaluation. The child has prominent epicanthal folds and is diagnosed with pseudostrabismus. On dilated fundoscopic examination, the optic nerves are found to have a cup-to-disc ratio of 0.6 in both eyes with otherwise normal appearance. The intraocular pressures are normal, and corneas are clear with normal corneal diameters. What component of the patient's medical history is most consistent with her examination findings?

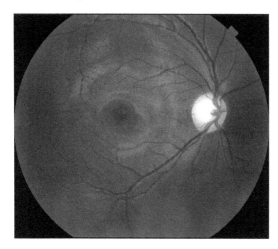

A. The child was born at 42 weeks and required resuscitation for less than 1 minute at birth due to meconium aspiration and was subsequently discharged after 48 hours.

B. There is a family history of glaucoma, and this child has infantile glaucoma.

C. The child was born at 28 weeks and had a history of intraventricular hemorrhage.

D. The child was born full term and was hospitalized at 3 weeks of age for fever when sepsis was ruled out.

2. A 5-year-old girl is referred for an eye examination due to a failed vision screening at school. The school form from the nurse's office states that the child has failed stereopsis testing. Why the testing of fusion and stereoacuity should be performed first during the eye examination?

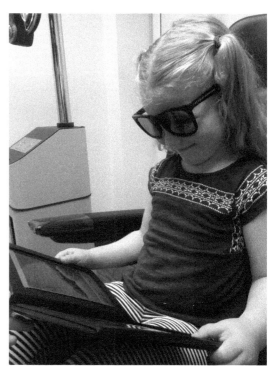

A. Testing of visual acuity and cover testing for strabismus may dissociate a patient with tenuous stereoacuity and underestimate the patient's fusion.

B. Stereoacuity testing is the only part of the examination that needs to be assessed with accuracy because of the reason for the referral.

C. Stereoacuity testing is the most engaging part of the examination for a child.

D. Strabismus measurements will be inaccurate if done prior to stereoacuity testing.

3. When evaluating the visual acuity of a preverbal infant, CSM (central, steady, and maintained) is one method of characterizing a patient's fixation behavior. Which section of this method is tested under binocular conditions?

A. Steady

B. Central and maintained

C. Maintained

D. All three sections

4. A 12-year-old healthy girl with nystagmus is reported by the technician to have decreased visual acuity of each eye compared to last year's examination. You recheck the visual acuity and find that it is actually unchanged. The remainder of the examination is stable, and there have been no new concerns voiced by her or her family. What is a potential explanation for this discrepancy in visual acuity at the same visit?

A. Technician checked vision only under binocular conditions.

B. You used a high plus power lens to blur the fellow eye during testing.

C. Technician used preverbal optotypes (i.e., Teller cards, matching optotypes).

D. You used optotypes with crowding bars.

5. A 10-year-old boy being treated for attention deficit disorder is referred to the eye clinic for concerns about difficulty with reading. He tells you that he needs glasses. Cycloplegic retinoscopy reveals +0.75 D of hyperopia in both eyes. What diagnostic testing can be done to determine if glasses may be helpful for the patient?

A. Assess visual acuity at near before dilation.

B. Refer the patient for comprehensive neuropsychological testing.

C. Dynamic retinoscopy.

D. No further testing is needed as he does not need glasses.

6. A 4-year-old girl with anisometropic amblyopia is not tolerating treatment of amblyopia with patching therapy. Atropine 1.0% as an eyedrop is suggested as an alternative treatment option for amblyopia. The child's father inquires about possible side effects of the drop. Which one of the following would you inform him?

A. There are no adverse effects of atropine if given as an eyedrop.

B. Possible side effects include fever, dry mouth, flushing of the face, tachycardia, delirium, and dizziness.

C. If severe adverse effects occur, accidental ingestion should be considered, and the child should be taken to the emergency room for evaluation and possible treatment with physostigmine.

D. Both B and C.

7. A 20-year-old woman is referred for a complete eye examination due to a history of strabismus. She states that she has a history of "infantile esotropia" and underwent strabismus surgery at 2 years of age. What was the likely age of onset of this patient's strabismus?

A. Two years old.

B. Less than 12 months of age.

C. Less than 6 months of age.

D. The age of onset cannot be determined.

8. A 2-year-old girl is referred to your office from the emergency room for vomiting and development of a new left head turn. She is esotropic in primary gaze. An MRI of the brain done in the emergency room shows a mass in the left pons. What other examination findings may be present?

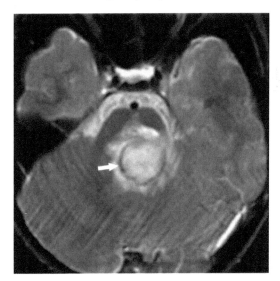

A. Incomitant esotropia that is larger in right gaze

B. A large secondary esotropia with fixation of the left eye

C. Limitation of adduction in the right eye

D. Limitation of abduction in the right eye

9. A 56-year-old woman presents with a long-standing alternating exotropia. She states that she had eye surgery in childhood to straighten the eyes but does not recall the type of strabismus she had. She has no history of diplopia. She also had pterygium excision surgery in both eyes 5 years ago. External and slit lamp examinations show conjunctival scarring both nasally and temporally in both eyes. What intraoperative finding would confirm the diagnosis of consecutive exotropia?

A. Lateral rectus muscles found to be inserted 14.5 mm posterior to the limbus

B. Medial rectus muscles found to be inserted 5.5 mm posterior to the limbus

C. Medial rectus muscles found to be inserted 12 mm posterior to the limbus

D. Lateral rectus muscles found to be inserted 7 mm posterior to the limbus

10. The insertions of which muscles comprise the spiral of Tillaux in order of proximity to the limbus (closest to farthest)?

A. Medial rectus, inferior rectus, superior rectus, lateral rectus

B. Inferior rectus, medial rectus, superior rectus, lateral rectus

C. Medial rectus, inferior rectus, lateral rectus, superior rectus

D. Inferior rectus, medial rectus, lateral rectus, superior rectus

11. Which of the following are correct statements about the anatomy of the extraocular muscles?

A. The superior rectus forms a 51-degree angle with the visual axis; the tertiary action of the superior oblique is abduction; the superior oblique passes inferior to the superior rectus muscle.

B. The superior rectus forms a 23-degree angle with the visual axis; the tertiary action of the superior oblique is abduction; the superior oblique passes inferior to the superior rectus muscle.

C. The superior rectus forms a 23-degree angle with the visual axis; the tertiary action of the superior oblique is depression; the superior oblique passes inferior to the superior rectus muscle.

D. The superior rectus forms a 23-degree angle with the visual axis; the tertiary action of the superior oblique is depression; the superior oblique passes superior to the superior rectus muscle.

12. How many bellies can the inferior oblique muscle have?

A. One

B. Two

C. Three

D. All of the above

13. A 62-year-old man presents with a large right exotropia following endoscopic ethmoid sinus surgery. He has −5 limitation of adduction of the right eye and is diplopic. What is the primary limiting factor to surgically improving the eye alignment?

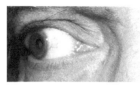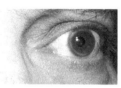

A. The medial rectus muscle cannot be identified on imaging due to the presence of blood and scar tissue.

B. The medial rectus muscle has no direct anatomic relationships with other extraocular muscles.

C. Only the lateral rectus has a direct anatomic relationship with the inferior oblique muscle.

D. The superior oblique muscle is composed of tendon anteriorly.

14. Which arterial branches give rise to the anterior ciliary arteries?

A. The lateral and medial muscular branches

B. The lacrimal artery

C. The infraorbital artery

D. The vortex artery

15. A 63-year-old woman undergoes strabismus surgery, including left inferior rectus muscle recession, for thyroid ophthalmopathy, which is causing diplopia. A large recession is required to resolve the diplopia in primary gaze. The patient should be made aware of what potential postoperative finding?

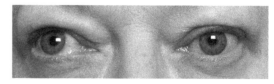

A. A persistent but comitant strabismus

B. Severe inflammation of the anterior segment

C. Left lower lid retraction and change in the palpebral fissure

D. Left lower lid elevation and change in the palpebral fissure

16. In the first year of life, the dimensions of the eye undergo rapid changes including which of the following?

A. Decrease in axial length

B. Flattening of keratometry

C. Thickening of the cornea

D. Increase in crystalline lens power

17. Based on the natural history of the refractive state in early childhood, how can you counsel the family on a 6-year-old boy with a refractive error of +0.25 D?

A. The refractive error will not change as the child gets older.

B. The child may become significantly more hyperopic as he gets older.

C. The child may become myopic as he gets older.

D. The future refractive state of the child cannot be predicted.

18. Which eye movement findings are normal in a 3-month-old infant?

A. Constant strabismus

B. Elevation deficit

C. Adduction deficit

D. Nystagmus

19. By what age is visual acuity estimated to reach 20/20?

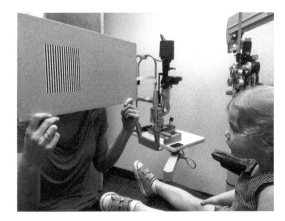

A. By 6 to 7 months of age based on visually evoked potential (VEP) studies

B. By 3 to 5 years of age based on method illustrated in the figure

C. By 6 to 7 years of age based on optotype testing

D. Both A and B

20. A 4-year-old girl presents with an anomalous head position and history of strabismus surgery for a right superior oblique paresis. You confirm the diagnosis on your examination. Her mother states that the head tilt initially improved after surgery but has recurred and worsened. She does all activities, including running, with a large left head tilt. Intraoperatively, forced ductions reveal 4+ tightness of the right inferior oblique and 1+ laxity of the right superior oblique. You identify the right inferior oblique inserted 2 mm posterior to the right inferior rectus insertion. What surgical procedure should be performed for this patient at this time to improve the head position?

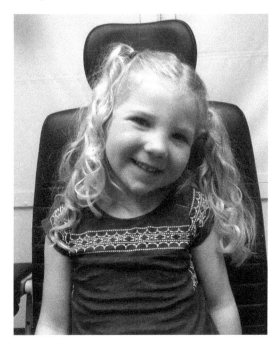

A. Further recess the right inferior oblique muscle.

B. Advance the right inferior oblique to the original insertion.

C. Recess the right inferior rectus muscle to the level of the current inferior oblique insertion.

D. Perform denervation and extirpation of the right inferior oblique muscle.

21. A 23-year-old woman with a history of infantile esotropia and strabismus surgery in early childhood presents to discuss treatment options for her eyes, which frequently drift up and out. Visual acuity is 20/25 in both eyes. On examination, you find a large left dissociated vertical deviation (DVD) that manifests without occlusion, as well as a small right DVD that is only evident with occlusion. There is 2+ inferior oblique overaction of both eyes. What surgical treatment would you recommend?

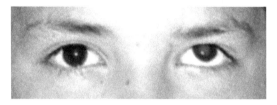

A. Left superior rectus muscle recession
B. Left inferior oblique muscle recession and anteriorization
C. Bilateral inferior oblique muscle anteriorization
D. Right inferior oblique muscle recession and anteriorization

22. A 9-year-old boy presents with high accommodative convergence-to-accommodation (AC/A) ratio esotropia (diagnosed when he was 2 years old) as mother would like a second opinion. She is concerned about whether he still needs his glasses. He appears to be orthotropic in his glasses. How would you counsel the mother?

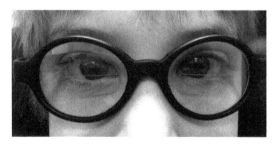

A. Proceed with strabismus surgery with posterior fixation sutures or bilateral medial rectus muscle recessions.
B. If the child is orthotropic in bifocals and tolerates spectacle wear, no change in management recommended.
C. Promptly discontinue his glasses as he is older now.
D. Convergence exercises.

23. A 79-year-old woman presents with oblique diplopia at distance and is found to have a 30Δ esotropia and 14Δ right hypertropia. Motility is full in both eyes. Torsion is detected neither on the fundus examination nor with double Maddox rod. Neuroimaging is normal. She strongly prefers that surgery only be done on one eye and that she can continue to wear glasses for reading only. What is the best surgical option for this patient?

A. Right medial rectus muscle recession, right lateral rectus muscle resection, right superior rectus muscle recession.
B. Inform the patient that bilateral medial rectus muscle recession is the only treatment option, and she will need prism glasses after surgery.
C. Right medial rectus muscle recession, right lateral rectus muscle resection with infraplacement of the muscles.
D. Right medial rectus muscle recession, right lateral rectus muscle plication, right superior rectus muscle recession.

24. A 20-year-old man presents with exotropia and undergoes strabismus surgery with bilateral lateral rectus muscle recessions. At postoperative week 1, the patient has a small esophoria in primary gaze. He complains of intermittent diplopia and would like to know what can be done about the diplopia. What do you tell him?

A. One of the risks of strabismus surgery is diplopia, of which he was informed preoperatively and nothing can be done to improve the diplopia at this time.
B. One of the risks of strabismus surgery is diplopia, but in his case, the diplopia will likely improve over time, and monitoring is recommended.
C. Prism glasses or a temporary prism will negatively affect the long-term outcome of the surgery and is not recommended.
D. Repeat surgery is recommended at this time.

25. A 12-year-old boy undergoes strabismus surgery using a fornix incision for intermittent exotropia. At postoperative week 1, the patient is brought to the eye clinic for redness, tearing, irritation, and mild lid edema of both eyes. He does not complain of pain. Visual acuity is unchanged, slit lamp examination demonstrates clear corneas, quiet anterior chamber, and fundus examination is normal. What is the likely etiology of the findings?

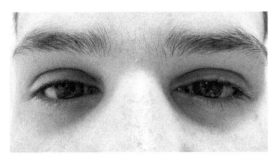

A. Allergy to the sutures

B. Dellen formation

C. Endophthalmitis

D. Severe conjunctival scarring

26. An 8-year-old boy undergoes strabismus surgery for esotropia. Intraoperatively, the patient's cardiopulmonary monitor shows the following. What should be done next?

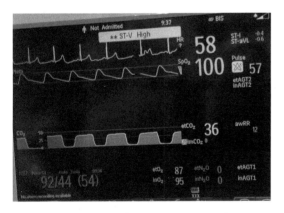

A. Cancel the surgery for the patient to undergo a full cardiac work-up.

B. Ask the anesthesiologist to administer an antiemetic medication.

C. Pause the surgery until the heart rate normalizes.

D. Proceed with the surgery uninterrupted.

27. A 34-year-old woman presents with intermittent esotropia of 12Δ associated with diplopia. She demonstrates excellent stereopsis at near. Motility is full in both eyes with good visual acuity and normal dilated fundus examination. She strongly prefers not to undergo incisional strabismus surgery and does not want to wear glasses. She asks if botulinum toxin can be used as a treatment alternative. What do you tell the patient about this treatment option?

A. Risks of the procedure include ptosis, overcorrection, development of vertical strabismus after injection of a horizontal muscle, all of which are permanent.

B. Scleral perforation is not a risk of this procedure, as it is with incisional surgery.

C. Repeated injections may be needed, but the injected muscle may lengthen while it is paralyzed and provide long-term improvement of alignment.

D. Only incisional surgery is recommended at this time.

28. A 4-year old girl presents with esotropia of 40 prism diopters at near and 20 prism diopters at distance with visual acuity of 20/60 in the right eye and 20/30 in the left eye. Motility is full. Cycloplegic refraction is +4.00 +3.00 × 90 in the right eye and +3 in the left eye. Eye examination is otherwise unremarkable including dilated fundus examination. Which one would be the most important recommended next step?

A. Brain MRI

B. Plano sphere +3.00 add bifocals

C. Patching

D. Full cycloplegic refraction

29. A 6-year-old boy presents with a diagnosis of strabismic amblyopia and 40 prism diopters of esotropia at distance and 40 prism diopters of esotropia at near. Visual acuity is 20/20 in the right eye and 20/200 in the left eye with no improvement in spite of 6 h/d patching for 2 years. Cycloplegic refraction is +1.00 in each eye. You obtain an optic nerve optical coherence tomography (OCT) of the left eye which reveals an optic nerve diameter of 400 μm. Which of the following would be appropriate next step?

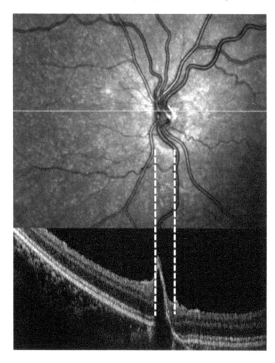

A. Full cycloplegic refraction
B. Bifocals
C. Endocrine consult
D. Resume patching 6 h/d

30. In a child with septo-optic dysplasia, a brain MRI is likely to show which of the following findings?

A. Abnormal decussation of the optic nerve fibers
B. Absent septum pellucidum
C. Optic nerve glioma
D. Basal encephalocele

31. A child with severe optic nerve hypoplasia of the left eye presents with 40 prism diopters of esotropia at distance and near and visual acuity of 20/20 in the right eye and 20/200 in the left eye. What surgical intervention would be recommended to address the strabismus?

A. Left medial rectus recession, left lateral rectus resection, because the left eye is the amblyopic eye and would therefore minimize risk.
B. Right medial rectus recession, right lateral rectus resection, because the right eye is the functioning eye therefore it is most likely to benefit from surgery.
C. Bilateral lateral rectus recession.
D. Strabismus surgery is unlikely to be beneficial in a case of unilateral optic nerve hypoplasia.

32. A 2-year-old girl presents with esotropia since birth with a small left face turn. Her nine cardinal positions of gaze are shown in the figure. Which of the following is true about this child's condition?

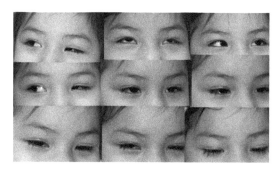

A. She likely has a small exotropia in right gaze.
B. She likely has poor fusion.
C. Her right cranial nerve VI nucleus is likely absent.
D. Her left cranial nerve III nucleus is firing during left gaze.

33. An 11-year-old otherwise healthy boy presents with 2 years of progressive ptosis of the left upper eyelid with a left hypotropia of 30 prism diopters and now ptosis of the right upper eyelid. He has a −3 supraduction deficit of the left eye and −1 supraduction deficit of the right eye. Pupils are equal. His findings do not fluctuate, his myasthenia panel is negative, and a rest test is negative. An MRI of the brain and orbit is unremarkable and a trial of high-dose corticosteroids does not improve his signs or symptoms. What do you consider the most reasonable next step?

A. Cerebral angiogram
B. Plasmapheresis
C. Electrocardiogram
D. Thyroid function tests

34. An 18-month old boy presents to your clinic with the following strabismus examination and another pertinent clinical examination finding. He has symmetric mild proptosis consistent with shallow orbits. What is likely true about this patient?

	XT 30	
XT 20	XT 20	XT 20
	XT 10	

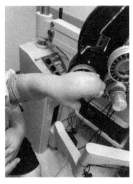

A. He has Crouzon's syndrome with associated craniosynostosis and syndactyly.

B. He has significant risk of optic nerve coloboma.

C. Elevated intracranial pressure is unlikely to result in papilledema.

D. He has a V-pattern strabismus due to rotated configuration of his extraocular muscles within his orbits.

35. A 6-year-old boy presented with 1 month of the left eye turning inward along with a face turn to the right. He had an upper respiratory infection prior to onset of the ocular symptoms. On his sensorimotor examination, he had 20 to 25 prism diopters of esotropia in primary gaze at near with 30 prism diopters of esotropia at distance. He had a −2 to −3 abduction deficit of the right eye. His optic nerves had cupping 0.55 on the right and 0.7 on the left with no pallor or edema. Intraocular pressures were normal. His brain MRI is shown in the figure. What is likely to be true about this patient?

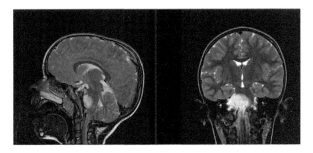

A. He likely had a left cranial nerve VI palsy due to a brain tumor.

B. He likely had an acute acquired comitant esotropia.

C. He likely had a viral cranial nerve VI palsy of the right eye.

D. He likely had a right cranial nerve VI palsy due to a brain tumor.

36. A 24-year-old woman with long-standing esotropia presents with crossed diplopia. You perform cover testing and identify 30 prism diopters of esotropia. The afterimage test results are shown in the figure part A. Which of the following is true about this patient?

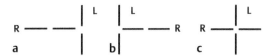

A. This patient has harmonious anomalous retinal correspondence.

B. This patient has paradoxical diplopia.

C. This patient has a dragged macula.

D. This patient has a pseudofovea located temporal to the actual fovea.

37. Among images shown in figure parts A to C, what likely represents what a healthy 3-month-old infant sees?

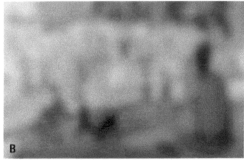

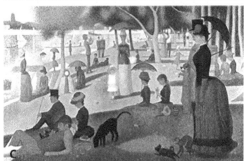

A. Image A.

B. Image B.

C. Image C.

D. The estimated vision of a 3-month-old infant is not known.

38. A 6-month-old ex-27-week gestational age male infant presents with exotropia. He had been screened for retinopathy of prematurity while in the neonatal intensive care unit, however, failed communication between the neonatal intensive care unit staff and the ophthalmology office led to his being lost to follow-up. Though no movement is seen on alternate cover testing with excellent fixation, he has 35 prism diopters of exotropia based on the Krimsky testing. Dilated fundus examination of the left eye is shown in the figure. (courtesy of Francine Baran, MD). Which of the following is most accurate about this patient?

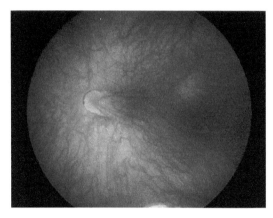

A. This patient has anomalous retinal correspondence.

B. This patient has eccentric fixation.

C. This patient has a positive angle kappa.

D. This patient has exotropia.

39. A 10-year-old boy underwent bilateral medial rectus recession when he was 1-year-old. He now presents with 5 prism diopters of constant esotropia. Visual acuity is 20/20 in the right eye and 20/25 in the left eye, and worth four dot testing at near is shown in part A of the figure and worth four dot testing at distance is shown in part B of the figure. What is most likely to be true about this patient?

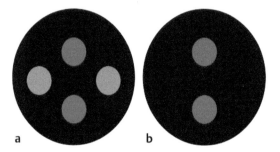

A. This patient has absent stereopsis.

B. This patient would benefit from strabismus surgery.

C. This patient has a suppression scotoma in monocular viewing conditions.

D. This patient has partial stereopsis.

40. A 9-month-old male infant with trisomy 21 presents with torticollis is shown in the figure. What would be an appropriate test to perform on this patient to confirm a congenital cranial nerve IV palsy?

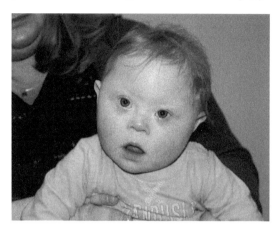

A. Double Maddox rod

B. 4 prism diopter base-out test

C. Hirschberg's test in right head tilt

D. Single Maddox rod in left gaze

41. A 7-year-old boy presents to your clinic with intermittent exotropia of 35 prism diopters at distance and orthophoria at near. You perform a 60-minute patch test to maximally dissociate his eyes. Immediately after removing the patch, you begin to perform alternate cover testing at near. What result would most closely correspond with tenacious proximal fusion?

A. 35 prism diopters of exophoria.

B. Orthophoria.

C. 15 prism diopters of esotropia.

D. This test cannot diagnose tenacious proximal fusion.

42. A 2-year-old girl is poorly cooperative in the clinic and will not tolerate cover testing; however, her parents are convinced that she crosses her eyes. Looking at her picture in the figure, what would you say is most likely true about this patient?

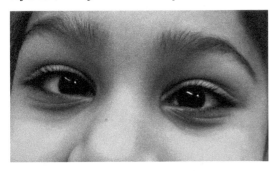

A. Pseudoesotropia only

B. Esotropia

C. Esophoria

D. Exotropia

43. A 4-year-old girl is undergoing evaluation for strabismus surgery. Her nine cardinal positions of gaze are shown in the figure. What surgical options would be most appropriate?

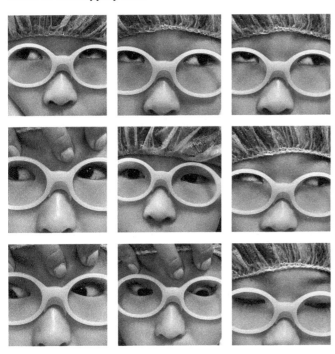

A. Left lateral rectus recession and left medial rectus resection with bilateral superior oblique tenotomies

B. Bilateral lateral rectus recession with inferior transposition

C. Bilateral medial rectus recession with inferior transposition

D. Right lateral rectus recession and right medial rectus resection with bilateral inferior oblique myectomies

44. A 10-year-old girl presents to your clinic with poor vision since birth and a previous diagnosis of optic nerve hypoplasia. She underwent bilateral medial rectus muscle recessions at 1 year of age for infantile esotropia. On examination, her visual acuity is 2/400 in each eye with a large angle jerk nystagmus. The optic nerve appears normally sized, and the fundus examination is unremarkable. The electroretinogram is shown in the figure. Which of the following is likely associated with this child's symptoms?

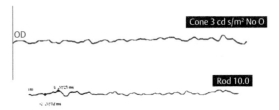

A. Optic nerve telangiectasias

B. Hypopituitarism

C. Autosomal recessive inheritance

D. Progressive external ophthalmoplegia

45. A 3-year-old ex-25-week premature infant has been diagnosed with retinopathy of prematurity, infantile exotropia, and blindness. He has never undergone retinal surgery or laser. Parents state that he has never been able to see since birth. Patient is alert and interactive. His visual acuity appears to be light perception only with either eye. Fundus examination is unremarkable in both eyes with normally sized optic nerves, and nystagmus is absent. His optical coherence tomography (OCT) is shown in the figure. Which of the following is the most likely diagnosis?

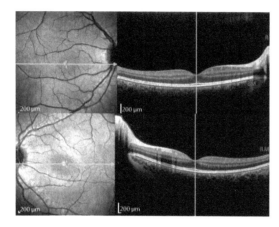

A. Cortical visual impairment

B. Optic nerve hypoplasia

C. Stage V retinopathy of prematurity

D. Leber's congenital amaurosis

46. A 3-year-old boy with no significant family history of blindness has been diagnosed with Usher's syndrome based on sensorineural deafness and vestibular abnormalities. His visual acuity is 20/40 binocularly using Allen optotypes, but he does not tolerate monocular testing. He has an intermittent exotropia of 30 prism diopters, and his fundus examination is unremarkable. His cycloplegic refraction is +1.00 sphere in each eye. He has no nystagmus. Which of the following would be a reasonable next step for diagnostic testing?

A. Double Maddox rod

B. Genetic testing

C. Brain CT

D. Fluorescein angiogram

47. A 2-month-old infant presents to your clinic with absent fix and follow response as well as intermittent, variable exotropia. His examination is unremarkable except for variable exotropia with a normal dilated fundus examination and absence of nystagmus. The infant fixes and follow your face but no toys or other objects. At what age would you consider obtaining additional work-up if vision does not improve?

A. Now

B. 3 to 5 months old

C. 6 to 9 months old

D. 3 to 4 years old

48. A 2-year-old girl presents with "abnormal movements" of her eyes since birth. Which of the following features distinguishes congenital motor nystagmus from fusion maldevelopment nystagmus syndrome (aka latent nystagmus)?

A. Nystagmus reverses direction depending on which eye is occluded.

B. There is a null point with corresponding head posture.

C. Nystagmus increases with an optokinetic nystagmus (OKN) drum moving in the opposite direction to the fast phase.

D. The velocity of the slow phase exponentially increases with distance from fixation.

49. A 6-month-old infant presents with bilateral, horizontal nystagmus and normal-appearing anterior and posterior segment examination. Pupillary examination revealed the findings shown in the figure. What other testing may aid in the diagnosis?

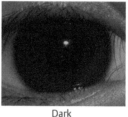

Dark   Light

A. Fluorescein angiography (FA)

B. Electroretinogram (ERG)

C. Magnetic resonance imaging (MRI)

D. Urine test for homovanillic acid (HVA) and vanillylmandelic acid (VMA)

50. A 15-month-old child presents to you with a small amplitude, high-frequency binocular nystagmus present for the past 6 months, right head tilt, and head nodding when attempting to follow a target. What would be an appropriate next step in management?

A. Baclofen

B. Eye muscle surgery

C. Urine test for homovanillic acid (HVA) and vanillylmandelic acid (VMA)

D. MRI neuroimaging

51. Which of the following is uncommon in patients with infantile esotropia with cross-fixation?

A. Amblyopia

B. Inferior oblique overaction

C. Dissociative vertical deviation

D. Latent nystagmus

52. A rambunctious 3-year-old boy presents to your clinic with a 25Δ comitant esotropia. Cycloplegic refraction was limited but showed roughly +3.00 diopters of hyperopic error in both eyes. The full hyperopic error was prescribed, and the patient returned for follow-up with good compliance. However, he continues to demonstrate 12Δ of intermittent esotropia. What would be the next step in his management?

A. Bilateral medial rectus recessions

B. Bilateral lateral rectus recessions

C. Repeat cycloplegic refraction

D. Alternate patching with close follow-up

53. A 4-year-old girl with accommodative esotropia presents for follow-up. With her +4.50 D lenses on, she has a 20Δ alternating esotropia. When she takes her glasses off, the deviation increases to a 45Δ esotropia. Repeat cycloplegic refraction reveals that she is wearing her full hyperopic correction. What would be the next step in her management?

A. Bilateral medial rectus recession 3.5 mm

B. Bilateral medial rectus recession 5.5 mm

C. Bilateral lateral rectus recession 5 mm

D. Bilateral lateral rectus resection 7 mm

54. Two weeks after bilateral medial rectus muscle recession surgery, a patient's parent urgently sends you the following picture of his eyes. On examination, there is significantly limited adduction of the right eye. Forced ductions were intact. Which of the following is the most likely diagnosis?

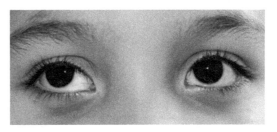

A. Anterior segment ischemia

B. Slipped muscle

C. Adherence syndrome

D. Consecutive exotropia

55. A 7-year-old boy comes to your clinic with his parents who report that occasionally his eye "drifts out" when he is tired. On your sensorimotor examination, he has the following findings: X(T) 45Δ and X(T)' 15Δ. The near deviation remains the same with a +3.00 lens but increases to X(T)' 37Δ after 1 hour of monocular occlusion. What is the diagnosis?

A. Intermittent exotropia with convergence insufficiency

B. Intermittent exotropia with true divergence excess

C. Intermittent exotropia with tenacious proximal fusion

D. Intermittent exotropia with a high accommodative convergence to accommodation (AC/A) ratio

56. Which of the following is not typically utilized in the management of intermittent exotropia?

A. Orthoptic exercises

B. Overminus glasses

C. Alternate patching

D. Base-out prisms ground into spectacles

57. Which of the following is the most common pattern of strabismus in patients with craniosynostosis?

A. A-pattern exotropia

B. V-pattern exotropia

C. A-pattern esotropia

D. V-pattern esotropia

58. A 9-year-old boy presents with the following examination. Forced duction testing in the office was noted to be negative in both eyes. Which of the following would be the best initial surgical option?

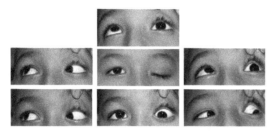

A. Left superior rectus recession

B. Left inferior rectus recession

C. Left frontalis sling surgery

D. Left medial rectus and lateral rectus superior transposition

59. A 4-year-old girl presents with the following examination. Which of the following is the most likely diagnosis?

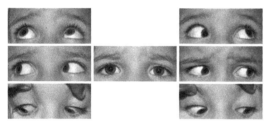

A. Brown's syndrome

B. Superior oblique palsy

C. Monocular elevation deficiency

D. Superior rectus palsy

60. You have been following a 5-year-old male patient who presents with the following motility examination since infancy. He has excellent stereoacuity with a compensatory head posture. Which of the following is his most likely head posture?

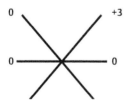 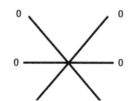

A. Right head tilt

B. Left head tilt

C. Right face turn

D. Chin down

61. A 65-year-old woman presents with left hypotropia and the following CT findings. Which of the following tests would most likely be abnormal in this patient?

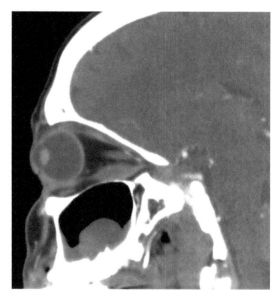

A. Complete blood count

B. Liver function tests

C. Thyroid function tests

D. Bone marrow biopsy

62. Which of the following is the most appropriate management for a patient with type I Duane's syndrome who is orthotropic in primary gaze but esotropic in left gaze?

A. Observation

B. Left medial rectus recession and lateral rectus resection

C. Left superior rectus lateral transposition and medial rectus recession

D. Right superior rectus lateral transposition and medial rectus recession

63. Which of the following is not a characteristic of Moebius' syndrome?

A. Inability to smile

B. Absent pectoralis muscle

C. Deficiency of upgaze

D. Limited horizontal motility

64. A 50-year-old woman presents with bilateral ptosis and limitation of movement of both eyes in all directions. She notes that she has had this problem since birth and it has been stable since then. Forced duction testing was positive for restriction. Which of the following is the most likely diagnosis?

A. Chronic progressive external ophthalmoplegia (CPEO)

B. Congenital fibrosis syndrome

C. Thyroid eye disease

D. Myasthenia gravis

65. A 6-year-old boy presents with a swollen right eyelid for the past 2 days. His mother does not recall any inciting factors such as blunt trauma or insect bites. What finding on examination would make you concerned for orbital cellulitis?

A. Conjunctival swelling and injection

B. Warmth and erythema of the eyelid

C. Tense eyelid

D. Decreased ocular motility

66. An 8-year-old boy who presents with mild erythema of the periorbital region with normal vision, intraocular pressure, color vision, pupils, and motility has been started on a course of oral Augmentin for presumed preseptal cellulitis.

A. His clinical appearance worsens over the next couple of days, and he now reports worsening pain with eye movement. What would be the next step?Switch to oral clindamycin.

B. Switch to oral cephalexin.

C. Add oral vancomycin for presumed methicillin-resistant *Staphylococcus aureus*.

D. Send to ER for CT scan.

67. A 6-month-old male infant presents urgently to your office because he has had sudden swelling and erythema of skin inferior to the medial canthus in his left eye. There is also tearing and some mucoid discharge in the affected eye. The child has also been running a low-grade fever at home. What do you suggest next for management of this patient?

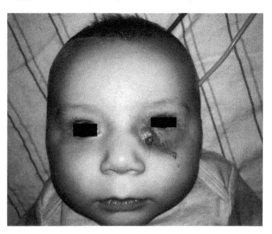

A. Treatment with oral antibiotics

B. Hospital admission for IV antibiotics

C. Immediate nasolacrimal duct probing and irrigation

D. Dacryocystorhinostomy

68. A 3-year-old girl was diagnosed with juvenile rheumatoid arthritis 3 months ago after having a couple of episodes of right knee pain and swelling. Blood testing reveals rheumatoid factor negative (RF−), antinuclear antibody positive (ANA+). No other joints have been affected. The pediatric rheumatologist has started her on Naprosyn. She has no ocular irritation or injection. How often should she undergo slit lamp examinations to rule out uveitis?

A. Every 3 months

B. Every 6 months

C. Every 6 months, sooner with ocular irritation or injection

D. Once a year

69. A 5-year-old girl with antinuclear antibody positive (ANA+) and juvenile idiopathic arthritis (JIA) oligoarthritis presents for her 3-month follow-up for uveitis screening. She is asymptomatic. What is the most likely type of uveitis in her condition?

A. Vitritis

B. Retinitis

C. Nongranulomatous anterior uveitis

D. Mutton-fat keratic precipitates

70. A 7-year-old girl is transferred to your clinic after moving from out of state. She is 5-foot 6 inches in height and has very long, slender extremities. She is wearing extremely thick glasses. Her slit lamp examination reveals bilateral lens subluxation superotemporally. Genetic testing will reveal an anomaly on what chromosome?

A. 11

B. 15

C. 17

D. 22

71. You evaluate a patient for the first time who has superotemporal lens subluxation of both eyes. In addition to genetic testing, what is the most important diagnostic testing this patient should undergo next?

A. Complete blood count

B. Stress test

C. Echocardiogram

D. Spirometry

72. A 10-year-old boy suffered blunt trauma to his right eye with a Nerf gun while playing at home. He presents to the emergency room, and slit lamp examination reveals a 1-mm layered hyphema with 4+ red blood cells in the anterior chamber and mild corneal edema of the affected eye. What should be part of the initial evaluation?

A. Dilated fundus examination

B. Intraocular pressure measurement

C. Fluorescein staining of the cornea

D. All of the above

73. You have diagnosed an 8-year-old African American boy with a traumatic hyphema. His intraocular pressure in the affected eye is measured to be 28 mm Hg, and that in the unaffected eye is 16 mm Hg. In addition to treating the elevated intraocular pressure, which of the following laboratory tests is recommended in this patient?

A. Beta-thalassemia testing

B. Rapid plasma reagin

C. Antinuclear antibody titers

D. Sickle cell screen

74. An 11-month-old male infant with a strong family history of a genetic condition presents for an evaluation because his mom has noticed drooping of his left upper eyelid for the past 3 months. He demonstrates normal and equal vision with each eye tested individually. He has a margin to reflex distance 1 of 4.5 mm on the right and 2.0 mm on the left. He has mild proptosis of the left eye with moderate resistance to retropulsion. There are no palpable masses of the periorbital region. Anterior segment and dilated fundus examination are unremarkable in either eye. Cycloplegic retinoscopy reveals moderate anisometropia. He has multiple flat, pigmented skin lesions on his trunk and extremities. An MRI of the orbits is ordered to further evaluate the proptosis, and the T1-weighted scan with fat suppression is depicted in the image . What is the next step in management?

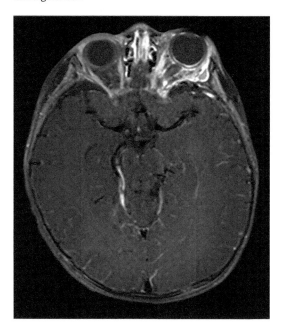

A. Close observation

B. Orbital biopsy

C. Orbital debulking

D. Enucleation

75. A 22-year-old man is diagnosed with vestibular schwannomas while being worked up for progressive hearing loss and tinnitus. A referral to genetics is placed. What chromosomal mutation is most likely to be found in his condition, and what is the most common mode of inheritance?

A. Chromosome 17, autosomal dominant

B. Chromosome 17, autosomal recessive

C. Chromosome 22, autosomal dominant

D. Chromosome 22, autosomal recessive

76. What is the appropriate management of a child with mild tearing secondary to bilateral epiblepharon causing trichiasis but no corneal or conjunctival abrasions?

E. Close observation

F. Lubrication eyedrops every 2 hours

G. Quickert's suture repair

H. Orbicularis muscle stripping surgery

77. The pediatric inpatient team consults you for a 3-month-old female infant who was admitted after being found unresponsive at home. Her dilated fundus examination is illustrated in the figures. What is the mortality rate of a child with this diagnosis?

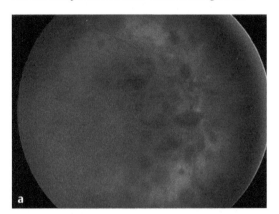

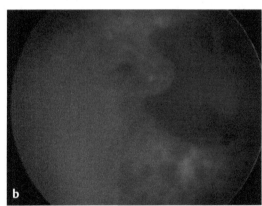

A. 5%

B. 30%

C. 50%

D. 70%

78. An 8-month-old female infant presents with a lesion on the right upper eyelid. Her mother has noticed the bump on the central right upper eyelid for the past several months. Warm compresses and lid hygiene are recommended. After 3 months, her mother returns reporting no change in the lesion. Tissue is sent for pathology at the time of incision and drainage of this presumed chalazion. The pathology slide is shown in the figure. What is the next step in management?

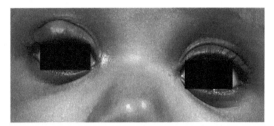

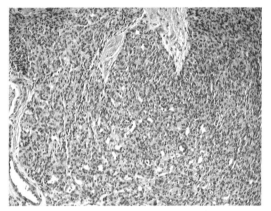

A. Steroid injection

B. Surgical debulking of lesion

C. Topical timolol ointment

D. Systemic propranolol

79. An 11-year-old boy presents urgently to clinic with history of blunt trauma to his left eye while on the trampoline. There was no loss of consciousness. On examination, he has a normal external examination, visual acuities, intraocular pressures, and unremarkable anterior segment and fundus examinations. The motility examination is challenging, as he reports reproducible eye pain and nausea when trying to elevate the left eye and refuses to cooperate with the motility examination. What is the next best step in evaluation?

A. Observation

B. Orbital imaging

C. Concussion work-up

D. Empiric treatment of pain and nausea

80. A 6-year-old girl is referred to your office for evaluation of discoloration of her left upper eyelid. On examination, she has mild edema of her eyelid with moderate ecchymosis and 2+ ptosis of the left upper eyelid. She has normal visual acuities, intraocular pressures, anterior segment examination, and fundus examination. Motility is full in both eyes, and she does not complain of any ocular pain or discomfort. Parents deny witnessing any recent trauma to the eye. There are no palpable masses in the periorbital region. She does not have any bruises on the remainder of her body, and she has not been more fatigued than usual. What is the next best step in her work-up?

A. Observation.

B. Orbital imaging.

C. Start oral antibiotics.

D. Obtain complete blood count.

81. A 14-year-old adolescent boy presents to your office with history of seizures and developmental delay. On initial glance at the patient, you notice that he has multiple hypopigmented macules on his extremities and what appears to be severe facial acne. What is the most likely finding on his ocular examination?

A. Retinal coloboma

B. Astrocytic hamartoma

C. Myelinated nerve fiber layer

D. Lisch nodules

82. What is the most common genetic mode of inheritance for tuberous sclerosis?

A. Autosomal dominant

B. Autosomal recessive

C. X-linked dominant

D. Sporadic

83. A 5-year-old girl with history of chronic kidney disease is referred for significant light sensitivity. Her best corrected visual acuity is 20/25 with both eyes. Slit lamp examination reveals significant iridescent corneal crystals in both eyes . The posterior examination is limited by her inability to cooperate given significant photophobia, but brief views of the fundus reveal a grossly normal posterior pole in both eyes. Which of the following is the best potential treatment to offer her?

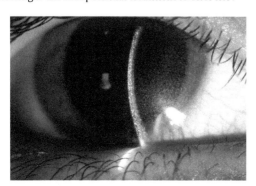

A. Oral cysteamine

B. Topical cysteamine every hour

C. Deep anterior lamellar keratoplasty

D. Serum copper and ceruloplasmin test

84. A 10-year-old boy is referred to your clinic by an optometrist for irregular pupils. His past medical history is significant for developmental delay, short stature, and umbilical hernia repair. On examination, his is vision is 20/60 in the right and 20/40 in the left eye with his −6.00 +4.00 × 113 OU glasses. His eye pressure is 32- and 35 mm Hg in the right and left eye, respectively, by Icare. His anterior segment examination is shown in the figure. Which gene mutation is identified with this disorder?

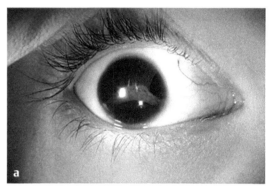

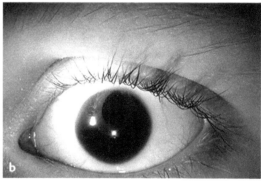

A. PITX2

B. PAX6

C. ACTA2

D. IKBG (previously NEMO) gene

85. A 5-year-old girl presents to your clinic with a "white bump" on her left eye, which has been present since birth. Her local optometrist has been treating her with glasses (+0.25 plano OD; −1.00 +4.00 × 65 OS) and patching. Her family is interested in surgical removal of the lesion. They also note that she has had a head tilt her entire life. On examination, her best corrected visual acuity is 20/20 and 20/25 with her right and left eye, respectively. Given the diagnosis of her corneal lesion and its most common associated type of strabismus, what would you expect on sensorimotor examination?

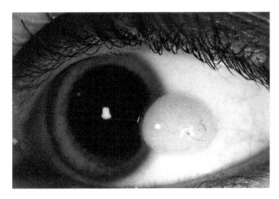

A. Chin-up position and small right head turn

B. Left head turn

C. Right head tilt

D. Left head tilt

86. A 10-year-old healthy child with a past medical history of skin rash 2 years ago presents with anisocoria. Mom reports that the anisocoria is more obvious when the child is watching television and less noticeable when reading his tablet. On examination, vision is 20/20 OU. The anterior segment is normal. Under lighted conditions, the right eye pupil measures 5 mm in diameter and left pupil 3 mm; in dim light, the right pupil is 6 mm and the left pupil is 5.5 mm. Based on the history and examination, what would you expect the results of your testing to be?

A. No testing; physiologic.

B. After 0.01% pilocarpine instillation OU, OD 2 mm and OS 3 mm.

C. After apraclonidine instillation OU, OD 3 mm OS 4.5 mm.

D. MRIs of brain, neck, chest, and abdomen reveal neuroblastoma.

87. A 4-week-old newborn is referred to you for port-wine stain involving the right face including the right upper and lower eyelids. Visual behavior is deemed appropriate with either eye occluded. Intraocular pressure is 30 mm Hg in the right eye and 12 mm Hg in the left eye. The anterior segment is notable for a corneal diameter on the right of 12 mm and 10 mm on the left. The posterior examination is shown in the figure. Her intraocular pressure of the right eye remains elevated on maximum glaucoma medications. The decision is made to provide glaucoma surgery. Because of her syndrome, what particular surgical complication is she at risk for?

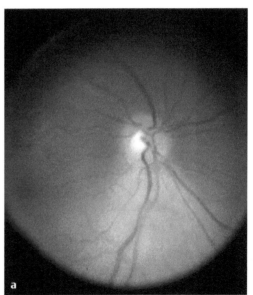

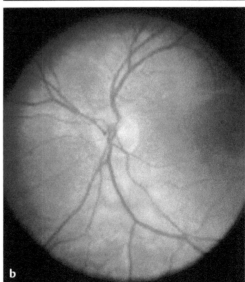

A. Intraoperative or postoperative exudation or hemorrhage

B. Difficult intraoperative visibility due to shallow anterior chamber

C. Robust postoperative inflammation

D. Endophthalmitis

88. Primary congenital glaucoma (PCG) is the most common nonacquired glaucoma of childhood. It most commonly presents in the first year of life. What constitutes the classic clinical triad of PCG?

A. Epiphora, photophobia, blepharospasm

B. Epiphora, photophobia, buphthalmos

C. Blurry vision, photophobia, blepharospasm

D. Epiblepharon, blepharospasm, buphthalmos

89. A 1-year-old boy with unilateral buphthalmos and elevated intraocular pressure (IOP) is scheduled for his examination under anesthesia and likely goniotomy in 1 week. You want to start him on topical drops to lower the IOP as much as possible to keep the cornea clear for surgery and prevent further glaucomatous damage. Which medication should be avoided in this child?

A. Betaxolol

B. Dorzolamide

C. Pilocarpine

D. Brimonidine

90. You are called to the NICU to examine this 1-week old newborn baby. The nurses have not placed any dilating drops. Careful screening must be performed to rule out which of the following systemic diseases?

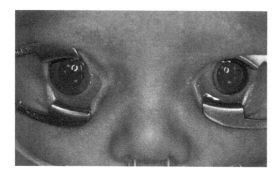

A. Retinoblastoma

B. Wilms' tumor

C. Pheochromocytoma

D. Rhabdomyosarcoma

91. A 12-year-old girl is referred for progressive myopia by her optometrist. She is 20/30 OU in −5.00 sphere glasses. Her intraocular pressure is 27 mm Hg OD and 26 mm Hg OS. Her anterior segment examination is normal. Her posterior examination is normal except for 0.7 cup to disc ratio of bilateral optic nerves. Her father had surgery as a teenager for "high eye pressures" and is doing reportedly well, although he admits he has not been evaluated by an eye care provider in 5 years. The genetics of this child's eye condition is most likely which of the following?

A. Autosomal dominant, *CLC1A/myocilin gene*

B. Autosomal recessive, *CYP1B1*

C. X-linked, *PITX2*

D. Autosomal dominant, *FOXC1*

92. What are the most common risk factors for developing glaucoma following cataract surgery?

A. Microcornea and early age of cataract surgery

B. Microcornea and pseudophakia

C. Microcornea and aphakia

D. Aphakia and family history of glaucoma

93. A 4-year-old boy referred for failed vision screen presents to the clinic for his first eye examination. Uncorrected visual acuity is 20/400 and 20/30 in the right and left eye, respectively. He has a small anterior polar cataract in the right eye. His examination is otherwise structurally normal. His refraction is +4.00 +2.50 × 90 in the right eye and +1.00 in the left eye. What is the most appropriate next step in the management of his condition?

A. Cataract surgery with an intraocular lens placement in the right eye

B. Amblyopia therapy with glasses and patching

C. TORCH laboratory screening

D. MRI brain and orbit scan

94. A 1-year-old boy had bilateral cataract surgery at age 3 months for dense nuclear cataracts. He has not tolerated contact lenses and parents elect for spectacles. His cycloplegic refraction is +18.00 +0.50 × 90 OD and +17.00 + 1.00 × 90 OS. What is the appropriate glasses Rx for him?

A. +20.00 × +0.50 × 90 OD and +19.00 +1.00 × 90 OS

B. +18.00 +0.50 × 90 OD and +17.00 + 1.00 × 90 OS

C. +16.00 +0.50 × 90 OD and +15.00 + 1.00 × 90 OS

D. +18.00 OD and +17.00 OS

95. Which of the following is a risk factor for developing uveitis in juvenile idiopathic arthritis (JIA)?

A. Oligoarthritis

B. Old age of onset of arthritis

C. Antinuclear antibody (ANA) negative

D. Rheumatoid factor (RF) positive

96. A neonate is born at 31 weeks 3 days weighing 1,453 g. The NICU would like to know when the next eye examination should be scheduled. What would be the most appropriate time frame?

A. Does not need follow-up; born after 30 weeks.

B. Needs follow-up; examination as soon as possible as baby is born after 30 weeks.

C. Needs follow-up; examination in 1 month.

D. Needs follow-up; examination in 2 weeks.

97. A 13-year-old adolescent girl is referred by her pediatrician after a failed vision screen. She is a refugee and has not received any health care previously. On examination, her vision is 20/20 and 20/200 in her right and left eye, respectively. Her examination is notable for optic nerve findings in the left eye shown in the figure. What is the next appropriate step in management?

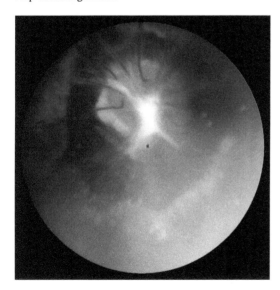

A. Brain MRI and MR angiogram

B. Referral back to pediatrician to evaluate for CHARGE syndrome

C. Goldman's visual field

D. MRI and referral to endocrinology

98. A 3-month-old male infant presents to your office for "eye shaking" since birth. He was born at 39 weeks and his birth was complicated by a prolonged NICU admission for neonatal jaundice and seizures. A brain MRI was performed in the NICU, which demonstrated absence of the septum pellucidum and agenesis of the corpus collosum. You are most concerned about which of the following eye conditions?

A. Morning glory disc anomaly (MGD)

B. Optic nerve hypoplasia

C. Foveal hypoplasia

D. X-linked congenital stationary night blindness (CSNB)

99. An 11-year-old boy is undergoing bilateral strabismus surgery for poorly controlled intermittent exotropia. The procedure, indication, risks, benefits, and alternatives are discussed with her mother, and she provides verbal and written consent to proceed with the procedure. At this time, what should the surgeon do?

A. Should proceed with scheduling the surgery.

B. Consent the child.

C. Ask the child what his thoughts and concerns are as he should be able to assent to the procedure.

D. Should refer to child psychiatry.

100. A 5-year-old girl presents with 7 months of redness of the left eye. She is otherwise healthy. On examination, visual acuity is 20/20 with both eyes, and the bulbar conjunctiva of the left eye is diffusely injected. There is 1+ follicular conjunctivitis of the inferior palpebral lid. On closer examination of her left eye, there is a 2-mm elevated round umbilicated lesion along her left lower lid. Her condition is most likely caused by which of the following?

A. DNA pox virus

B. Adenovirus

C. DNA herpes virus

D. *Chlamydia* bacteria

6.2 Answers and Explanations

Easy	Medium	Hard

1.   Correct: The child was born at 28 weeks and had a history of intraventricular hemorrhage (C)

In pediatrics, prenatal and perinatal history, including pregnancy complications, gestational age at birth, birth weight, and developmental history are critical components of the past medical history. Resuscitation without complications (**A**) and potential sepsis (**D**) are not associated with optic nerve cupping. Her examination findings of normal intraocular pressures and normal corneas (**B**) are inconsistent with infantile glaucoma, although it is not unreasonable to continue monitoring the child for progression of optic neuropathy.

2.   Correct: Testing of visual acuity and cover testing for strabismus may dissociate a patient with tenuous stereoacuity and underestimate the patient's fusion (A)

Since evaluation of fusion is done under binocular condition, stereopsis should be evaluated first, as monocular testing (i.e., visual acuities of each eye) may dissociate the two eyes and potentially lead to underestimation of the presence of fusion in a child with tenuous binocularity. Evaluation of stereopsis is part of a comprehensive vision evaluation in children, and the entire eye examination should be completed for all new patients (**B**). While stereoacuity testing may be interesting for the child (**C**), methods of engaging the child during the entire examination, such as using appropriate vocabulary and playing games, should be used. There are various methods of evaluating stereopsis including the Frisby and the Lang stereotest, which do not require the use of polarized lenses. Identifying the best method for each individual and his or her ability to cooperate is critical in obtaining accurate data. Strabismus measurements are not affected by stereoacuity testing (**D**).

3.   Correct: Maintained (C)

"Maintained" refers to fixation that is preserved when both eyes are uncovered. "Central" (**B**) refers to foveal fixation with a central corneal light reflex during monocular fixation. "Steady" refers to the absence of nystagmus or other motor disturbances of fixation and is also assessed during monocular fixation (**A**). If an eye does not maintain fixation under binocular conditions, the visual acuity of that eye is presumed to be lower than the fellow eye.

4.   Correct: You used a high plus power lens to blur the fellow eye during testing (B)

A high plus power lens, or an opaque occluder should be used to fog one eye instead of complete occlusion as nystagmus often worsens under monocular conditions. Visual acuity would actually have tested better under binocular conditions, as nystagmus often increases with one eye occluded (**A**). Preverbal optotypes would have been an inappropriate method of assessing visual acuity in a developmentally normal 12-year-old patient. Age-appropriate optotypes should be used (**C**). Isolated optotypes without crowding bars may overestimate the visual acuity if amblyopia is present (**D**).

5.   Correct: Dynamic retinoscopy (C)

Dynamic retinoscopy assesses the retinoscopic reflex with the patient fixating on a distant target and then quickly switching to a near fixation target. The near target should be at the same distance from the patient as the retinoscope, and the patient should be in his appropriate refractive correction. The "with" movement of the retinoscopic reflex should rapidly neutralize or become "against" with appropriate accommodation to a near fixation target. Hypoaccommodation results in persistent "with" movement of the reflex and may be an indication for reading glasses. Some medications and medical conditions (i.e., post-concussion, Down's syndrome) may affect accommodation. Visual acuity at near may be normal, but often, prolonged duration of near work is necessary in order to elicit asthenopia (**A**). While learning disabilities such as dyslexia, which are diagnosed by neuropsychological testing (**B**), may contribute to reading difficulties, a complete ophthalmologic examination is warranted in the assessment of reading difficulties. Some children may arrive to the office voicing a desire for glasses, and it is important to assess for any indication for glasses before determining whether glasses are needed, as glasses may pose a financial burden as well as time commitment to a patient's family and should only be prescribed if needed (**D**).

6.   Correct: Both B and C (D)

Atropine given as an eyedrop is relatively safe but can have systemic side effects (**A**). One drop of atropine 1.0% is equivalent to 0.5 mg of atropine. Occlusion of the punctum after instillation can decrease systemic absorption of the medication. Other possible side effects include nausea and erythema (**B**). A severe adverse reaction to atropine may require treatment with physostigmine. Guardians of the patient should be counseled that as with all medications, ophthalmic drops should also be stored in a secure location away from children (**C**).

7.   Correct: Less than 6 months of age (C)

Infantile esotropia is defined as an esodeviation that occurs before 6 months of age. Accommodative strabismus often occurs around the age of 2 years (**A**). Examination findings and history from parents can also be helpful in diagnosis (**D**). Lack of significant hyperopia and her mother reporting that she was "crossed basically since birth" would be consistent with infantile esotropia.

8. Correct: A large secondary esotropia with fixation of the left eye (B)

This patient's presentation is suspicious for an incomitant strabismus due to an abducens nerve paresis affecting the left eye, prompting an anomalous head position. Fixation with the paretic eye may induce a large secondary deviation due to *Hering's law*. The incomitant strabismus in this case would be larger in left gaze (**A**) with limitation of abduction of the left eye (**C, D**).

9. Correct: Medial rectus muscles found to be inserted 12 mm posterior to the limbus (C)

Consecutive strabismus is defined as a deviation that occurs following strabismus surgery for strabismus in the opposite direction. A consecutive exotropia may occur after medial rectus muscle recessions for esotropia especially in patients with poor fusion and early onset of strabismus. Evidence of a previous lateral rectus muscle recession in a patient with exotropia would indicate a recurrent exotropia (**A**). Evidence of prior strabismus surgery in rectus muscles (i.e., surrounding fibrotic adhesions) that are inserted along the spiral of Tillaux (**B, D**) may indicate that resection of the rectus muscles was performed or may possibly be related to previous surgeries (i.e., pterygium surgery).

10. Correct: Medial rectus, inferior rectus, lateral rectus, superior rectus (C)

Starting at the insertion of the medial rectus muscle and continuing to the inferior rectus, lateral rectus, and superior rectus muscles, the tendons insert on the sclera progressively farther from the limbus. The medial rectus muscle inserts 5.5 mm posterior to the limbus; the inferior rectus muscle inserts 6.5 mm posterior to the limbus; the lateral rectus muscle inserts 6.9 mm posterior the limbus; and the superior rectus muscle inserts 7.7 mm posterior to the limbus.

11. Correct: The superior rectus forms a 23-degree angle with the visual axis; the tertiary action of the superior oblique is abduction; the superior oblique passes inferior to the superior rectus muscle (B)

The superior and inferior rectus muscles form a 23-degree angle with the visual axis, while the superior and inferior oblique muscles form a 51-degree angle with the visual axis (**A**). These angles affect the primary, secondary, and tertiary actions of the cyclovertical muscles. The primary action of the superior oblique is incyclotorsion; the secondary action of the superior oblique is depression; and the tertiary action of the superior oblique is abduction (**C, D**). The superior and inferior oblique muscles pass inferior to the superior and inferior rectus muscles, respectively (**D**).

12. Correct: All of the above (D)

While most inferior oblique muscles have one belly (**A**), approximately 10% have two (**B**), and rarely, three (**C**) have been reported. Thus, during surgery on the inferior oblique muscle, the muscle is carefully inspected to ensure that the entire muscle is identified in the inferolateral quadrant. Repeat exaggerated traction test (retroplacement and torsion of globe in depression) after weakening the inferior oblique muscle can be helpful in confirming that the entire muscle was addressed.

13. Correct: The medial rectus muscle has no direct anatomic relationships with other extraocular muscles (B)

While the lateral rectus muscle has associated anatomic structures including the inferior oblique muscle (**C**), the inferior rectus muscle has a close anatomic relationship with the inferior oblique, and the superior rectus muscle has a close anatomic relationship with the superior oblique tendon (**D**), the medial rectus muscle has no direct anatomic relationship with other extraocular muscles, making its recovery more challenging in a case of a lost or slipped medial rectus muscle. Motility is routinely documented using a scale with 0 representing normal (full motility) and −4 representing inability to move the eye beyond midline. If the eye cannot even move to midline, then negative numbers even lower than −4 are used. If the eye is overacting in a certain direction (i.e., inferior oblique overaction), then a "+" is used to notate the overaction (i.e., +1). Each eye should be tested individually to assess full range of motility or ductions in contrast to versions (convergence and divergence to be tested under binocular condition).

14. Correct: The lateral and medial muscular branches (A)

The lateral muscular branch supplies the lateral rectus, superior rectus, superior oblique, and levator palpebrae superioris muscles. The medial muscular branch, which is larger than the lateral branch, supplies the inferior rectus, medial rectus, and inferior oblique muscles. The muscular branches of the ophthalmic artery give rise to the anterior ciliary arteries, which accompany the rectus muscles and supply the anterior segment. The lateral rectus muscle is partially supplied by the lacrimal artery (**B**), and the infraorbital artery partially supplies the inferior oblique and inferior rectus muscles (**C**). The vortex veins are located posterior to the equator and empty into the superior and inferior orbital veins (**D**). Unintentional severing of the vortex veins is possible during strabismus surgery due to their locations just posterior to the superior and inferior oblique muscles, especially in surgery involving the cyclovertical muscles.

15. Correct: Left lower lid retraction and change in the palpebral fissure (C)

Because of the association of the inferior rectus muscle to the lower eyelid by its fascial extension and the Lockwood ligament, recession of the inferior rectus recession muscle can result in lower lid retraction and widening of the palpebral fissure. Lower lid elevation may occur after inferior rectus resection surgery (**D**). Changes in the lower lid position can be mediated by intraoperative techniques during strabismus surgery, or the patient may be referred for lid surgery postoperatively. Thyroid ophthalmopathy almost always causes an incomitant strabismus, and the patient should be counseled that the goal of strabismus surgery is to improve diplopia in primary and downgaze in most cases and that strabismus may be persistent in some gaze positions (**A**). Severe postoperative inflammation after strabismus surgery in patients with thyroid ophthalmopathy has been reported (**B**); thus, strabismus surgery is not recommended until the thyroid ophthalmopathy is in remission.

16. Correct: Flattening of keratometry (B)

Keratometry values start at 52.00 D at birth and flatten to 46.00 D by 6 months of age. From birth to 2 years of age, the axial length increases rapidly by about 6 mm (**A**). The average corneal thickness at 30 to 32 weeks' gestation is 691 μm and decreases to 564 μm at birth and then 553 μm by 1 year of age (**C**). Mild corneal haze may be seen in healthy newborns and is common in premature infants. The power of the lens decreases over the first several years of life, which is taken into consideration when planning for intraocular lens implantation for a young patient who is undergoing cataract surgery (**D**).

17. Correct: The child may become myopic as he gets older (C)

As the eye's axial length increases and the cornea and lens flatten, eyes are typically hyperopic at birth, become slightly more hyperopic until approximately 7 years of age, and then experience a myopic shift, which is thought to be the course to emmetropia. However, if a young child has a plano refraction prior to the myopic shift, it is more likely that the child will eventually become myopic. The refractive error is likely to continue to change as the child gets older (**A**). The child may become slightly more hyperopic until 7 years of age, but this is unlikely to be significant (**B**). The future refractive state of a young child is somewhat predictable based on what is known about the natural history of an eye's axial length, cornea, and lens, although precise predictions cannot be made (**D**).

18. Correct: Elevation deficit (B)

Vertical gaze may not fully develop until 6 months of age. Conjugate horizontal gaze is present at birth (**C**).

Nystagmus is not normal at any age (**D**). Intermittent strabismus occurs in approximately two-thirds of young infants but should resolve by 2 to 3 months of age (**A**).

19. Correct: Both A and B (D)

The discrepancy between measurements of visual acuity by VEP studies (**A**) and by preferential looking (PL) studies (**B**) may be due to the higher cortical processing required for PL compared to VEP. While VEP and PL may overestimate visual acuity, optotype testing is age-dependent and may sometimes underestimate visual acuity if the child is not engaged or if optotypes inappropriate for age are used during the examination (**C**).

20. Correct: Perform denervation and extirpation of the right inferior oblique muscle (D)

Denervation and extirpation involve ablation of the entire accessible portion of the inferior oblique muscle, as well as ablation of the neurofibrovascular bundle containing the nerve to the inferior oblique. It must be ensured that the entire inferior oblique, including all bellies, is identified to provide the anticipated weakening of the muscle. With 4+ tightness of the inferior oblique and a large head tilt, further recession of the inferior oblique is unlikely to provide sufficient improvement (**A**). The inferior oblique muscle requires weakening rather than tightening in this case (**B**). Recession of the right inferior rectus muscle would not be indicated in a right superior oblique paresis with which there is a right hypertropia (**C**).

21. Correct: Bilateral inferior oblique muscle anteriorization (C)

DVD defies Hering's law and is often present in the setting of childhood strabismus. On examination, DVD can be best detected through a translucent occluder, as the hyperdeviation of the occluded eye can be easily visualized. Often DVD is bilateral, and either eye will manifest a hyperdeviation upon occlusion. DVD can also manifest without occlusion affecting patients' confidence in maintaining eye contact. In this case, although the DVD is more obvious on the left, bilateral surgery is recommended, as surgery on only the left eye is likely to result in the right DVD becoming more obvious. Anteriorizing the inferior oblique muscles is an effective procedure to address the inferior oblique overaction as well as the DVD. In the absence of inferior oblique overaction, large superior rectus muscle recessions are recommended.

22. Correct: If the child is orthotropic in bifocals and tolerates spectacle wear, no change in management recommended (B)

Normal AC/A is approximately 3:1. Clinically, patients with a high AC/A will have a larger deviation at near with accommodation than at distance. The goal of management for accommodative esotropia is for the child to be orthotropic with spectacles. If there is residual esotropia even in their full cycloplegic refraction, then surgical interventions are considered. Since the child is orthotropic in his bifocals, the recommendation would be to remain in spectacles (**B**). Often the hyperopic correction in the spectacles can be decreased over time if the child can demonstrate stable alignment with less hyperopic correction in the clinic. However, spectacles are not typically promptly discontinued in this condition as esotropia may recur (**C**). Convergence exercises are often utilized for convergence insufficient pattern intermittent exodeviations (**D**). With distance–near incomitance, deciding on the amount of muscle surgery can be challenging. Both bilateral medial rectus muscle recessions and posterior fixation sutures are reasonable options to surgically manage residual esotropia despite full correction of cycloplegic refractive error (**A**).

23. Correct: Right medial rectus muscle recession, right lateral rectus muscle plication, right superior rectus muscle recession (D)

Plication of a rectus muscle tendon is an alternative to resection and provides a relatively vessel-sparing approach to muscle tightening. While some surgeons prefer symmetric surgery for horizontal strabismus, it is important to consider the patient's preferences in surgical planning (**B**). Disinsertion of three rectus muscles in an older patient poses a higher risk of anterior segment ischemia due to disruption of the anterior ciliary arteries, which accompany the rectus muscles (**A**). Infraplacement of the horizontal muscles may improve the right hypertropia but is likely to be insufficient for the 14Δ vertical deviation (**C**). Even disinsertion of only two rectus muscles in patients with poor circulation can lead to anterior segment ischemia. In high-risk cases, meticulous surgical techniques to spare the anterior ciliary vessels should be used to decrease the risk of anterior segment ischemia. Staging muscle surgeries may also decrease the risk of anterior segment ischemia when multiple vertical muscles need to be manipulated.

24. Correct: One of the risks of strabismus surgery is diplopia, but in his case, the diplopia will likely improve over time, and monitoring is recommended (B)

Following strabismus surgery, patients with long-standing strabismus may develop diplopia, which typically improves in the weeks to months following surgery by restoration of fusion or development of a new suppression scotoma. Diplopia can be very bothersome for a patient, and although it is a known complication of strabismus surgery, treatment options and expectations should be discussed with the patient preoperatively (**A**). If the diplopia persists, prism glasses or a temporary prism can be provided to alleviate the diplopia (**C**). Unless there is concern for a lost or slipped muscle, reoperations are typically considered several months after surgery if diplopia persists.

25. Correct: Allergy to the sutures (A)

Bilateral symptoms of redness and irritation may be due to an allergic reaction to the sutures. Exposed sutures alone can cause significant irritation and tearing. Exposed conjunctival sutures should be identified on examination and trimmed if possible, and often this alone will provide immediate relief. Burying conjunctival sutures intraoperatively can prevent much postoperative ocular surface irritation. Extending the course of postoperative topical steroids in combination with artificial tears can improve symptoms. Dellen are more likely to occur with limbal incisions or large resections of recti muscles (**B**). Endophthalmitis and/or retinal detachment are possible complications if scleral perforation occurred intraoperatively (**C**). A spatulated needle should be used to decrease the risk of scleral perforation. Conjunctival scarring occurs to some degree in all strabismus surgery, but significant scarring typically does not occur within the first week after surgery (**D**). Conjunctival scarring may cause persistent hyperemia due to advancement of thickened Tenon's capsule too close to the limbus in resections or advancement of the plica semilunaris.

26. Correct: Pause the surgery until the heart rate normalizes (C)

The oculocardiac reflex is a slowing of the heart rate caused by tension on the extraocular muscles, particularly the medial rectus muscle, and is a known physiologic occurrence (**A**). In extreme cases, asystole can also occur. Tension on the muscle should be released if bradycardia is noted, and the surgeon should work with the anesthesiologist to determine when to proceed with the surgery (**D**). Administration of an anticholinergic such as atropine may be necessary if the bradycardia persists or occurs repeatedly. Antiemetic medications are not indicated in this situation (**B**).

27. Correct: Repeated injections may be needed, but the injected muscle may lengthen while it is paralyzed and provide long-term improvement of alignment (C)

Botulinum toxin was originally developed for strabismus treatment and can be used to treat specific forms of strabismus. A patient with intermittent esotropia and good fusion is a candidate for botulinum as an alternative to incisional strabismus surgery (**D**). While the effect of botulinum toxin wears off after 6 to 10 weeks and repeated injections are usually needed in adults, the injected muscle may lengthen while it is paralyzed and eventually provide good long-term alignment. Rare complications of botulinum toxin injection include scleral perforation (**B**), retrobulbar hemorrhage, pupillary dilation, and permanent diplopia. The more common risks of ptosis, initial overcorrection, development of vertical strabismus after injection of a horizontal muscle are typically transient and improve a few weeks after botulinum toxin injection for strabismus (**A**).

28. Correct: Full cycloplegic refraction (D)

This child has refractive and strabismic amblyopia of the right eye with a likely accommodative esotropia with high accommodative convergence-to-accommodation (AC/A) ratio that would benefit from full cycloplegic refraction to treat the refractive error, anisometropia, and accommodative esotropia. A brain MRI (**A**) is not necessary in this case, because the patient has significant anisometropia to account for the strabismus and full extraocular motility without abduction deficit to suggest cranial nerve VI palsy. Although patching (**C**) may be a necessary component of therapy, it may not be the most appropriate first step, since correction of refractive error and strabismus alone may resolve the amblyopia. Although the patient has a high AC/A ratio, bifocals with only plano distance correction (**B**) would not resolve the distance deviation, and also would not resolve the anisometropia.

29. Correct: Endocrine consult (C)

This child likely has unilateral optic nerve hypoplasia, which was misdiagnosed as strabismic amblyopia, but really represented a sensory strabismus. Optic nerve hypoplasia associated with septo-optic dysplasia or de Morsier's syndrome is usually bilateral; however, highly asymmetric forms can occur presenting unilaterally like this patient in 25% of cases. Because septo-optic dysplasia may be associated with hypopituitarism in 6 to 71% of cases, an endocrine consultation is recommended to evaluate for pituitary hormone deficiencies. Wearing the full cycloplegic refraction (**A**) is unlikely to correct the strabismus nor help with amblyopia because the refractive error is only +1.00 sphere in each eye. While bifocals (**B**) can be helpful in cases of high accommodative convergence-to-accommodation (AC/A) ratio esotropia, in this case there is no high AC/A ratio since distance and near deviation are identical. After 2 years of extensive patching, this patient is unlikely to benefit from further patching (**D**), particularly since there was no improvement in visual acuity during that time, and the OCT of the optic nerve demonstrates an extremely hypoplastic optic nerve.

30. Correct: Absent septum pellucidum (B)

With optic nerve hypoplasia, damage to optic nerve axons early in development leads to a small optic nerve diameter and impaired visual acuity. Septo-optic dysplasia or de Morsier's syndrome is on the differential diagnosis, even in highly asymmetric cases such as this one. For this reason, absence of the septum pellucidum and other midline structures may be visible on brain MRI. Abnormal decussation of the optic nerve fibers may be visible in cases of albinism with foveal hypoplasia; however, it is not associated with optic nerve hypoplasia and is also not typically visible on brain MRI (visual evoked potential should show this). Optic nerve glioma (**C**) can lead to optic atrophy and decreased visual acuity; however, the diameter of the optic nerve is usually not diminished because it impacts the optic nerve after complete development. Basal encephalocele (**D**) is associated with morning glory disc anomaly but not with optic nerve hypoplasia.

31. Correct: Left medial rectus recession, left lateral rectus resection, because the left eye is the amblyopic eye and would therefore minimize risk (A)

The left eye has significant amblyopia and visual deficit due to the unilateral optic nerve hypoplasia, therefore strabismus surgery in the left eye would minimize risk by operating on an already poorly seeing eye. Unilateral strabismus surgery on the eye with 20/20 visual acuity (**B**) would not be recommended as the initial surgery, because there is no particular surgical benefit to operating on that eye, and although risk is not significant, a postoperative endophthalmitis or orbital cellulitis would potentially impact the child's only well-seeing eye. Bilateral lateral rectus muscle recessions (**C**) would be the appropriate surgery for an exotropia but not for an esotropia as in this case. Strabismus surgery may have a higher likelihood of recurrence in the future due to poor visual acuity in the amblyopic eye; however, optic nerve hypoplasia does not otherwise increase the risk of failure of the surgery (**D**).

32. Correct: She likely has a small exotropia in right gaze (A)

Based on the narrowing left eye palpebral fissures in right gaze and the diminished abduction of the left eye in left gaze, this patient most likely has a Duane syndrome. Patients with Duane's syndrome may manifest a small exotropia on adduction of the affected eye, because cranial nerve III is innervating both the lateral rectus and medial rectus, leading to some deficit in complete adduction along with the palpebral fissure narrowing as the globe is pulled back into the orbit. On abduction of the left eye, cranial nerve VI should be firing, however the left cranial nerve VI nucleus and nerve are usually missing during this condition, causing the eye to stop at midline. The right cranial nerve VI nucleus should be intact (**C**). The nucleus of the left cranial nerve III should not fire on left gaze (**D**). Because the innervation of the lateral rectus with cranial nerve III gives the muscle some tone, the degree of esotropia is smaller than patients with complete cranial nerve VI palsies. Hence, patients with Duane's syndrome can adapt a small face turn to achieve fusion (**B**).

33. Correct: Electrocardiogram (C)

This patient's findings are suspicious for chronic progressive external ophthalmoplegia (CPEO), a mitochondrial disease characterized by progressive extraocular muscle paralysis with ptosis. Kearns–Sayre syndrome is a variant of CPEO that includes pigmentary retinopathy and heart block; therefore, prompt electrocardiogram is recommended. A cerebral angiogram (**A**) would be recommended to rule out aneurysm causing cranial nerve III palsy, however, lack of pupillary involvement, bilateral involvement, and exotropia all make cranial nerve III palsy from a compressive lesion less likely. Also, usually a less-invasive CT or MR angiogram can be performed instead to rule out aneurysm. Plasmapheresis (**B**) may be considered as a treatment for myasthenia gravis, however, this patient has not been given that diagnosis, and you would likely want to have a more definitive finding, such as a positive Tensilon test, before undergoing this treatment. Thyroid function tests (**D**) would be reasonable if you were concerned about thyroid eye disease; however, this patient does not have typical findings for thyroid eye disease with progressive ptosis rather than eyelid retraction. It is also highly unusual for a male of this age to develop thyroid eye disease associated with strabismus.

34. Correct: He has a V-pattern strabismus due to rotated configuration of his extraocular muscles within his orbits (D)

This patient has craniosynostosis with Apert's syndrome, associated with significant syndactyly as shown in the second figure. Typical features include shallow orbits and V-pattern exotropia with an appearance similar to inferior oblique overaction but due to rotation of the orbit rather than true inferior oblique overaction. Crouzon's syndrome is not typically associated with significant syndactyly, although it shares other features with Apert's syndrome (**A**). Children with Apert's syndrome are not at any particular increased risk of optic nerve coloboma (**B**). They can get optic atrophy or papilledema due to elevated intracranial pressure, making (**C**) false.

35. Correct: He likely had a right cranial nerve VI palsy due to a brain tumor (D)

This patient had a diffuse pontine glioma visible on brain MRI. He presented with a left esotropia, however, it is his right eye that had the abduction deficit, therefore the right eye had the cranial nerve VI palsy, not the left (A). With a significant abduction deficit, an acute acquired comitant esotropia (B) would be the incorrect diagnosis. His left esotropia was likely due to fixation preference from underlying optic neuropathy (has increased optic nerve cupping on the left) or some other cause. Although viral cranial nerve VI palsy (C) is very common in children, having a viral illness prior to onset of cranial nerve VI palsy does not guarantee that the patient's symptoms are caused by the virus. In this case, the unexplained optic neuropathy was suspicious, and therefore an MRI was obtained and clearly shows a large pontine glioma.

36. Correct: This patient has paradoxical diplopia (B)

A patient with esotropia measured by cover testing would be expected to have uncrossed diplopia, however, this patient has crossed diplopia, which is unexpected and paradoxical. The reason for this paradoxical diplopia is anomalous retinal correspondence, whereby a pseudofovea has developed to create binocularity under strabismic conditions. This is confirmed based on the afterimage test, whereby the true fovea is marked by bleaching the photoreceptors, and it shows that the cortical correspondence is extrafoveal since the true foveas are not aligned (as they should be as shown in figure part C. This patient's anomalous retinal correspondence is non-harmonious rather than harmonious (**A**), because the strabismus has now moved so that the pseudofovea is no longer aligned with the fovea of the opposite eye, and for this reason she has developed diplopia. The pseudofovea identified by the afterimage test is a cortical change rather than an anatomic retinal change, therefore it would be inaccurate to say that this patient had a dragged macula (**C**). For esotropia, the pseudofovea develops in the retina nasal to the true fovea to develop binocularity, not temporal to the true fovea (**D**).

37. Correct: Image B (B)

A 3-month-old infant has not completed visual development, with myelination of optic nerves starting from the brain and completing throughout the optic nerves in early childhood. Foveal development is also still in progress at 3 months and likely does not reach completion until 15 months. For these reasons, the expected visual acuity at 3 months is diminished from adult visual acuity (**C**), although it should be adequate for fix and follow; therefore (**A**) is not correct. We are able to estimate visual acuity in infants using Teller's preferential looking test and visual evoked potentials (**D**).

38. Correct: This patient has a positive angle kappa (C)

A dragged macula may occur as a consequence of retinopathy of prematurity, particularly if there is inadequate follow-up and treatment due to miscommunication. Positive angle kappa leads to the appearance of exotropia due to misalignment of the fovea with the central pupillary axis. This appearance takes place even though there is no true exotropia (no movement on cover testing) (**D**). Anomalous retinal correspondence involves a cortical change in binocular linkage between retinal loci, and differs from the physical retinal change that occurs with positive angle kappa (**A**). Eccentric fixation involves use of extrafoveal fixation due to obliteration of the fovea and is generally a monocular behavior that does not create the appearance of strabismus (**B**).

39. Correct: This patient has partial stereopsis (D)

This patient fits a classic presentation for monofixation syndrome. Monofixation syndrome often occurs as a consequence of corrected infantile esotropia, which is most likely what occurred with this patient. Low levels of monocular amblyopia are typical along with a microtropia (i.e., 5 prism diopters) and partial but not absent stereopsis (A). There is a monocular facultative central suppression scotoma that appears under binocular conditions rather than monocular conditions (**C**). At near, the Worth four dot shows fusion (four dots), because the larger relative size increases peripheral viewing of the Worth four dot. At distance, there is suppression (two red dots or three green dots) because the Worth four dot falls within the suppression scotoma. These patients should not undergo strabismus surgery, because they do not have complete fusional potential and therefore the microtropia cannot be improved with surgery (**B**).

40. Correct: Hirschberg's test in right head tilt (C)

Since the patient is adopting a left head tilt to alleviate his strabismus, a right cranial nerve IV palsy should result in worse hypertropia of the right eye on right head tilt. At 9-months' old with Down's syndrome, it would be appropriate to first attempt the Hirschberg test in right head tilt to identify the presence of a right hypertropia. The double Maddox rod (**A**) is helpful to look for torsion but impossible to perform for this age group. The 4 prism diopter base-out test (**B**) is an appropriate test to diagnose monofixation syndrome but is not helpful for diagnosing cranial nerve IV palsy. A single Maddox rod test in left gaze (**D**) may identify a deviation, however, this requires cooperation and a verbal response from the patient, which is not possible at this age. Furthermore, deviations in side gaze are easiest to determine with cover testing and/or corneal light reflex rather than the Maddox rod test.

41. Correct: 35 prism diopters of exophoria (A)

Tenacious proximal fusion eliminates an intermittent exotropia at near because fusion at near is so strong that the patient can overcome latent exotropia. It is important to identify tenacious proximal fusion in order to determine the most appropriate amount of surgery to perform. The patch test can help break fusion and determine the latent exotropia or exophoria

at near. Orthophoria (**B**) at near immediately following the 60-minute patch test would suggest a true high accommodative convergence-to-accommodation (AC/A) ratio and would not support tenacious proximal fusion. 15 prism diopters of esotropia (**C**) would not support tenacious proximal fusion and would be an unexpected result. The 60-minute patch test should identify tenacious proximal fusion, and therefore (**D**) is incorrect.

42. Correct: Esotropia (B)

The Hirschberg test shows a well-centered corneal light reflex in the right eye and a temporally deviated corneal light reflex in the left eye, supporting the presence of esotropia. The Hirschberg test is an alternative to the cover test in an uncooperative child, particularly one with pseudoesotropia. Pseudoesotropia is the illusion of strabismus due to prominent epicanthal folds or a wide nasal bridge. This patient has an abnormal Hirschberg test, which is inconsistent with pseudoesotropia (**A**). Because the patient is exhibiting esotropia under binocular conditions, her finding also cannot be defined as an esophoria (**C**) as phorias should be absent in binocular conditions. Finally, the corneal light reflex is falling temporally rather than nasally consistent with esotropia rather than exotropia (**D**).

43. Correct: Right lateral rectus recession and right medial rectus resection with bilateral inferior oblique myectomies (D)

The nine cardinal positions of gaze show a V-pattern exotropia, as visible by an increasing outward deviation in upgaze compared to downgaze. Although the patient has a pseudoesotropia with prominent epicanthal folds, the corneal light reflex supports an exotropia. The patient also has bilateral inferior oblique overaction, with an upward deviation on adduction. Together, these findings support performing a two-horizontal muscle surgery (unilateral recession–resection or bilateral recession) along with inferior oblique weakening procedure. Bilateral superior oblique tenotomies (**A**) would not be helpful since the inferior oblique is overacting, *not* the superior oblique. Bilateral lateral rectus recession with inferior transposition (**B**) moves the muscles in the wrong direction to address a V pattern. The MALE acronym (medials toward the apex, laterals toward the empty space) is helpful to remember that the lateral rectus should be transposed to the empty space, or superiorly in the case of a V pattern. While (**C**) has the medial recti muscles being transposed in the correct direction, the incorrect horizontal rectus muscles are being recessed given this patient has an exotropia rather than an esotropia.

44. Correct: Autosomal recessive inheritance (C)

The electroretinogram shows both flat scotopic and photopic waveforms. Along with poor visual acuity since birth with associated nystagmus with an unremarkable fundus examination, this is more likely to represent Leber's congenital amaurosis than optic nerve hypoplasia, particularly since the size of the optic nerve appears normal on examination. Infantile esotropia requiring strabismus surgery is common in children with diminished visual acuity of any cause, but can also be seen in children with normal vision. Optic nerve telangiectasias (**A**) are associated with Leber's hereditary optic neuropathy *not* Leber's congenital amaurosis. Hypopituitarism (**B**) can be associated with septo-optic dysplasia in optic nerve hypoplasia, however, this is unlikely to represent optic nerve hypoplasia with this electroretinogram and optic nerve appearance. Finally, chronic progressive external ophthalmoplegia (CPEO) (**D**) may be associated with retinal dystrophy and decreased waveforms on electroretinogram; however, profound vision loss with nystagmus since birth would be unexpected as CPEO typically presents later in life.

45. Correct: Cortical visual impairment (A)

Although this child is at risk for retinopathy of prematurity, a normal-appearing fundus examination and OCT make blindness due to retinopathy of prematurity extremely unlikely. Premature infants are also at risk for cortical visual impairment due to periventricular hemorrhage and other intracranial processes. Neurologic changes can also contribute to infantile exotropia as can poor visual acuity. Furthermore, blindness in the newborn period from retinopathy of prematurity (**C**) or any other ocular (**D**) or optic nerve process (**B**) would be expected to result in nystagmus, which this patient does not have. Optic nerve hypoplasia (**B**) would also be visible on fundus examination with small optic nerves, which were not seen.

46. Correct: Genetic testing (B)

Usher's syndrome is associated with retinitis pigmentosa (RP) with childhood onset. His visual acuity could be normal for his age although it is borderline low. Intermittent exotropia is nonspecific. Genetic testing for Usher's syndrome can be helpful to make a more definitive diagnosis, guide family planning, and allow for participation in future clinical trials. It is a reasonable first step to determine whether the child requires work-up such as an electroretinogram. Double Maddox rod (**A**) testing is typically performed to measure torsion, which is not particularly of concern for this child and is difficult to measure in an uncooperative 3-year old. A brain CT (**C**) is not particularly revealing in Usher's syndrome and would expose the child to unnecessary radiation. A fluorescein angiogram (**D**) is not particularly diagnostic of RP and difficult to perform in this age group.

47. Correct: 6 to 9 months old (C)

This child may or may not have delayed visual maturation, a finding characterized by delay in visual behavior without any associated ocular pathology. Normal infants start to fix and follow faces before objects, as in this case, therefore this child may be normal. Infants with delayed visual maturation or normal development prior to fixation often also have a variable strabismus, as in this case. Delayed visual maturation is often associated with developmental delay although it can be a normal variant. Normal infants are expected to develop fix and follow behavior with orthophoric alignment between 6 weeks and 3 months, therefore performing any further testing now (**A**) would be inappropriate. Delayed visual maturation can occur with onset of visual behavior between 3 and 6 months. If there are no abnormal ocular findings or risk factors, it is reasonable to observe during this period (**B**). Waiting until the child is 3 to 4 years old (**D**) would be an inappropriate delay in work-up for a child with persistently low vision. Options for additional work-up include MRI of the brain, optical coherence tomography of the retina and optic nerve, visual evoked potential, and/or electroretinogram.

48. Correct: The velocity of the slow phase exponentially increases with distance from fixation (D)

Congenital motor nystagmus and fusion maldevelopment nystagmus are both forms of infantile nystagmus syndrome. They both are present early in childhood and are not associated with oscillopsia or central nervous system abnormalities. While the pattern of nystagmus in both forms are characteristically bilateral, horizontal, and uniplanar, there are significant differences between the two. Congenital motor nystagmus differs from fusion maldevelopment nystagmus, as there is an exponential increase in the velocity of the slow phase with distance from fixation in the former (**D**) compared to an exponential decrease in the velocity of the slow phase in the latter. Furthermore, there is an inversion of the OKN response in patients with congenital motor nystagmus, which means that the nystagmus decreases or is dampened when the patient is presented with an OKN drum moving in the opposite direction of the fast phase (**C**). Both fusion maldevelopment and congenital motor nystagmus have a null point (**B**), and fusion maldevelopment nystagmus demonstrates reversal of the direction of the fast phase with occlusion of the contralateral eye (**A**).

49. Correct: Electroretinogram (ERG) (B)

The figure shows a paradoxical pupillary response. The normal pupillary response is immediate dilation in dark conditions and constriction in light conditions. A paradoxical pupillary response is characterized by constriction of the pupil in darkness and dilation in the light. This response in addition to sensory nystagmus can be seen with several retinal or optic nerve diseases, such as congenital stationary night blindness, congenital achromatopsia, Leber's congenital amaurosis, retinitis pigmentosa, Best's disease, albinism, and optic nerve hypoplasia. As the dilated funduscopic examination can often appear to be normal in several of these retinal dystrophies, ERG is used to aid in their diagnosis (**D**). FA (**A**) is not helpful in the diagnosis of retinal dystrophies associated with nystagmus, and MRI (**C**) is usually not required in congenital, binocular, horizontal nystagmus. Urine testing for HVA and VMA (**D**) is used for the diagnosis of neuroblastoma, which can present with opsoclonus, which is not a true nystagmus.

50. Correct: MRI neuroimaging (D)

This patient presents with the classic triad seen in spasmus nutans syndrome: nystagmus, head nodding, and torticollis. The nystagmus is acquired and presents during the first 2 years of life. It is usually characterized as a bilateral, conjugate, small-amplitude, high-frequency "shimmering" nystagmus, though it can also present asymmetrically between the two eyes. Spasmus nutans is a benign, idiopathic disorder that often resolves by 3 to 4 years of age. However, it can also be associated with chiasmal or suprachiasmal tumors, and neuroimaging is recommended (**D**). Baclofen (**A**) is used in the treatment of periodic alternating nystagmus, which can also present with abnormal head posturing away from the null point, though the head position often alternates with the direction of the nystagmus, and there is no head nodding seen in this condition. Eye muscle surgery is not indicated for spasmus nutans (**B**). Urine testing for HVA and VMA (**C**) is used in the diagnosis of neuroblastoma, which can present with opsoclonus or saccadomania. There is no abnormal head bobbing in this condition.

51. Correct: Amblyopia (A)

Infantile esotropia is characterized by the presence of esotropia by 6 months of age in addition to signs of early loss of binocularity, such as dissociative vertical deviation (**C**) and latent nystagmus (**D**), which often develop later. Inferior oblique muscle overaction (B) is also seen in greater than 50% of patients with infantile esotropia. As the angle of the esotropia is often large, cross-fixation, or the use of the adducted eye for fixation in the contralateral temporal field is observed. This allows for equal visual development in each eye, and thus a lower likelihood for amblyopia (**A**).

52. Correct: Repeat cycloplegic refraction (C)

The first line of treatment for accommodative esotropia is full hyperopic correction. The average amount of hyperopia seen in patients with accommodative esotropia is +4.00 diopters. This patient has a residual small-angle intermittent esotropia despite good compliance with the hyperopic correction. However, as the initial cycloplegic refraction was noted to be difficult due to his inability to cooperate, repeat cycloplegic refraction is indicated as the next step to assess for any residual uncorrected hyperopia to

address this residual esodeviation (**C**). A cycloplegic agent may sometimes be prescribed to parents to administer prior to the appointment to ensure full cycloplegia. Repeat cycloplegic refraction should be done prior to committing to eye muscle surgery, such as bilateral medial rectus muscle recessions (**A**). Bilateral lateral rectus muscle recessions (**B**) are used for the treatment of exodeviations, and alternate patching (**D**) is not indicated in the treatment of accommodative esotropia.

53. Correct: Bilateral medial rectus recession 3.5 mm (A)

Surgical correction is indicated for partially accommodative esotropia. In these cases, there is a reduction in the angle of esotropia with full hyperopic correction (i.e., the accommodative component), but there is still a residual nonaccommodative esodeviation. The goal of surgery is to correct *only* the nonaccommodative portion of the esotropia, or the residual esotropia with full hyperopic correction. Parents of children undergoing this surgery should be counseled that the child will still continue to have an esodeviation without glasses, and that he/she will still need to continue full-time hyperopic correction after the surgery. In this case, the patient has a residual 20Δ esotropia with her hyperopic correction, which can be corrected with small bilateral medial rectus muscle recessions of 3.5 mm (**A**). A large bilateral medial rectus muscle recession of 5.5 mm to correct her deviation without her glasses (45Δ) is not indicated, as the accommodative component of her esotropia can be corrected with glasses alone (**B**). Bilateral lateral rectus muscle recessions (**C**) are used in the management of exodeviations. Finally, while bilateral lateral rectus muscle resections can be used for the treatment of esodeviations, a large 7-mm resection would correct for 50Δ of esotropia (**D**).

54. Correct: Slipped muscle (B)

This patient demonstrates moderate angle exotropia of the right eye along with limited adduction. As he presents with this finding only 2 weeks following bilateral medial rectus muscle recessions, this patient most likely has a slipped medial rectus muscle (**B**). Slipped muscle is the result of inadequate suturing of the muscle to the sclera, causing it to retract posteriorly in the postoperative period and thereby weakening it. One must always suspect slipped muscle if a large-angle "overcorrection" in the setting of limited motility in the field of action of the operated muscle is seen postoperatively. Reoperation should be performed as soon as possible to retrieve the muscle before it recedes further back and scarring occurs. Anterior segment ischemia (A) is a rare complication that occurs when three or more rectus muscles are operated on the same eye and is characterized by anterior chamber reaction, corneal edema, and conjunctival injection. Adherence syndrome (**C**) results from orbital fat exposure during eye muscle surgery, resulting in a restrictive pattern of strabismus postoperatively. Consecutive exotropia (**D**) is considered if the patient presents with an exotropia greater than 1 month after surgery for esotropia. There is usually no motility limitation in consecutive deviations.

55. Correct: Intermittent exotropia with tenacious proximal fusion (C)

This patient presents with an intermittent exotropia of 45 prism diopters at distance and 15 prism diopters at near, which are notated as "X(T) 45Δ" and "X(T)' 15Δ," respectively. Intermittent exotropia can be classified into several groups. Basic type exotropia is present when the deviation at distance and near are approximately the same. Convergence insufficiency (**A**) is seen when the exodeviation is greater at near than at distance. True divergence excess (**B**) is seen when the exodeviation is greater at distance than at near. However, "pseudo-divergence excess" can be seen in the setting of a high AC/A ratio or tenacious proximal fusion. The former can be tested for by using a +3.00 D lens at near to relax the accommodative drive. If the exotropia at near then increases with this lens to a deviation to close to what is seen at distance, the diagnosis of high AC/A ratio is made (**D**). Tenacious proximal fusion (**C**) is due to a fusion mechanism at near that prevents intermittent exotropia from manifesting with brief alternate cover testing. It can be unmasked with prolonged monocular patching, after which the angle of exotropia at near increases to that of distance.

56. Correct: Base-out prisms ground into spectacles (D)

There are several nonsurgical options in the management of intermittent exotropia, though most are felt to be temporizing measures to promote fusion at an early age and delay surgery. One such option is orthoptic exercises (**A**), consisting of antisuppression therapy, diplopia awareness, and fusional convergence training. Overminus glasses (**B**), or the addition of 2 to 3 diopters of minus power to a patient's current cycloplegic refraction, can stimulate accommodative convergence thereby improving control of an exodeviation. Finally, alternate patching (**C**) may be beneficial by disrupting suppression. While some may use base-in prisms to promote fusion in intermittent exotropia, ground in base-out prisms are not typically used in the treatment of exotropia (**D**). Prisms displace images to the apex; hence a base-in prism would displace images temporally so that the exotropic eye can perceive the displaced image promoting fusion. A base-out prism would displace images nasally, which would make it more challenging to fuse the images in the setting of exotropia.

57. Correct: V-pattern exotropia (B)

V-pattern exotropia, or an exodeviation that increases on upgaze and decreases on downgaze, is the most common strabismus pattern seen in patients with craniosynostosis. This pattern is often seen in conjunction with marked "inferior oblique muscle overaction" due to orbital and globe excyclotorsion. The other patterns listed in the answer choices (**A, C, D**) are less commonly seen in craniosynostosis.

58. Correct: Left medial rectus and lateral rectus superior transposition (D)

This patient presents with monocular elevation deficiency (previously referred to as double elevator palsy) in the left eye. This motility abnormality is characterized by hypotropia, limitation of elevation in both abduction (i.e., field of action of the superior rectus muscle) and adduction (i.e., field of action of the inferior oblique muscle), and true ptosis in 50% of cases. The condition may be due to restriction of the inferior rectus muscle or weakness of both elevator muscles, the superior rectus and inferior oblique muscles. Forced duction testing is critical in distinguishing between the two. If restriction of the inferior rectus is present, forced duction in elevation would be positive, but if the etiology is elevator muscle weakness, forced duction testing would be negative, as is in this case. Forced duction testing also guides the surgical approach. If forced ductions are free and elevator weakness is suspected, the appropriate surgical management is medial and lateral rectus transposition to the superior rectus muscle (Knapp's procedure) (**D**). However, if a restrictive etiology is suspected, inferior rectus muscle recession (**B**) on the affected eye is the appropriate management. Left superior rectus muscle recession (**A**) would not be the appropriate surgical choice in this case, as it would make the ipsilateral hypotropia worse. Finally, ptosis repair (**C**) would need to occur after the hypotropia is corrected, as strabismus surgery on the vertical muscles can alter lid position.

59. Correct: Brown's syndrome (A)

This patient's motility photographs demonstrate deficiency in elevation on adduction that improves on abduction in the right eye. This pattern may be due to inferior oblique muscle paralysis, which is quite rare (some even question its true existence), or Brown's syndrome (**A**). Brown's syndrome is secondary to various abnormalities of the superior rectus tendon or trochlea, resulting in a pattern of restrictive strabismus. Inferior oblique muscle paralysis presents with an A-pattern deviation, superior oblique muscle overaction, and free forced duction testing. Brown's syndrome, on the other hand, presents with a V-pattern deviation, no evidence of superior oblique muscle paralysis, and positive forced duction testing. Superior oblique palsy (**B**) would present with deficiency in depression on adduction, often in conjunction with inferior oblique muscle overaction. Monocular elevation deficiency (**C**) would present with deficiency of elevation both on adduction and abduction. Superior rectus palsy (**D**) would present with deficiency of elevation on abduction that improves on adduction.

60. Correct: Left head tilt (B)

This motility pattern demonstrates weakness in the field of action of the right superior oblique muscle and overaction of the right inferior oblique muscle. As the patient has had this deviation since infancy, this is most likely a right congenital superior oblique palsy. Superior oblique palsy manifests with an ipsilateral hyperdeviation that increases on gaze opposite of the affected eye and on head tilt in the direction ipsilateral to the deviated eye. In this patient's case, as there is a *right* superior oblique palsy, the patient would have a right hypertropia that increases on left gaze and right head tilt. Patients with congenital superior oblique palsy often take on a compensatory head posture to minimize their deviation and allow for the development of stereopsis. Thus, this patient with a right superior oblique palsy would adapt with a left head tilt (**B**) and left face turn to keep his eyes in dextroversion. The patient would not take on a right head tilt (A) or right face turn (C), which would keep his eyes in levoversion, as the deviation would be greatest in these positions. Finally, as patients with superior oblique palsy often also demonstrate V-pattern horizontal deviations, they may also demonstrate chin-up posturing, rather than chin down (**D**).

61. Correct: Thyroid function tests (C)

The CT scan of the orbit shows inferior rectus muscle enlargement that spares the tendon. This finding is classic for thyroid eye disease, in which there is inflammation and fibrosis of the extraocular muscles, resulting in a restrictive pattern of strabismus with positive forced duction testing. The most commonly affected muscle is the inferior rectus muscle, followed by the medial rectus, superior rectus, lateral rectus, and oblique muscles in descending order of frequency (mnemonic: "IMSLO"). Thyroid function testing (**C**) is important in patients with thyroid eye disease to help determine the activity of the disease. Euthyroid or hypothyroid patients can also develop thyroid eye disease, so testing for thyroid-stimulating immunoglobulins is also recommended. Complete blood count (**A**), liver function tests (**B**), and bone marrow biopsy (**D**) are less relevant.

62. Correct: Observation (A)

Type I Duane's syndrome is characterized by poor abduction with or without esotropia in primary position. Type II Duane's syndrome is characterized by poor adduction and exotropia. Type III Duane's syndrome is characterized by poor abduction and adduction with variable deviation in primary position. Surgical management for type I Duane's syndrome involves ipsilateral or bilateral medial rectus recessions (based on the size of the deviation) and ipsilateral superior rectus muscle transposition to the lateral rectus muscle. Indications for eye muscle surgery for Duane's syndrome are deviations in primary position, significant face turn, globe retraction, or large upshoots or downshoots. However, if none of these indications are present, as is the case in our patient, observation is indicated as the appropriate management (**A**). Answer choices (**B–D**) are all surgical options that would not be considered in this case.

63. Correct: Deficiency of upgaze (C)

Moebius' syndrome is characterized by congenital sixth and seventh nerve palsies, resulting in limited abduction, masked facies, and an inability to smile (**A**). Patients with Moebius' syndrome may manifest esotropia in primary position. They may also have limitation to adduction (**D**) that improves with convergence, similar to other gaze palsies, due to abnormalities in the pontine paramedian reticular formation or the nucleus of the sixth cranial nerve. There are several systemic abnormalities associated with Moebius' syndrome, including limb abnormalities, tongue defects, and absent pectoralis muscle (Poland's syndrome) (**B**). The vertical extraocular muscles are generally not involved, so we should not expect to see a deficiency of upgaze (**C**).

64. Correct: Congenital fibrosis syndrome (B)

This patient's presentation of bilateral ptosis and ophthalmoplegia since birth in the setting of restricted motility as demonstrated by forced duction testing is most consistent with the diagnosis of congenital fibrosis syndrome (**B**). This is a rare, autosomal dominant disorder in which there is extraocular muscle restriction due to the replacement of normal muscle fibers with fibrous tissue. It may involve one muscle, or it can be more generalized and involve all the extraocular muscles and the levator palpebrae. It is distinguished from CPEO (**A**) by positive forced duction testing, congenital origin, and its stability. CPEO, on the other hand, may begin in childhood but progresses slowly throughout life. Thyroid eye disease (**C**) is also absent at birth and usually does not result in ptosis, rather eyelid retraction. Finally, while myasthenia gravis (**D**) may present with ptosis and weakness of all the extraocular muscles, pattern of strabismus usually fluctuates, and the patient typically has negative forced duction testing.

65. Correct: Decreased ocular motility (D)

With any cellulitis involving the eyelid, you must determine if the infection is preseptal or postseptal (i.e., orbital cellulitis). Conjunctival swelling and injection, eyelid warmth and erythema, and tense eyelids can be seen in both preseptal and orbital cellulitis. Decreased ocular motility, anisocoria, proptosis, and decreased vision should promptly raise suspicion for orbital cellulitis.

66. Correct: Send to ER for CT scan (D)

The patient may have orbital cellulitis and needs to be referred for urgent CT scan and possible admission for IV antibiotics. If there is a concurrent orbital abscess, it may require surgical drainage. Two of the most common causes of an orbital cellulitis in children are ethmoid sinus disease that tracks into the orbit and direct trauma to the orbit.

67. Correct: Hospital admission for IV antibiotics (B)

This is a presentation of acute dacryocystitis. Given the low-grade fever and significantly inflamed appearance with extrusion of discharge through the external skin, it is best to admit the child for initiation of broad-spectrum IV antibiotics first. Once the inflammation has clinically improved, it is appropriate to plan for nasolacrimal duct probing and irrigation. Since most of these cases are associated with formation of intranasal cysts, it may be helpful to coordinate nasal endoscopy and intranasal cyst marsupialization at the time of the probing procedure to prevent future recurrences.

68. Correct: Every 3 months (A)

Juvenile idiopathic arthritis (JIA) can be associated with a "silent" uveitis that does not present with ocular pain, photophobia, or injection. Girls under the age of 6 years who have had less than a 4-year duration of the disease with pauciarticular involvement (< four joints) and with RF−, ANA+ laboratory markers have the highest risk for development of uveitis, and they should be monitored by an ophthalmologist every 3 months to rule out intraocular inflammation. Though frequently asymptomatic, JIA-related uveitis can present with significant findings such as band keratopathy, iris adhesions, cataract, and glaucoma. Management of these patients frequently requires close coordination between the pediatric ophthalmologist and rheumatologist to control the disease.

69. Correct: Nongranulomatous anterior uveitis (C)

The intraocular inflammation in JIA is usually bilateral and nongranulomatous with fine keratic precipitates as opposed to mutton fat (**D**). Posterior segment inflammation is rare in these cases (**A and B**).

70. Correct: 15 (B)

Children with Marfan's syndrome typically have a mutation in the fibrillin 1 (*FBN1*) gene on chromosome 15. Most cases are inherited in an autosomal dominant fashion, but some cases can be secondary to a new mutation. This disorder will cause connective tissue changes involving the skeletal system (long limbs), heart (aortic aneurysm), and lens (zonular fiber instability). Zonular stretching will lead to lens subluxation classically in a superotemporal direction.

71. Correct: Echocardiogram (C)

Superotemporal lens subluxation is associated with Marfan's syndrome. These patients have an increased risk of developing aortic aneurysms due to the connective tissue disorder. These patients should undergo a cardiac echocardiogram to monitor for aortic changes.

72. Correct: All of the above (D)

During the work-up of a patient for ocular trauma, assessment of the fundus is important to rule out retinal detachment, tears, and hemorrhage, as well as signs of commotio retinae. A hyphema can be associated with fluctuations in intraocular pressure, so measurement of intraocular pressures by Tonopen or Icare is also necessary. Fluorescein staining is helpful to assess the extent and size of any traumatic epithelial defects. Gonioscopy and/or scleral depressed examination are not recommended at the initial evaluation of an acute hyphema, as compression of the globe can further exacerbate bleeding inside the eye. Since traumatic hyphemas do have an association with angle recession, it is important to perform gonioscopy at future visits once the hyphema has cleared. A repeat dilated examination is often useful, as the view to the fundus is often much clearer after the hyphema has resolved.

73. Correct: Sickle cell screen (D)

In African American patients with traumatic hyphema and elevated intraocular pressure, it is important to rule out sickle cell anemia or trait. He should undergo a sickle cell screen and concurrent management of the increased intraocular pressure with topical glaucoma medications. He should be followed closely on a daily basis especially for the first 72 hours to monitor for late complications such as rebleeds or elevated intraocular pressures.

74. Correct: Close observation (A)

This scan shows a plexiform neurofibroma of the left orbit with proptosis of the left globe. His clinical examination and findings, including diffuse café-au-lait spots, are most suggestive of neurofibromatosis 1 (NF1). Since the neurofibroma itself is benign, it is best to monitor closely for signs of any optic nerve compromise (relative afferent pupillary defect, optic nerve pallor, etc.). Though orbital biopsy may be pursued if the diagnosis remains unclear, biopsy is not necessary

205

to confirm the diagnosis with radiologic findings consistent with neurofibroma in the setting of likely NF1 (**B**). Orbital debulking procedures are reserved for the most advanced cases as they have been associated with significant postoperative swelling and may actually increase the risk for amblyopia, offering very limited benefit in regaining any vision in patients (**C**). Enucleation would be inappropriate in this case (**D**).

75. Correct: Chromosome 22, autosomal dominant (C)

Neurofibromatosis 2 (NF2) is caused by a microdeletion on the long arm of chromosome 22. It is often inherited in an autosomal dominant fashion, resulting in a strong family history of the condition in multiple generations. Neurofibromatosis 1 (NF1) is caused by a gene mutation on chromosome 17. Café-au-lait spots, Lisch nodules, plexiform neurofibromas, and optic nerve gliomas are all potential features of NF1. Findings in NF1 are thought to be caused by defective neurofibromin protein and also inherited most commonly in an autosomal dominant fashion.

76. Correct: Close observation (A)

If there is minimal to no irritation of the ocular surface with negative fluorescein staining, then observation is best. Most cases of epiblepharon usually resolve spontaneously as children grow.

77. Correct: 30% (B)

There is a 30% mortality rate in cases of nonaccidental trauma, also known as shaken baby syndrome. Often, there is evidence of intracranial hemorrhage and other systemic injuries. In many cases, when the child does survive, there are frequently lasting neurologic impairments and developmental delays.

78. Correct: Systemic propranolol (D)

The pathology slide shows many endothelial and epithelial cells with capillary formations throughout. There are not many inflammatory cells seen. This is consistent with a diagnosis of capillary hemangioma. The next recommended step in management would be systemic propranolol, usually coordinated with the care of a hematologist or dermatologist to monitor for systemic side effects from the medication. As in all fields of medicine, other differential diagnoses should be considered especially when a condition, which normally resolves with time or with other conservative treatment modalities, persists. Steroid injections were more frequently used in the past to treat capillary hemangiomas, but due to their associations with causing skin necrosis, fat atrophy, and central retinal artery occlusions, they are no longer considered first line for treatment (**A**). Topical timolol ointment has been shown to be effective in treatment of superficial cutaneous

capillary hemangiomas. However, given the deeper appearance of the lesion in this patient's case, topical timolol ointment is unlikely to be effective (**C**). Surgical debulking may be considered as a last resort if the lesion is not responding to other medications but has been reportedly difficult and unsatisfactory since hemangiomas are not encapsulated and tend to bleed profusely during surgery (**B**).

79. Correct: Orbital imaging (B)

The patient's symptoms are concerning for a whiteout orbital fracture and muscle and/or other soft-tissue entrapment causing pain with certain eye movements. It is recommended that he undergo orbital imaging (i.e., CT) to evaluate for orbital fracture and referral for surgical repair if confirmed. Sinus precautions should be provided and the child should be instructed not to blow his nose.

80. Correct: Orbital imaging (B)

This is a case of spontaneous and painless periorbital ecchymosis and edema without inciting trauma for which observation would not be recommended (**A**). Antibiotics would only be indicated if the etiology was thought to be infectious (**C**). Though cellulitis is a differential diagnosis for eyelid edema, the lack of pain or discomfort makes infection unlikely. The lack of fatigue and other bruising on her body make anemia or thrombocytopenia as the cause of ecchymosis less likely (**D**). There was no recent trauma to explain her findings. Though the remainder of the ocular examination is unremarkable, the unusual history and presentation should prompt raised suspicion for an underlying malignancy. Orbital imaging by CT or MRI is recommended to evaluate for orbital malignancies such as rhabdomyosarcoma. If a lesion is detected on orbital imaging, a biopsy of the lesion should be obtained as soon as possible.

81. Correct: Astrocytic hamartoma (B)

Patients with tuberous sclerosis often manifest with hypopigmented macular lesions on their skin, also known as ash-leaf spots, which are best visualized under a Wood lamp. These patients frequently have adenoma sebaceum (facial angiofibromas) that are often mistaken for facial acne. Patients often have multiple systemic growths (cardiac rhabdomyomas, renal angiomyolipomas, bone cysts, and oral fibromas). Cortical tubers and subependymal astrocytomas are associated with seizure activity and developmental delay. One of the most common ocular findings in tuberous sclerosis is retinal astrocytic hamartomas of the flat and translucent type or of the multinodular "mulberry" configuration. Hypopigmented lesions are frequently noted in the retinal periphery in these patients. Retinal colobomas are not typically seen in tuberous sclerosis and would be more characteristic of conditions like CHARGE (Coloboma, Heart defects, Atresia of nasal choanae, Retardation of growth and/or development, Genitourinary abnormalities, Ear anomalies) syndrome (**A**). Myelinated nerve fiber layers have been associated with GAPO (Growth retardation, Alopecia, Pseudoanodontia, Ocular manifestations) syndrome, Turner's syndrome, and Down's syndrome but not with tuberous sclerosis (**C**). Lisch nodules are characteristic of patients with neurofibromatosis type 1 (**D**).

82. Correct: Sporadic (D)

Phakomatoses are a group of disorders, including tuberous sclerosis, with abnormalities affecting two or more organ systems (including skin and central nervous system). Most cases (approximately up to two-thirds) of tuberous sclerosis, also known as Bourneville's disease, are associated with sporadic mutations. Autosomal dominant inheritance patterns have been reported in a minority of cases. Sturge–Weber syndrome and Wyburn–Mason syndrome are other phakomatoses secondary to sporadic mutations (**D**). Patients with Sturge–Weber syndrome have varying levels of mental deficits, seizure activity, cutaneous angiomas (port-wine stains), and choroidal angiomatosis. They are more prone to develop glaucoma. Wyburn–Mason syndrome presents with arteriovenous malformations of the brain and retina. Patients with this diagnosis often have tortuous and dilated retinal vessels on their fundus examination. Neurofibromatosis (NF) types 1 and 2 are both inherited in an autosomal dominant fashion. NF 1 is more common and is due to a defect in chromosome 17, resulting in formation of Lisch nodules, plexiform neurofibromas, optic nerve gliomas, axillary and inguinal freckling, and café-au-lait spots. NF 2 is less common, due to a defect in chromosome 22, and often manifests with bilateral acoustic neuromas. von Hippel–Lindau disease is another phakomatosis that is inherited in an autosomal dominant manner and is due to a defect in chromosome 3. This disease manifests with vascular tumors (hemangioblastomas) affecting the retina and central nervous syndrome. It is also associated with pheochromocytomas and renal cell carcinomas. Ataxia–telangiectasia is a phakomatosis characterized by autosomal recessive inheritance (**B**), associated with progressive ataxia during childhood and increased susceptibility to infections and cancers due to a deficient immune system. Incontinentia pigmenti is inherited in an X-linked dominant fashion (**C**). It is lethal in males and therefore only manifests in viable females. Clusters of small hyperpigmented macules along the trunk can be seen, along with a proliferative retinal vasculopathy resembling retinopathy of prematurity.

83. Correct: Topical cysteamine every hour (B)

This child has cystinosis, a rare metabolic disease characterized by elevated levels of cystine within the cell. In the infantile form, children present with failure to thrive, rickets, and renal failure. The corneal crystals appear at 1 year of age initially in the periphery but progress to involve the entire cornea. Treatment is typically with oral cysteamine for the systemic problems but has no effect on the corneal crystals. Topical cysteamine is available but requires hourly application, and the crystals return when treatment stops. Given the good vision, corneal transplant is not appropriate (**C**). Serum copper and ceruloplasmin test refers to the diagnostic tests for Wilson's disease (**D**).

84. Correct: PITX2 (A)

Axenfeld–Rieger syndrome can be caused by a mutation in the *PITX2* gene as well as *FOXC1*. *FOXC1* mutations can also cause heart abnormalities and iris hypoplasia. The iris can present with a wide spectrum of abnormalities from only posterior embryotoxon to nearly complete malformation of the iris that can be mistaken for aniridia. Commonly there is a smooth, cryptless iris surface, high iris insertions, corectopia, and posterior embryotoxon. It is a bilateral condition with an associated 50% risk of glaucoma. There can be associated dental abnormalities (small pointed teeth), redundant periumbilical skin (that can be mistaken for an umbilical hernia), hypospadias, and pituitary abnormalities. Treatment includes correction of any refractive errors and frequent monitoring for glaucoma. Glaucoma treatment usually begins with topical treatment, as the shallow anterior segment and high iris insertions make angle procedures and anterior segment glaucoma drainage devices challenging surgeries with risk for complications. *PAX6* is associated with aniridia (**B**), and *ACTA2* is associated with congenital mydriasis (**C**). *IKBG* is associated with incontinentia pigmenti (**D**). Incontinentia pigmenti is an X-linked dominant condition in which all affected persons are female. This condition involves the skin, brain, and eyes. Children develop erythema and bullae in the first few days of life, which evolve into clusters of small hyperpigmented macules on the trunk. Children can also develop proliferative retinal vasculopathy that closely resembles retinopathy of prematurity.

85. Correct: Left head turn (B)

This photograph demonstrates a classic epibulbar dermoid. This is a choristoma that can contain hair follicles (as seen in the photograph), sebaceous glands, or sweat glands. They typically straddle the limbus and are in the inferotemporal position. They are often seen in children with Goldenhar's syndrome, which can include other anomalies such as ear deformities, maxillary or mandibular hypoplasia, eyelid colobomas, and Duane's retraction syndrome. For type I Duane (the most common form), you would expect limitation in abduction of the affected eye (left) with resulting esotropia in left gaze, a preference for a left head turn and eyes in right gaze. Choice (**A**) describes

207

a head position frequently seen in a left Brown syndrome. Choices (**C**) and (**D**) refer to head tilts, which are commonly seen in fourth nerve palsies.

86. Correct: After 0.01% pilocarpine instillation OU, OD 2 mm and OS 3 mm (B)

This child appears to have a tonic pupil. The anisocoria is greater in bright light than dark indicating that the affected eye does not constrict normally. The affected eye also tends to have sluggish response to light but be more responsive with accommodation (anisocoria improves with reading at near). Greater than normal constriction to dilute pilocarpine is diagnostic. Possible etiologies include varicella-zoster virus. With Horner's syndrome, the miotic eye would demonstrate mild ptosis. Degree of anisocoria is also usually greater in the dark than in light. With apraclonidine drops, reversal of anisocoria is demonstrated (**C**). MRI of brain, neck, chest, abdomen is the appropriate next step for Horner's syndrome (**D**).

87. Correct: Intraoperative or postoperative exudation or hemorrhage (A)

This newborn child has infantile glaucoma related to Sturge–Weber syndrome (SWS). Eyelid involvement by the large port-wine stain is concerning for increased risk of glaucoma. She also has a buphthalmic right eye. Her fundus examination demonstrates "tomato-catsup" fundus caused by choroidal hemangioma on the right. She also has a cupped nerve on the right compared to the left. SWS glaucoma is difficult to manage and fraught with surgical challenges. SWS glaucoma is bimodal in incidence and often presents in infancy or in older childhood. Topical glaucoma medication can be effective especially in late-onset glaucoma. Surgery is indicated in early-onset cases, and multiple operations are often necessary. Many surgeons begin with angle procedures, but adequate control often requires glaucoma drainage devices. SWS children are at risk for massive intraoperative and postoperative exudation and hemorrhage from the anomalous choroidal vessels secondary to acutely decreased intraocular pressure. Special care must be taken to prevent early postoperative hypotony.

88. Correct: Epiphora, photophobia, blepharospasm (A)

The classic triad is epiphora, photophobia, and blepharospasm. PCG should be on the differential for any child presenting with those symptoms. Although not part of the classic triad, buphthalmos is an important sign of congenital glaucoma. Any child with large eyes should be evaluated for congenital glaucoma.

89. Correct: Brimonidine (D)

The α_2-adrenergic agonist, brimonidine, can effectively reduce IOP in some cases but can cause profound systemic adverse effects in infants and small children. It is contraindicated in children less than 2 years of age. It should be used as a last resort and with strong side effect precautions in older children. Beta blockers, topical carbonic anhydrase inhibitors, and miotics are all safe to use in the treatment of congenital glaucoma. Prostaglandins are considered to be safe for children. They are often used as first-, second-, or third-line medications in juvenile open-angle glaucoma, and typically second- or third-line medication in other forms of childhood glaucoma. As with all medications, parents should be informed of potential side effects including lengthening of lashes and change in iris pigmentation. Providers may avoid prostaglandins in uveitic glaucoma cases due to the potential risk of worsening inflammation.

90. Correct: Wilms' tumor (B)

Children with sporadic aniridia should be screened for Wilms' tumor with renal ultrasounds. The combination of aniridia and Wilms' tumor represents a genetic syndrome in which PAX6 and Wilms' tumor genes are both deleted. Some deletions result in the WAGR complex (Wilms's tumor, aniridia, genitourinary malformations, and mental retardation). Retinoblastoma typically presents with an abnormal red reflex and is not associated with aniridia (**A**). Pheochromocytomas can be found in von Hippel–Lindau disease (VHL) (**C**). Children with retinal angiomatosis and VHL should undergo annual comprehensive physical examinations, dilated eye examinations, renal ultrasonography, and 24-hour urine collection for vanillylmandelic acids as well as neuroimaging. Rhabdomyosarcoma, a cancer of the soft tissues, occurs with greater frequency in those with neurofibromatosis type 1 (**D**).

91. Correct: Autosomal dominant, CLC1A/ myocilin gene (A)

This child has juvenile open-angle glaucoma. It is often inherited as an autosomal dominant trait and been linked to *CLC1A*/myocilin gene. *CYP1B1* is associated with primary congenital glaucoma and is autosomal dominant (**B**). *PITX2* and *FOXC1* are associated with Axenfeld–Rieger anomalies (**C, D**). Axenfeld–Rieger syndrome tends to be autosomal dominant.

92. Correct: Microcornea and early age of cataract surgery (A)

Glaucoma following pediatric cataract surgery is a common and important complication of childhood cataract surgery. The most common risk factors for developing glaucoma following cataract surgery are microcornea and cataract surgery performed at an early age. Glaucoma can occur in aphakic and pseudophakic eyes (**B, C**). Although a family history of glaucoma following cataract surgery is a risk factor, especially for families with congenital cataracts, the most common risk factors are microcornea and young age at the time of cataract surgery (**D**). This risk of glaucoma is lifelong following cataract surgery in children, so regular monitoring is necessary. Intraocular pressure lowering medications are the first-line treatment for glaucoma following cataract surgery. Surgical therapy is indicated if medications are insufficient, but there is no consensus on the preferred approach.

93. Correct: Amblyopia therapy with glasses and patching (B)

Anterior polar cataracts are common and usually less than 3 mm in diameter. They often present as a "small white dot" on the center of the anterior lens. They are usually nonprogressive and not visually significant opacities. However, they can cause anisometropic amblyopia. The first step is glasses and amblyopia therapy.

94. Correct: +20.00 × +0.50 × 90 OD and +19.00 +1.00 × 90 OS (A)

For infants with bilateral aphakia, spectacles are the safest and simplest method of refractive correction available. The prescription can be easily altered to accommodate the refractive shifts that occur with growth. Until the child can use a bifocal lens, the power selected should make the child myopic because most of an infant's visual activity occurs at near. Therefore, answer (**A**) is correct. Choices (**B–D**) will all leave the child with residual hyperopia, which may be potentially amblyogenic.

95. Correct: Oligoarthritis (A)

RF is usually negative in oligoarthritis, which is the most common type of chronic arthritis in children in the United States and Europe. The four factors that predispose children with JIA to uveitis are category of arthritis (oligo > polyarthritis), age of onset (young > old), ANA positivity, and female gender.

96. Correct: Needs follow-up; examination in 1 month (C)

Retinopathy of prematurity (ROP) screening examinations are indicated in infants who were born at 30 weeks' gestational age or less or birth weight less than 1,500 g. Also, examinations may be requested by the pediatrician at their discretion if a child has significant comorbidities that may place the child at higher risk for developing ROP despite not meeting gestational age or birth weight criteria. The first examination should be performed at 4 weeks of chronologic age or 31 weeks corrected gestational age, whichever is later. Follow-up examinations are performed every 1 to 2 weeks until retinal vessels have grown normally into zone 3. If ROP begins to develop, examinations are performed more frequently, either weekly or twice-weekly.

97. Correct: Brain MRI and MR angiogram (A)

This child has morning glory disc (MGD) anomaly of the left optic nerve caused by an abnormality in embryonic fissure closure or maldevelopment of the distal optic stalk into the primitive optic vesicle. The photograph highlights the funnel-shaped excavation of the posterior fundus involving the optic disc. MGD occurs more commonly in females, tends to be unilateral, and typically results in visual acuity of around 20/200. MGD has been associated with PHACE syndrome (posterior fossa malformations, hemangiomas, arterial lesions, cardiac and eye anomalies) as well as abnormalities in the carotid circulation. An MRI and MRA of the brain should be obtained in all children with MGD. Patients with coloboma of the optic nerve should be worked up for CHARGE syndrome (**B**). Visual field testing can be helpful in characterizing defects in the visual field but is not the most appropriate next step in managing this condition which can be affiliated with significant central nervous system findings (**C**). Children with optic nerve hypoplasia need endocrinology work-up, as it can be associated with pituitary dysfunction (**D**).

98. Correct: Optic nerve hypoplasia (B)

Optic nerve hypoplasia is characterized by a decreased number of optic nerve axons. It can be unilateral or bilateral (with considerable asymmetry). It can be associated with a yellow/white ring around the disc (double-ring sign). Visual acuity ranges from normal to no light perception, which often does not correlate with the appearance of the disc. Bilateral disease presents with congenital sensory nystagmus or nystagmoid roving eye movements if vision is severely affected. Midline central nervous system (CNS) abnormalities are often visualized on MRI. Optic nerve hypoplasia in addition to CNS midline anomalies is referred to as de Morsier's syndrome or septo-optic dysplasia. Children with de Morsier's syndrome often have pituitary abnormalities including hypothyroidism (presenting as neonatal jaundice in infancy) and hypoglycemia (presenting with seizures). MGD is typically unilateral and does not typically present with nystagmus (**A**). MGD is also not associated with pituitary abnormalities. Foveal hypoplasia and CSNB can also cause sensory nystagmus but not associated with the mentioned MRI findings.

99. Correct: Ask the child what his thoughts and concerns are as he should be able to assent to the procedure (C)

In general, children younger than 18 years of age cannot legally consent to procedures on their own. However, children between the age of 10- and

209

18-years often demonstrate the capacity to understand the indications, alternatives, risks, and benefits associated with the proposed procedure and should be allowed the opportunity to assent to the procedure. Patients should be allowed to ask questions and discuss the decision with their parents to ensure that they are comfortable with the decision.

100. Correct: DNA pox virus (A)

Based on her presentation, she is most likely affected by molluscum contagiosum, which is a DNA pox virus that demonstrates a volcano-like crater within a thickened epidermis; molluscum bodies, or viral inclusions within central epithelial cells, are initially eosinophilic and become increasingly basophilic toward the surface (refer to the figure). Adenovirus is a common cause of viral conjunctivitis (**B**). Blepharoconjunctivitis and keratitis can be caused by herpes simplex virus, which is a DNA herpes virus (**C**). Trachoma is caused by *Chlamydia trachomatis* (**D**).

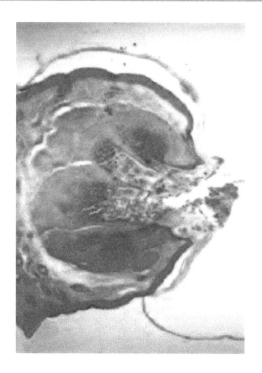

Chapter 7

Refractive Management and Optics

John Gorfinkel, John Lloyd, Craig W. See

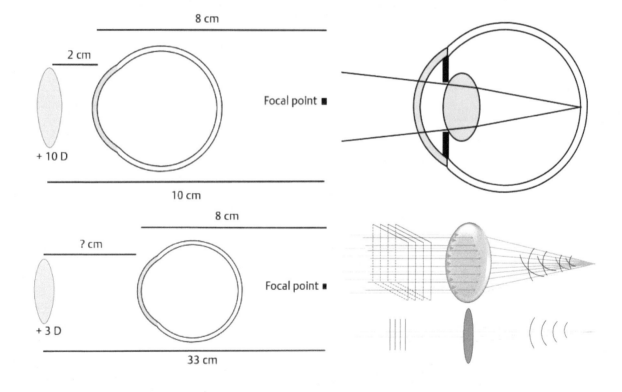

7.1 Questions

Easy	Medium	Hard

1. Which of the following is correct regarding light waves?

A. Light rays from a point source are parallel in uniform media.

B. A light ray is a vector parallel to a wavefront surface.

C. Uniform heating of air causes a desert mirage.

D. Light waves maintain an identifiable direction during specular reflection.

2. Which of the following is correct regarding magnification?

A. Transverse magnification can be calculated by dividing object distance by image distance.

B. Linear magnification is synonymous with transverse magnification.

C. Axial magnification refers to the area of the image perpendicular to the optical axis.

D. Longitudinal magnification is equal to the square of the transverse magnification.

3. Which of the following is true regarding the concept of refractive index?

A. The refractive index (n) of a medium is the ratio of the speed of light in air to the speed of light in that medium.

B. Silicone has a different index of refraction at room temperature than at body temperature.

C. Dispersion of light occurs in a vacuum.

D. Cornea has a lower index of refraction than water.

4. Which of the following is correct regarding Snell's law?

A. The refractive index of both incident and transmitted medium must be known to calculate a transmission angle.

B. The Fermat principle was derived from Snell's law.

C. Snell's law relates the cosine of the incidence angle to the transmission angle.

D. Snell's law is insufficient to calculate the critical angle of an interface.

5. An object is 10 cm to the left of a +6 D lens. A +4 D lens is 25 cm to the right of the +6 D lens. Which of the following is true regarding the image of the object?

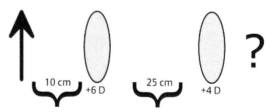

A. The image is 50 cm to the right of the +4 D lens, upright, and smaller.

B. There is no image formed by this system.

C. The image is 50 cm to the right of the +4 D lens, inverted, and larger.

D. The image is 50 cm to the left of the +4 D lens, inverted, and smaller.

6. Which of the following is true about the central or chief ray in an optical system?

A. In ray tracing optics, the central ray is required to locate the image of an object.

B. In thin lens systems in uniform media, the central ray passes undeviated through the lens.

C. In lens systems with different media on alternate sides, the nodal point(s) are shifted toward the less dense medium.

D. The central ray may pass through one of the focal points in thick lens optics.

7. Which of the following is true regarding Knapp's law?

A. Knapp's law is applicable at standard spectacle vertex distances of 10 to 15 mm.

B. The Badal principle is Knapp's law applied to lensometers.

C. The optometer principle does not relate to Knapp's law.

D. Knapp's law is clinically very useful when prescribing spectacles.

8. Which of the following correctly describes the parameters in a focal system?

A. +2 D objective, −5 D eyepiece, 30 cm apart, Keplerian, transverse magnification −0.4 ×

B. +2 D objective, +5 D eyepiece, 70 cm apart, Keplerian, transverse magnification +2.5 ×

C. +2 D objective, −5 D eyepiece, 30 cm apart, Galilean, transverse magnification +2.5 ×

D. +2 D objective, + 5 D eyepiece, 70 cm apart, Galilean, transverse magnification +0.4 ×

9. Which of the following is correct regarding the power for a cornea with a radius of curvature of 10 mm? Use the standardized cornea index of refraction of n = 1.3375.

A. Refracting power +43.75 D

B. Reflecting power +200 D

C. Refracting power +33.75 D

D. Reflecting power −250 D

10. If a 20 D posterior-chamber intraocular lens (IOL) is tilted 20 degrees around its horizontal axis, what is the functional power when viewing obliquely through the IOL?

A. +19.50 +1.50 × 090

B. +19.50 +2.00 × 180

C. +20.75 +2.75 × 180

D. +21.25 +3.50 × 090

11. Regarding aberrations of ophthalmic lenses, which of the following is a correct pairing?

A. High minus lenses–pincushion distortion

B. Object off-axis–coma

C. Aspheric lenses–field curvature

D. High plus lenses–barrel distortion

12. You stand 1 m from a concave "shaving" mirror with a 1-m radius of curvature. Which of the following is correct?

A. Your image is real and not magnified.

B. The reflecting power of the mirror is −2 D.

C. Your image is 100 cm behind the mirror.

D. Your image is erect.

13. What is the result of combining the following spherocylindrical lenses?

+2.00 −3.00 × 180 and +3.00 +5.00 × 090

A. +5.00 +2.00 × 180

B. +1.00 +2.00 × 090

C. Plano −8.00 × 180

D. +2.00 +8.00 × 090

14. Which of the following is true regarding Jackson's cross cylinders?

A. A cross cylinder of ± 0.50 D is appropriate for a patient with 20/70 best visual acuity (VA).

B. The spherical equivalent of a ±1.00 D Jackson cross cylinder is +0.50 D.

C. It is usually ground as a combination of two cylinders.

D. The spherocylinder +0.25 −0.50 × 180 is equivalent to a ±0.50-D Jackson cross cylinder.

15. When the approximation of sin θ = θ is used in optical calculations, which of the following is not a correct notation of this?

A. Small-angle approximation

B. Paraxial approximation

C. First-order approximation

D. Radian approximation

16. A patient is phakic and emmetropic in the right eye and aphakic in the left. With an aphakic contact lens with power +15.00, they report symptomatic aniseikonia. The patient refuses surgery. What should be done to improve the aniseikonia?

A. Reduce contact lens power to +12.00, wear +3.00 in spectacles over contact lens.

B. Increase contact lens power to +18.00, wear −3.00 in spectacles over contact lens.

C. Discontinue use of contact lenses and use full correction in spectacles.

D. Investigate other causes as contact lenses do not induce symptomatic aniseikonia.

17. An eye focuses light on the fovea only when the inbound rays of light have positive vergence (see diagram). Where is the far point of the eye?

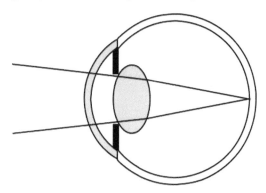

A. At infinity

B. In front of the eye

C. Behind the eye

D. There is insufficient information to determine the far point

18. You are looking at the letter "E" on a street sign 20 m away. The letter is 1 m in height. The nodal point of your eye is 20 mm anterior to your retina. How large is the image on your retina?

A. 2.0 mm

B. 1.8 mm

C. 1.0 mm

D. 0.8 mm

19. A person with myopia of 10 D has +48 D corneal power at the anterior surface and −5 D power at the posterior surface. If the refractive index of cornea = 1.37 and that of water = 1.33, which of the following ametropic results would you expect this person to have underwater?

A. +58 D hyperopia

B. 58 D myopia

C. +43 D hyperopia

D. +33 D hyperopia

20. Which of the following applies to the two diagrams of the same eye shown below looking at a point of light far away without accommodating? Assume the light rays are colored as shown.

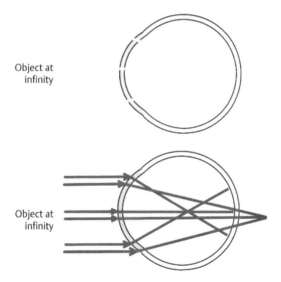

Object at infinity

Object at infinity

A. The eye is myopic.

B. The eye is emmetropic.

C. The eye is hyperopic.

D. The eye is astigmatic.

21. A patient's retinas are conjugate with a plane 1/3 m in front of the eyes. Which of the following diagnoses is correct? Assume the patient is not wearing any refractive correction.

A. The patient is emmetropic and is accommodating 2 D.

B. The patient is myopic and is accommodating 2 D.

C. The patient is hyperopic and is accommodating 2 D.

D. The patient emmetropic and is not accommodating.

22. You are performing retinoscopy on a pseudophakic patient. Without any lens in place, you notice a wide bright reflex with fast "with" movement in all directions. What is the patient's approximate refraction?

A. −3.00

B. −2.00

C. −1.00

D. Plano

23. You are measuring the manifest refraction of a pseudophakic patient using a Jackson cross cylinder. You start by correcting their sphere. Next, you determine the axis and then the magnitude of their astigmatism using the Jackson cross. What is the next step you should perform?

A. Refine the axis of cylinder with the Jackson cross.

B. Refine the spherical correction.

C. Use a duochrome red-green chart to ensure you haven't overminused the patient.

D. Record their visual acuity.

24. You want to measure the accommodative convergence to accommodation (AC/A) ratio in a child. You decide to use the gradient method. Which of the following is true of the gradient method?

A. You need to measure interpupillary distance.

B. You need to measure phorias at 6 m and again at 0.33 m.

C. You need to measure phorias at 6 m with and without −1.00 correction in front of both eyes.

D. None of the above.

25. You perform manifest refraction on yourself in clinic. After you correct sphere, cylinder axis, cylinder power, and refine sphere, you see the following image on duochrome test. What is the correct next step, and why?

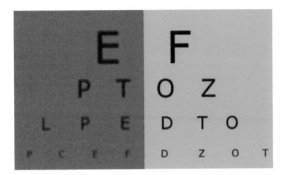

A. Add plus; the red light is focused in front of the retina.
B. Add plus; the red light is focused behind the retina.
C. Add minus; the red light is focused in front of the retina.
D. Add minus; the red light is focused behind the retina.

26. A patient reads a letter E that is 4 mm in size and subtends an angle of 30 minutes of arc. What is the Snellen acuity?

A. 20/120
B. 20/600
C. 3/4
D. 0.5 M

27. A hyperopic patient has right hypertropia. One may correct the deviation by decentering the lens correction by which of the following?

A. Right optical center downward
B. Left optical center downward
C. Right and left optical centers temporally
D. Right and left optical centers downward

28. A young myopic patient complains of uncomfortable, new −1.50 OU glasses. The refraction has been verified. Optical centers are centrally placed. The lenses are ground correctly. Which of the following one may consider?

A. Aniseikonia
B. Meridional magnification
C. Pincushion distortion
D. Facial asymmetry

29. Where should a +3 D lens be placed to correct a patient who can be corrected with a +10 D lens at vertex distance of 20 mm?

A. 10 cm in front of the cornea
B. 25 cm in front of the cornea
C. 33 cm in front of the cornea
D. 35 cm in front of the cornea

30. The light filament in the retinoscope must be conjugate with which of the following?

A. The subject's retina
B. The far point of the patient
C. The far point of the observer
D. None of these

31. When neutrality is achieved in retinoscopy, which of the following is true?

A. The far point of the subject's eye is at the observer's pupil.
B. The far point of the subject's eye is at infinity.
C. The far point of the subject's eye is at the retinoscopy filament.
D. The far point of the subject's eye is anywhere behind the observer.

32. When does the "with-motion" in cycloplegic retinoscopy occur?

A. The observer's far point is beyond the subject.
B. The subject's far point is beyond the observer.
C. The observer's far point is in front of the subject.
D. The subject's far point is in front of the observer.

33. You refract a patient in your phoropter and find a correction of −10.0 D. Assuming a vertex of 11 mm, what would you expect his or her contact lens prescription to be?

A. −10.0 D
B. −9.5 D
C. −9.0 D
D. −8.5 D

34. You need to increase the sagittal depth of a contact lens. Which of the following would achieve this?

A. Increasing the lens diameter

B. Increasing the base curve

C. Increasing the minus power of the lens

D. Increasing the plus power of the lens

35. You see a 44-year-old patient in consultation for refractive surgery. You would like her to try contact lenses first. Which of the following is true regarding accommodation?

A. Hyperopic patients will lose some accommodative range going from glasses to contact lenses.

B. Myopic patients will lose some accommodative range going from glasses to contact lenses.

C. Toric contact lenses do not affect accommodative range as much as spherical ones.

D. None of the above.

36. A patient with a manifest refraction of −4.00 +2.00 × 180 has keratometry measuring 45.00 D @ 180 and 47.00 D @ 90. Which of the following lenses would be easiest to fit?

A. Spherical rigid gas permeable (RGP)

B. Toric RGP

C. Soft toric contact lens

D. Scleral lens

37. Which statement about scleral lenses is true?

A. Scleral lenses may be therapeutic in severe ocular surface disease.

B. Keratoconus patients who fail rigid gas permeable (RGP) lenses are not good candidates for scleral lenses.

C. Air bubbles between the lens and the cornea are usually well-tolerated.

D. Soft contact lenses can be placed over scleral lenses as a "piggyback."

38. You are fitting a rigid gas permeable (RGP) lens. The patient reports good vision with the lens. At the slit lamp, you see the following fluorescein pattern. What is the best next step?

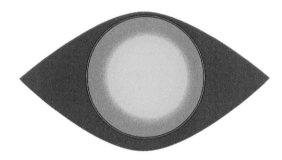

A. Order this lens, the fit is correct.

B. Place a large-diameter soft lens as a piggyback to improve fit.

C. Increase the diameter of the lens.

D. Increase the base curve of the lens.

39. You place fluorescein in the eye of a patient wearing rigid gas permeable (RGP) lenses and see the pattern below. Which of the following is most likely to be true?

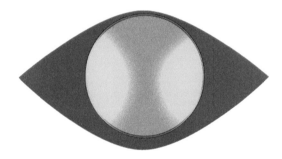

A. The contact lens rocks vertically during blink.

B. Keratometry may indicate 44.00 D @ 90, 46.00 D @ 180.

C. Vision would be poor with glasses.

D. The patient would be more comfortable in the RGP lens than a soft contact lens.

40. You are examining a patient with cataract in the right eye. The appearance of the cataract is shown. What is true regarding lens calculations for this patient?

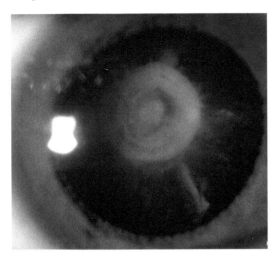

A. Optical axial length measurement is likely to be the most accurate for this eye.

B. Applanation A-scan measurement may result in a hyperopic visual outcome.

C. Manual keratometry measures the anterior and posterior corneal curvatures.

D. None of the above.

41. Your attending breaks capsule during cataract surgery. The surgical plan was for a one-piece lens with an A constant of 119. The attending asks you to pick out a three-piece lens for placement in the sulcus. The three-piece lens has an A constant of 118. How do you need to adjust lens power?

A. Difference in A constant: lower power lens. Sulcus lens placement: lower power lens.

B. Difference in A constant: lower power lens. Sulcus lens placement: higher power lens.

C. Difference in A constant: higher power lens. Sulcus lens placement: lower power lens.

D. Difference in A constant: higher power lens. Sulcus lens placement: higher power lens.

42. You are seeing a 68-year-old patient for cataract evaluation. She has keratoconus and wears gas permeable lenses. Which of the following is true for this patient?

A. Multifocal lens can be offered because the gas permeable lenses correct any astigmatism.

B. Toric lens can be offered because the gas permeable lens will help to correct the astigmatism.

C. Simultaneous penetrating keratoplasty can be considered to improve the refractive outcome.

D. None of the above.

43. You perform cataract surgery and place a toric intraocular lens. You measure 4.00 D of corneal astigmatism. Calculations indicate a desired lens axis of 100 degrees, with an expected refractive outcome of −0.50 +0.25 × 100. Postoperatively, you note the lens to be positioned at 115 degrees. Which of the following refractive outcomes would you expect?

A. −0.50 +0.25 × 100

B. −1.00 +2.00 × 125

C. −1.00 +2.00 × 85

D. −2.00 +4.00 × 125

44. Following refractive surgery, what is the name of the intraocular lens calculation error in which the effective lens position is incorrectly assumed?

A. Instrument error

B. Index of refraction error

C. Capsular error

D. Formula error

45. Which factor is thought to reduce the incidence of posterior capsular opacification?

A. Single-piece lens design

B. Three-piece lens design

C. Round edges on the lens optic

D. Square edges on the lens optic

46. You are performing cataract surgery on a high myope. Your lens calculations indicate you should place a 0.0 D lens. Is there an advantage to implanting this lens over leaving the patient aphakic?

A. Yes, it may reduce the rate of retinal tear or detachment.

B. Yes, it may reduce the rate of endothelial failure.

C. Yes, it may reduce the rate of postoperative cystoid macular edema.

D. No, there is no advantage.

47. You are planning cataract surgery for a patient with a history of retinal detachment and silicone oil placement. The silicone oil cannot be removed. How should you adjust lens power?

A. Decrease power by 6 to 8 D.

B. Decrease power by 3 to 5 D.

C. Increase power by 3 to 5 D.

D. Increase power by 6 to 8 D.

48. After myopic laser vision correction, keratometry power (K) readings result in which of the following errors when calculating intraocular lens (IOL) power for cataract surgery?

A. The posterior cornea is flatter than estimated.

B. The total corneal power is less than estimated.

C. The emmetropic IOL power is less than calculated.

D. The effective lens position is less than estimated.

49. Diffractive multifocal intraocular lenses (MFIOLs) have which of the following properties?

A. Contrast sensitivity is increased compared to monofocal lenses.

B. Blur circles with a uniform intensity are formed by different diffractive rings.

C. Apodization of diffractive MFIOL rings may allow for a smoother transition between distance and near images.

D. Regular corneal astigmatism may improve near image clarity with MFIOLs.

50. Negative dysphotopsias from intraocular lenses (IOLs) are created by which of the following mechanisms?

A. Light reaches the retina directly, without passing through the IOL

B. Reflection of light from the retina

C. Reflection of light from the anterior surface of the IOL

D. Reflection of light from the posterior surface of the IOL

51. You are screening a 25-year-old patient for refractive surgery. Her manifest refraction is −10.00 and cycloplegic refraction −9.50. The corneas are sufficiently thick. Your laser is approved for treatments up to −10.00. Keratometry by multiple methods measures 39.0 centrally without any irregularity. What is the recommended treatment for this patient?

A. Perform LASIK correcting for −10.00.

B. Perform LASIK correcting for −9.75.

C. Perform LASIK correcting for −9.50.

D. This patient is not a candidate for LASIK.

52. You are examining a 55-year-old patient who had LASIK in both eyes at age 35. He reports difficulty reading street signs at night. His right eye has uncorrected vision of 20/25, which corrects to 20/20 with −0.50. His left eye has uncorrected vision of 20/60, which corrects to 20/20 with −1.50 correction. He does not use any glasses currently. A sagittal curvature map for his left eye is displayed below. Which of the following is the most appropriate management for this patient?

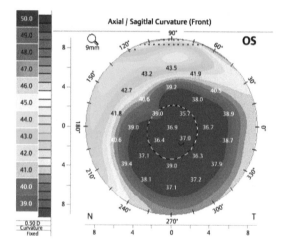

A. Dispense spectacles.

B. Retreat the left eye with PRK to correct −1.50.

C. Fit a rigid gas permeable lens in the left eye to correct his decentered ablation.

D. Perform cataract surgery in the left eye to correct his myopic shift.

53. You are reviewing the topography of a patient who had previous laser keratorefractive surgery. He is currently 20/25 uncorrected and happy with his vision. Which of the following is true?

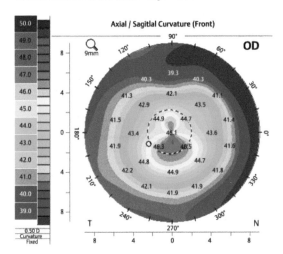

A. PRK will reduce higher-order aberrations in this eye.

B. This cornea probably has less spherical aberration than a typical cornea.

C. Keratorefractive surgery should never have been performed in this patient.

D. It is unlikely that a rigid gas permeable lens would fit on a cornea as irregular as this.

54. A patient with −7.00 D of myopia has a relatively thin cornea but normal topography. You are concerned about leaving enough residual tissue. Your laser defaults to a 7.0-mm optical zone. Which of the following is true?

A. LASIK will leave a thicker stromal bed than PRK.

B. Reducing the optical zone to 6.0 mm will leave more residual tissue than reducing treatment power to −6.00.

C. Wavefront-guided treatment will leave a thicker stromal bed than wavefront optimized.

D. None of the above.

55. Which of the following is true regarding the asphericity factor (Q) and spherical aberration?

A. As corneal Q becomes more negative, the corneal spherical aberration increases.

B. The Q factor for the average human cornea is −0.50.

C. Aspheric intraocular lenses should not be used in post-myopic LASIK patients.

D. A hyperopic LASIK treatment results in a more negative Q factor.

56. A hyperopic patient being evaluated for LASIK is noted to have an increased angle kappa. Which of the following is most correct?

A. The treatment should be centered on the geometric center of the cornea.

B. Centering the treatment on the midpoint of the entrance pupil is ideal.

C. Monocular diplopia is likely if the treatment is centered on the visual axis.

D. When the corneal apex is decentered from the pupillary axis, significant angle kappa occurs.

57. A patient interested in LASIK is noted to have "large" pupils in dim light. Which of the following is correct regarding such patient?

A. Large pupils are defined as 7.0 mm.

B. The transition zone between ablated and unablated cornea should be 1.5 mm larger than the pupil.

C. Older generation lasers used larger optical zones without transition zones.

D. Brimonidine 0.2% may help with postoperative night vision issues.

58 Following refractive surgery, a patient has uncorrected visual acuity of 20/25 but complains of poor quality of vision. Which of the following is most likely correct regarding this patient?

A. Autorefraction may show a high degree of cylinder.

B. Retreating residual cylinder will likely resolve the symptoms.

C. Corneal topography may show a symmetrical bow tie pattern.

D. The Jackson cross cylinder will be very helpful in refraction.

59. Which of the following is a third-order wavefront aberration?

A. Horizontal coma

B. Secondary astigmatism

C. Spherical aberration

D. Defocus

60. Which of the following would be least likely to cause irregular astigmatism?

A. PRK treatment centered on the pupillary axis

B. Epithelial basement membrane dystrophy

C. LASIK flap microstriae

D. LASIK with nonuniform stromal bed hydration after flap lift

61. Which of the following is correct when viewing an emmetropic patient's retina using an indirect ophthalmoscope and a 20 D lens? Assume the clinician has an interpupillary distance of 60 mm, which is effectively reduced to 15 mm by the ophthalmoscope.

A. The image of the retina is virtual and inverted.

B. The perceived axial magnification is 2.25 ×.

C. The retinal image is 5 cm further from the observer than the 20 D lens.

D. The transverse magnification is 15 ×.

62. A rectangular postage stamp which is 1 cm in height and 2 cm wide is 50 cm from a +3 D convex lens. Which of the following is true about the image of the stamp?

A. The image of the stamp is real and upright.

B. The transverse magnification is 0.4 ×.

C. The image size is 2 × 4 cm.

D. The image of the stamp is virtual and minified.

63. How much accommodation is required for an emmetropic eye to view an object at 33 cm through a 2 X telescope?

A. 3 D

B. 6 D

C. 9 D

D. 12 D

64. Which of the following pairings is correct when referring to an optical system?

A. Aperture stop–minimum size opening for system to function.

B. Entrance pupil–the eye's aperture stops.

C. Field of view–the range of object space visible in the image plane.

D. Depth of focus–distance the object can be moved without noticeable image blurring.

65. When performing direct ophthalmoscopy on an aphakic eye with refractive error of +12 D, what would be the approximate simple angular magnification?

A. 3 ×

B. 12 ×

C. 15 ×

D. 18 ×

66. When viewing the patient's eye at the slit lamp, which type of illumination best allows the observer to see the corneal endothelial cell pattern?

A. Direct illumination

B. Retroillumination

C. Specular reflection

D. Sclerotic scatter

67. You have a patient look at a distant light source. They look through an occluder with two pinholes, one above the other. The patient reports seeing two spots of light. When you cover the upper light, the patient reports that the bottom spot disappears. From this test, what can you infer about the patient's refractive error?

A. The patient is emmetropic.

B. The patient is hyperopic.

C. The patient is myopic.

D. To make a determination, you need to repeat the test covering the other pinhole.

68. Which of the following is true regarding manual keratometry?

A. The instrument directly reads the refractive power of the cornea.

B. It measures the central corneal power at a 2-mm diameter.

C. It relies on the cornea's reflective power.

D. It provides reliable measurements of irregular astigmatism.

69. Which of the following is true regarding simple magnifiers when used as low-vision aids?

A. A +4 D hand magnifier can have 2 × magnification.

B. A +28 D hand magnifier is a good choice for those with hand tremors.

C. The common range for hand magnifiers is +20 to +30 D.

D. Continuous text reading is difficult with lower power hand magnifiers.

70. Which of the following is true regarding telescopic visual aids?

A. Near vision loupes provide a narrow field of view but good depth of field.

B. Distance telescopic aids enhance contrast.

C. Bioptic spectacle-mounted telescopes are allowed for driving in certain regions.

D. Telescopic spectacles require a casing.

71. Which is the most suitable option for a +2.00 hyperopic patient with symmetric binocular visual loss to the 20/120 level?

A. +2.00 bifocals with a +6.00 add

B. +8.00 single vision reading glasses without prism

C. +12.00 monocular reading glass without prism for the dominant eye

D. +6.00 laptop computer reading glasses with 8 prism diopter (PD) base-in OU

72. Which of the following is the least appropriate low-vision aid when visual loss becomes more profound?

A. Video magnifiers

B. Tactile aids/Braille

C. Optical character recognition with audio output

D. Mobility training

73. The indirect ophthalmoscope must meet which of the following requirements for even illumination?

A. Observer and patient pupils are conjugate.

B. Observer pupil and patient retina are conjugate.

C. The far point of the patient is in front of the observer.

D. All of these.

74. The direct ophthalmoscope gives a more magnified view of a myopic fundus than an emmetropic one because of which of the following?

A. The effect of a simple magnifier

B. The effect of a telescope

C. The effect of pincushion distortion

D. The effect of all of these

75. There is an optimal pupil size to maximize the resolution of the eye and make the smallest possible point-spread function (PSF). Which of the following is true of the optimal pupil size, which has the smallest possible PSF?

A. Diffraction plays a larger role than aberration.

B. Aberration plays a larger role than aberration.

C. There is no diffraction or aberration.

D. Diffraction and aberration play an equal role.

76. The green-colored appearance of the reflections in this lens is caused by which of the following mechanisms?

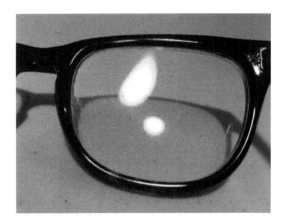

A. Diffraction

B. Dispersion

C. Interference

D. Refraction

77. Polarizing lenses are used in sunglasses because of which of the following properties?

A. They diminish the brightness of images.

B. They reduce reflected light.

C. They reduce refracted light.

D. They reduce reflected and refracted light.

78. Rainbows are caused by which physical process?

A. Dispersion

B. Diffraction

C. Scatter

D. Absorption

79. The scratches on a pair of glasses degrade vision because of which optical phenomenon?

A. Refraction

B. Diffraction

C. Reflection

D. Prismatic deviation

80. Orange-tinted sunglasses may sharpen distance vision because of which of the following?

A. Short-wavelength light scatter between subject and object is screened out.

B. Long-wavelength light scatter between subject and object is screened out.

C. Short-wavelength light scatter at the subject is screened out.

D. Long-wavelength light scatter at the subject is screened out.

81. You see a patient who reports seeing rainbow halos around lights. On examination you note corneal edema. Which process is most likely causing the colored halos?

A. Total internal reflection

B. Absorption

C. Diffraction

D. Refraction

82. The red appearance of the retina is caused by what?

A. Dispersion

B. Reflection

C. Refraction

D. Absorption

83. What is the optimal pupil size with respect to chromatic aberration?

A. 4.4 mm

B. 2.4 mm

C. 3.4 mm

D. 1.4 mm

84. What is the pupil size which will optimize the point-spread function (PSF) in an emmetropic eye?

A. 1.4 m

B. 2.4 mm

C. 3.4 mm

D. 4.4 mm

85. This is a picture of a dust storm. Why is the sky red and not blue?

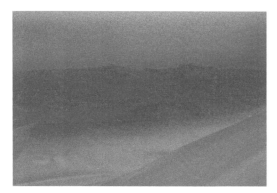

A. Short-wavelength light penetrates lower in the atmosphere than longer wavelengths.

B. Short-wavelength light is scattered by dust particles more than longer wavelengths.

C. Long-wavelength light is scattered more in the atmosphere than short-wavelength light.

D. Long-wavelength light penetrates lower in the atmosphere and is scattered by dust particles.

86. Your technician refracts a patient without realizing that he or she is wearing toric soft contact lenses. The over-refraction was −1.00 +1.00 × 90. The contact lens they are wearing is −3.00 −1.00 × 180. What would the true refraction be in this instance, assuming the contact lens was oriented properly?

A. −4.00 +2.00 × 180

B. −4.00 −2.00 × 180

C. −5.00 +2.00 × 90

D. −5.00 −2.00 × 90

87. Which of the following is an example of the particle nature of light?

A. Interference patterns produced by a double slit

B. Blue light creating images in fluorescein angiography

C. Glare being reduced by polarized sunglasses

D. Antireflective coating applied to camera lenses to improve low-light image quality

88. What is the correct description of accommodation in the human lens?

A. The ciliary muscle contracts, which loosens the zonular fibers.

B. The ciliary muscle relaxes, which loosens the zonular fibers.

C. The ciliary muscle contracts, which tightens the zonular fibers.

D. The ciliary muscle relaxes, which tightens the zonular fibers.

89. Which of the following is true about the attached diagram of a wavefront?

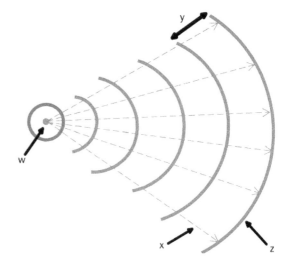

A. "w" represents an image point.

B. "x" represents the direction of travel of the wavefront.

C. "y" represents the frequency of the wavefront.

D. "z" represents a ray of light.

90. Which of the following is true about the diagram below? The diagram demonstrates both two- and three-dimensional representations of the same optical system.

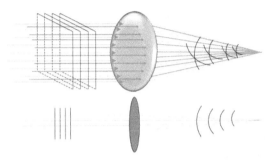

A. The planar wavefronts must have originated from a distance approximating infinity.

B. The lens material must have higher refractive index than the surrounding medium.

C. The light leaving the lens will have zero vergence at the focal point of the lens.

D. The vergence of light is uniform on both sides of the lens.

91. Which of the following accurately describes the power and/or direction of induced prism in the lens shown?

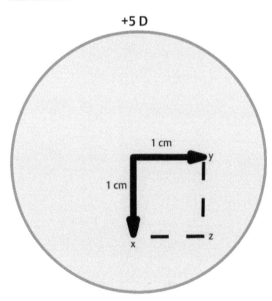

A. The lens induces 5 prism diopters base down at point *x*.

B. The lens induces √2 prism diopters with base toward the center of the lens at point *z*.

C. The lens induces 5 prism diopters base down at point *y*.

D. The lens induces base-down prism in the upper half of the lens.

92. A wavefront has vergence of −4 when it strikes a 5 D lens. What is the transverse magnification created by the 5-D lens?

A. 0.8

B. −0.8

C. −2

D. −4

93. You have a patient who complains that the world appears tilted when he or she wears his or her glasses. You look at your computer screen and see the first image. You then put on the glasses and the screen appears tilted, as in the second image. What is most likely to be the patient's wearing prescription?

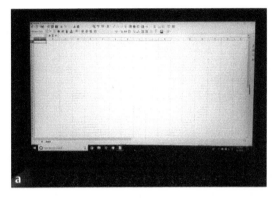

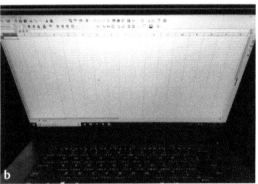

A. −1.00 +2.00 × 090 OD -1.00 +2.00 × 180 OS

B. −1.00 +2.00 × 075 OD -1.00 +2.00 × 165 OS

C. −1.00 +2.00 × 135 OD -1.00 +2.00 × 045 OS

D. −1.00 +2.00 × 180 OD -1.00 +2.00 × 180 OS

94. Which of the following is true regarding real versus virtual images?

A. Real images are always formed by converging rays.

B. Virtual images are always formed by converging rays.

C. Virtual images are always upright.

D. Real images are always upright.

95. You have a lens of unknown power. You hold it in sunlight and find that the lens creates the finest point of sunlight when you hold it 20 cm from the ground. What is the magnification of this lens when used as a simple magnifier?

A. 0.2 ×

B. 1 ×

C. 1.25 ×

D. 10 ×

96. Which of the following is true regarding conjugacy in optics?

A. The conjugate plane to the fovea in a cyclopleged eye is at the far point of the eye.

B. Every lens has two planes which are conjugate.

C. The focal points of a lens are conjugate.

D. The nodal point is unrelated to the concept of conjugacy.

97. You learned about the Airy disk and that the pupil size which allows best resolution is 2.4 mm. You take the pinhole occlude in your office and bore out each hole to 2.4 mm. What would you expect the result to be?

A. The larger pinhole is more effective at improving uncorrected vision, because it reduces the amount of diffraction.

B. The larger pinhole is more effective at improving uncorrected vision, because it reduces the amount of aberration.

C. The larger pinhole is less effective, because it increases the amount of diffraction.

D. None of the above.

98. An object is 5 m to the left of a +5.2 D lens. There is a +10 D lens 30 cm to the right of the first lens. Where is the image formed by the system?

A. Minus infinity

B. Infinity

C. 10 cm to the right of the minus lens

D. At the +5.2 D lens

99. You have a patient who is an engineer and spends a lot of time on the computer. She reports that at the end of the day, her eyes become misaligned and she sees double. Using a ruler, she measured the image displacement, and knows the right eye image is shifted 10 cm to the left. She measured the distance from her eye to the computer screen as 50 cm. What prism correction would resolve the diplopia?

A. 5 PD base out both eyes

B. 10 PD base out both eyes

C. 5 PD base in both eyes

D. 10 PD base in both eyes

100. You are trying to perform laser retinopexy in a patient with a dispersed vitreous hemorrhage. Which laser would be most effective and why?

A. Blue: highest energy per photon

B. Red: less absorption by hemoglobin

C. Green: less scatter from hemoglobin

D. Yellow: more absorption by retinal pigment

7.2 Answers and Explanations

Easy	Medium	Hard

1. Correct: Light waves maintain an identifiable direction during specular reflection (D)

Diffuse reflection does not have an identifiable direction, but specular refraction (as occurs with a mirror) does have an identifiable direction. (**A**) Light wavefronts from a point source are spherical in uniform media, not parallel. (**B**) Light rays are perpendicular to the wavefront and are rays, not vectors (a vector has a magnitude and a light ray does not). Variations in the medium density cause nonspherical wavefronts. (**C**) In the case of a desert mirage, there are variations in air temperature, and therefore density causes light to be refracted.

2. Correct: Longitudinal magnification is equal to the square of the transverse magnification (D)

Longitudinal magnification is approximately equal to the square of the transverse magnification when the thickness of an object is small compared to the object distance. Axial magnification and longitudinal magnification can be used interchangeably. Clinically, axial magnification is important when considering the height of a retinal lesion. For example, when performing indirect ophthalmoscopy, the transverse magnification can be calculated by taking the refracting power of the eye (60 D) and dividing by the power of the condensing lens. For a 20 D lens, this magnification is 60/20 = 3 ×, versus a 30 D lens, which is

60/30 = 2 ×—only a small difference. However, the axial magnification is 3^2 versus 2^2 (9 × vs. 4 ×), which means a retinal lesion would look 2.25 × more elevated with the 20 D lens. Transverse magnification is equal to image height/object height. (**A**) In most situations, this can also be calculated by image distance/object distance, the inverse of the answer choice. It is (+) if upright, and (−) if inverted. (**B**) Some authors do use linear magnification synonymously with transverse or lateral magnification, but in the current AAO manual, it is used to refer to the area of the image. (**C**) Axial magnification denotes magnification along the optical axis, not perpendicular to it.

3. Correct: Silicone has a different index of refraction at room temperature than at body temperature (B)

Silicone has an index of refraction that is sensitive to temperature changes. Manufacturers account for this when designing contact lenses or intraocular lenses. (**A**) The refractive index (n) refers to the ratio of the speed of light in a vacuum, not air, compared to the speed in the medium. Dispersion is the variation of the speed of light by wavelength. It causes chromatic aberration. Dispersion is due to interactions between light and its medium. (**C**) Dispersion does not occur in a vacuum. (**D**) The cornea has a higher index of refraction than water. It is worth memorizing the refractive index of various common medium of clinical relevance (i.e., air 1.000, water 1.333, aqueous/vitreous 1.336, cornea 1.376, silicone 1.438, acrylic 1.460, crown glass 1.523).

4. Correct: The refractive index of both incident and transmitted medium must be known to calculate a transmission angle (A)

Snell's law states that $n_i \sin \theta_i = n_t \sin \theta_t$, where i = incident and t = transmitted. Solving this for a transmission angle requires knowing the angle of incidence and both indices of refraction. Fermat's principle (that light travels from one point to another along the path that takes the shortest time) applies to both reflected and refracted light. (**B**) Snell's law can be derived from Fermat's principle, but not the other way around. (**C**) Snell's law relates the sine, not the cosine, of the involved angles. (**D**) The critical angle, at which total internal reflection occurs, can be calculated by using Snell's law and setting θ_t to 90 degrees (or, setting $\sin \theta_t = 1$).

5. Correct: The image is 50 cm to the right of the +4 D lens, inverted, and larger (C)

The first image created is 25 cm to the left of the first lens (see diagram). The magnification of this step is −25/−10 cm = 2.5 ×. This image forms the object for the second image. The final image is created 50 cm to the right of the +4 D lens. The magnification of this step is 50/−50 cm = −1 ×. Total magnification is the product of

the magnification of each step, (2.5) (−1) = −2.5 ×. The negative magnification indicates an inverted image.

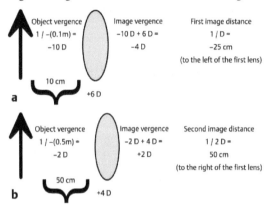

6. Correct: In thin lens systems in uniform media, the central ray passes undeviated through the lens (B)

The central or chief ray passes from the edge of the object through the center of the lens. In a thin lens system with uniform media, the central ray is not deviated as it passes through the lens. This is convenient when doing manual ray tracing, because no calculation is necessary to draw this ray. (**A**) In ray tracing, two rays are required, but the central ray does not have to be used. (**C**) Nodal points are shifted toward the denser, not the less dense, media in lens systems with variable media. (**D**) It is not possible for the central ray to pass through the focal points, because it passes from the edge of the object through the center of the lens.

7. Correct: The Badal principle is Knapp's law applied to lensometers (B)

Knapp's law states that the retinal image size will remain the same despite varying axial lengths if the correcting lens is placed at the anterior focal point of the eye. It is not clinically very useful because refractive error may not be purely axial. Also, the anterior focal point of most eyes is around 17 mm, which is farther than the usual spectacle vertex distance of 10 to 15 mm. Knapp's law is known as the Badal principle when applied to lensometers. (**A**) Vertex distances of 10 to 15 mm are most commonly used for spectacles, but Knapp's law only applies at the anterior focal point of the eye. (**C**) The optometer principle is another application of Knapp's law. (**D**) Because spectacles are usually not prescribed at 17-mm vertex and refractive error may not be purely axial, it is of limited clinical usefulness in prescribing glasses.

8. Correct: +2 D objective, −5 D eyepiece, 30 cm apart, Galilean, transverse magnification +2.5 × (C)

Galilean telescopes have a (+) objective and (−) eyepiece and are separated by the difference in their focal lengths. Astronomical (Keplerian) telescopes have a (+) objective and (+) eyepiece and are separated

225

by the sum of the focal lengths. The formula for the transverse magnification of a telescope is –Peye/Pobj. Given this formula, the (–) eyepiece for the Galilean telescope results in an erect image, whereas the (+) power in the Keplerian gives an inverted image. (**A**) With a +2 D objective and –5 D eyepiece, the telescope would be Galilean, not Keplerian, and magnification would be –(–5)/2 = +2.5. (**B**) With a +2 D objective and +5 D eyepiece, the telescope magnification would be –(5)/2 = –2.5 indicating an inverted image. (**D**) With a +2 D objective and +5 D eyepiece, the telescope would be Keplerian, not Galilean. The magnification would be –(5)/(2) = –2.5.

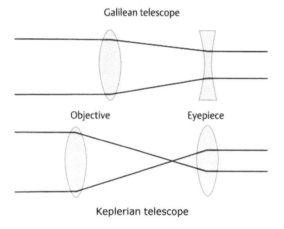

Galilean telescope

Objective   Eyepiece

Keplerian telescope

9. Correct: Refracting power +33.75 D (C)

The refracting power of a spherical surface is found by the formula P = (n′ – n)/r. For this cornea, that is (1.3375 – 1)/0.01 = +33.75 D. The reflecting power is P = –2/r = –2/0.01 = –200 D. The other answers either have incorrect signs (**B**) or have incorrectly applied the formulas (**A, D**).

10. Correct: +20.75 +2.75 × 180 (C)

When a plus lens is tilted around its horizontal axis and objects are viewed obliquely through it, both some additional plus sphere and plus cylinder with axis matching the angle of rotation are induced. The formula for the additional sphere is D × 1/3 sin² θ and the cylinder D × tan²θ, where θ is the angle of tilt, and D is the power of the tilted lens. For 10-, 20-, and 30-degree tilts, the calculations yield the following table. Note that you have to multiply these values by lens power.

Tilt (θ)	Sphere = 1/3 sin²θ	Cylinder = tan²θ
10°	0.010	0.031
20°	0.039	0.132
30°	0.083	0.333

Therefore, in this question, a 20-D IOL tilted 20 degrees about the horizontal would have effective power of (20) + (20 × 0.039) = 20.78 sphere and 0 + (20 × 0.132) = 2.64 cylinder. The total power would be 20.78 + 2.64 × 180. You will likely not be expected to perform these calculations on the examination. It is important that you understand that it induces additional plus sphere and that the axis is 180 degrees. Note that in plus cylinder, a lens with astigmatism at axis 180 has its additional plus power in the 90-degree meridian. The other answer choices either involve a reduced spherical power (**A, B**) or they have the induced cylinder in the wrong direction (**A, D**).

11. Correct: Object off-axis–coma (B)

Coma can result from off-axis viewing. When viewing light passing through high minus (**A**) or high plus (**D**) lenses respectively, the peripheral rays are bent differently than the central rays, which results in barrel or pincushion distortion, respectively. (**C**) Curvature of field refers to curvature of the depth of field, that is, the space which is in focus is not a plane but is curved. It is primarily a problem with spherical lenses, not aspheric lenses.

12. Correct: Your image is real and not magnified (A)

The reflecting power of the mirror is 2/r, with convex mirrors giving divergent or (–) power, and convex mirrors giving convergent or (+) power. Therefore, the power of this "shaving" mirror is 2/1 = +2 D. Using U + P = V gives –1 + 2 = +1 image vergence, but mirrors reverse the image space so that your image is 1 m in "front" of the mirror rather than "behind" it. The magnification is –1 ×, therefore your image is neither magnified nor minified, but it is inverted. Because the rays forming the image are converging, it is a real image. (**B**) The power is +2 D, not –2 D as per the calculation above. (**C**) Because the mirror inverts the image space, the image is in front of the mirror, not behind. (**D**) For a "shaving" mirror to give a virtual, erect, and magnified image, you need to be within its focal length which is r/2.

13. Correct: +2.00 +8.00 × 090 (D)

Both lenses must be expressed in the format with the same axis. To convert a spherocylinder, first add the cylinder to the sphere, then flip the sign of the cylinder, and finally change the axis by 90 degrees. Rearranging the first spherocylinder gives –1.00 +3.00 × 090 The second is +3.00 +5.00 × 090 Simple addition gives +2.00 +8.00 × 090

14. Correct: A cross cylinder of ± 0.50 D is appropriate for a patient with 20/70 best visual acuity (VA) (A)

The standard Jackson cross cylinder of ±0.25 D is best used for patients with best corrected VA of 20/30 or better. A ±0.50 is more appropriate for patients with VA 20/40 – 20/70, and even larger cross cylinders like ±1.00 D for patients with worse VA. The spherical equivalent of any Jackson's cross cylinder is always zero, since this allows changing of the cylinder without altering the spherical equivalent during refraction (**B**). It is usually ground as a cylinder on one side, and a sphere with opposite sign and one-half the power of the cylinder on the other (**C**). The spherocylinder in (**D**) is equivalent to a ±0.25 D Jackson cross, not a ±0.50 D cross. To see why this is the case, draw a power cross of a Jackson cross with +0.25 D in one direction and −0.25 D in the other. The spherocylindrical notation will be some variation on (**D**).

15. Correct: Radian approximation (D)

Radians are often used, but "radian approximation" is not a term used in optics. First-order optics is the general term for optics calculations, where the simplification of $\sin \theta = \theta$ is used (where θ is measured in radians). The full polynomial expansion for the sine function is $\sin \theta = \theta − \theta^3 3! + \theta^5/5! − \theta^7/7!...$ Third-order optics uses the third-order term $\theta^3/3!$. When the angle θ is small, the higher-order terms are insignificant. First-order optics is also called the small-angle approximation or paraxial approximation (**A–C**).

16. Correct: Increase contact lens power to +18.00, wear −3.00 in spectacles over contact lens (B)

A plus power corrective lens will tend to increase image size, so the solution for the left eye needs to decrease image size to account for this. Of the options available, (**B**) has a negative power lens with a greater vertex distance, which will decrease image size. "Minus lenses will minimize an image," or you can think of (**B**) as a reversed Galilean telescope. (**A**) Putting a plus lens in spectacles would worsen aniseikonia. (**C**) The degree of refractive aniseikonia is related to the vertex distance of the corrective lens, which is why contact lenses create less disparity than spectacles. (**D**) However, with high corrections, a contact lens can still cause symptoms.

17. Correct: Behind the eye (C)

There are multiple ways to come to this answer. The first is to consider which situations would cause the light entering the eye to have positive vergence.

Vergence is a measure of spread of light rays. Vergence is positive when the rays are traveling toward a single point and negative when the rays are spreading out and will not intersect. Positive vergence cannot occur without an optical system, such as a plus power lens or concave mirror. In other words, there must be a plus power lens in front of this eye, which means the eye is hyperopic. Hyperopic eyes have far points behind the retina. Another way to answer this problem is to remember that the far point is where an image would form *if you reverse the optical system and make the fovea the object.* You can extend the ray *exiting* the eye in either direction to see where it converges. See the diagram below.

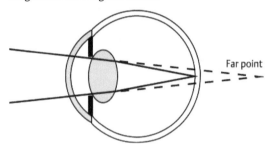

18. Correct: 1.0 mm (C)

Remember that the size of an image is directly proportional to its distance. In this case, the object distance is 20 m (20,000 mm) and the image distance is 20 mm. The object distance (distance from nodal point to the street sign) is 1,000 times greater than the image distance (distance from nodal point to retina), so the image will be 1,000 times smaller than the object. You can also use the formula:

$$\text{Transverse magnification} = \frac{\text{image height}}{\text{object height}} = \frac{\text{image distance}}{\text{object distance}}$$

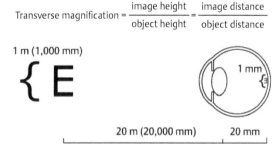

19. Correct: +33 D hyperopia (D)

The anterior refracting power of 48 D is reduced in water since $P = (n' − n)/r$, and $(n' − n)$ is reduced to about one-tenth of the amount in air from $0.37/r$ (= 1.37 − 1.00) to $0.04/r$ (= 1.37 − 1.33). The anterior corneal power is thus reduced from 48 to about 5 D. The loss of anterior corneal power is 48 − 5 = 43 D, and this person would be hyperopic by 43 D if not for this person's 10 D of myopia that reduces the total to 33 D hyperopia. (**A**) Only net corneal power (43 D) is lost but not lens power. (**B**) Refractive power is lost underwater and not gained by eliminating the air–cornea interface of the anterior cornea and replacing it with a water–cornea interface. So, a myopic shift is not possible. (**C**) The corneal power is not eliminated entirely.

20. Correct: The eye is emmetropic (B)

Standard measurements of the eye are done with yellow light. Since the light is conjugate on the retina with yellow light, the eye is emmetropic. (**A, C**) It is expected that chromatic aberration will result in blue light being focused in front of the retina and red light behind, but those do not make the eye myopic or hyperopic. (**D**) There are two points of focus shown in the lower diagram, but there is no conoid of Sturm or any of its components shown. Thus, there is no evidence one way or the other of astigmatism.

21. Correct: The patient is myopic and is accommodating 2 D (B)

This is possible if the patient is myopic by 1 D and accommodates by 2 D for a total of 3 D. The retina is then conjugate with the plane 1/3 m away. (**A**) If the patient were emmetropic and accommodating 2 D, the conjugate plane would be 1/2 m away. (**C**) If the patient were hyperopic and accommodating 2 D, the closest possible conjugate plane would be ½ m away. (**D**) If the patient were emmetropic and not accommodating, the conjugate plane would be at infinity.

22. Correct: −1.00 (C)

A useful approach to retinoscopy questions is to think through the steps of retinoscopy. You start by overminusing until you get "with" movement in all directions. Next, you add plus power until you neutralize in one meridian. Then you add plus cylinder in the direction which still has "with" movement until you neutralize in the other meridian. Last, you subtract your working distance, usually +1.50, from your correcting lenses. Performing retinoscopy without any lens is like testing a refraction of −1.50. In this situation, you have "with" movement in all directions. That means you need to add plus power to neutralize. Because the reflex is wide, bright, and fast-moving, you are likely close to neutralization. Of all the options, (**C**) is the most suitable. (**A, B**) If the patient were more myopic than −1.50, it would mean you are effectively underminused while performing retinoscopy. You would expect to see "against" movement. (**D**) Plano would also yield a "with" movement, but it would be less wide and bright because you are further from neutralization.

23. Correct: Refine the spherical correction (B)

The Jackson cross cylinder method is a very effective means of performing manifest refraction. The order of adjustment is sphere, axis, cylinder power, refine sphere, and then check visual acuity. Performing the correct order is essential. If you have not approximated the patients' sphere, they will be unable to notice small changes in cylinder axis. If you have not determined cylinder axis, the cylinder power added is meaningless because it is a vector quantity. While you are adding cylinder power, you should be compensating to maintain the same spherical equivalent (typically −0.25 sphere for every +0.50 cylinder). After you finish adjusting cylinder, you can refine sphere with progressively smaller letters, adjusting sphere by 0.25 increments, being sure not to overminus. At this point, the patient should be reading their best. If there is any doubt, you can repeat the steps as needed. Because you just determined the cylinder axis and power, the next step is refining the sphere. (**A**) This patient may need refining of his or her cylinder later, but first you should refine the sphere and check the vision. (**C**) A duochrome test may be helpful to ensure you are not overminusing your patients. In this case, the patient is unable to accommodate due to his or her pseudophakia, so this step is unnecessary. You should not record his or her visual acuity (**D**) until you have refined his or her sphere.

24. Correct: You need to measure phorias at 6 m with and without −1.00 correction in front of both eyes (C)

The gradient method involves placing lenses in front of both eyes to change the accommodative state of the eye and measure AC/A. One way is to measure phorias at near (0.33 m) with and without a +3.00 lens. The +3.00 lens will relax accommodation at near. With this method, you take the difference in phorias and divide by 3 (the difference in accommodation). The gradient method can also be performed by measuring phorias at distance (6 m) with and without a −1.00 lens. This will induce accommodation. You take the difference in phorias and it will give the AC/A ratio (**A**). With this method, you don't have to divide by anything at the end because the difference in accommodation is 1 D. (**A**) You don't need to know interpupillary distance with the gradient method. (**B**) Measuring at distance and again is the phoria method, not the gradient method. With this method, measure phorias at 6 m and again at 0.33 m. Use the equation

$$\frac{AC}{A\ ratio} = PD\ \frac{(difference\ in\ phorias)}{accommodation}$$

25. Correct: Add plus; the red light is focused behind the retina (B)

The duochrome test uses chromatic aberration to fine-tune spherical correction. Red light is refracted less than green light. In this example, the green light is in focus on the retina. Because red light is refracted less, you are effectively hyperopic for red light. (**A, C**) Hyperopia results in light being focused behind the retina. (**D**) You have overminused your-self and need to add plus. You can use the mnemonic RAM-GAP: Red Add Minus, Green Add Plus. This mnemonic describes the side of the chart which is in better focus. Remember that in refraction we are always asking which is clearer, not which is blurrier. It is the same for RAM-GAP.

26. Correct: 20/120 (A)

Remember that we measure angular resolution when checking acuity. 20/20 vision corresponds to a resolution of 1 minute of arc (MOA). For a Snellen letter, the letter has to be five times the size of the resolution to be visible (see diagram). In this case, a 30 MOA letter has resolution 6 MOA, so the acuity is six times worse than 20/20, or 20/120. The additional information given regarding the size of the letter is irrelevant because distance is not specified. The angular resolution is specified, so additional calculations are not necessary.

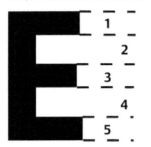

A single letter will subtend five times the angle of resolution. 20/20 acuity corresponds to a resolution of 1 minute of arc.

27. Correct: Right optical center downward (A)

Moving the right optical center downward places the upper half of the convex lens with base-down prism over the pupil. This shifts images upward to match the hypertropic eye. (**B**) Shifting the left optical center downward would induce base-down prism in the left eye and worsen the hypertropia. (**C**) Shifting the optical centers temporally would induce base-out prism, which is not helpful to correct hypertropia. (**D**) Shifting both optical centers downward would cause image displacement in both eyes but would not correct hypertropia.

28. Correct: Facial asymmetry (D)

Facial asymmetry may place the pupils in different vertical as well as horizontal positions that, when not aligned with the optical centers of the glasses, may induce prism. Centration should be marked with the patient wearing the glasses, then optical centration should be compared with these marks. (**A**) Aniseikonia would not be expected with a symmetric −1.50 correction. (**B**) Without astigmatic correction, there should be no meridional magnification (**B**). (**C**) Pincushion distortion occurs with plus power lenses. Barrel distortion occurs with minus power lenses. With −1.50 correction, neither would be significant for this patient.

29. Correct: 25 cm in front of the cornea (B)

If +10 D corrects at 2 cm from the cornea, and its secondary focal point is 10 cm behind this lens, the far point of the eye must be 10 − 2 = 8 cm behind the cornea. If a +3 D lens were placed so that its secondary focal point overlaps the far point, it must be 1/3 = 0.33 m = 33 cm in front of this far point which is 33 − 8 = 25 cm in front of the eye.

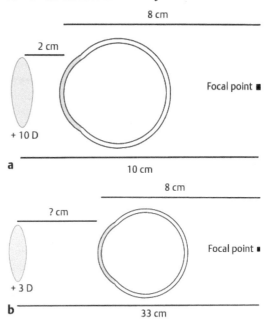

30. Correct: None of these (D)

The light filament need not be focused on any one structure (i.e., need not be conjugate with any one). The focus of the filament is adjusted by sliding the sleeve up and down the retinoscope. For most retinoscopy, the filament should be defocused (broad beam when shining at the wall). Focus adjustment can be useful when using "enhancement" to gauge the approximate ametropia before adding trial lenses in refraction.

31. Correct: The far point of the subject's eye is at the observer's pupil (A)

The far point is the point that is conjugate to the fovea when the eye is not accommodating. It indicates where an object would need to be located to create a focused image on the retina. Emmetropes have a far point at infinity, myopes in front of their eye, and hyperopes behind their eye. The far point of the patient's eye (i.e., the image of the patient's retina) is brought to the aperture of the retinoscope (almost at the observer's pupil) in retinoscopy. At this plane, the light band fills the pupil evenly, and no longer appears to move; it has been "neutralized." (**B**) If the far point were infinity, the observer would see "with" movement. This is the same reason you need to adjust for your working distance in retinoscopy. (**C**) The filament of the retinoscope illuminates the subject's retina but does not have to be conjugate with the far point, the pupil, or the retina. The focus of the filament can be adjusted with the sleeve on the retinoscope to refine cylinder axis. (**D**) If the far point were behind the observer, "with" movement would be observed.

32. Correct: The subject's far point is beyond the observer (B)

The far point is the point that is conjugate to the fovea when the eye is not accommodating. It indicates where an object would need to be located to create a focused image on the retina. Emmetropes have a far point at infinity, myopes in front of their eye, and hyperopes behind their eye. In this case, remember that with motion means the streak is focused behind the retina, so more plus power must be applied to bring the focus forward. In other words, the subject's eye is hyperopic relative to the position of the retinoscope. The subject's far point could be behind the observer at a finite distance, behind the observer at infinity, or beyond infinity (i.e., behind the subject as is the case for a hyperope). (**A, C**) The observer's far point is not relevant here. (**D**) The subject's far point will be in between the observer and subject only if there is residual myopia, in that case we would expect to see "against" motion.

33. Correct: −9.0 D (C)

Vertex distance refers to a change in effective lens power based on the distance between the lens and the cornea. Typically, we check refractions at the spectacle plane, usually 12 to 16 mm from the cornea. Contact lenses have zero vertex distance. When adjusting between glasses and contact lens prescriptions, this vertex distance can introduce error (usually for corrections stronger than 4 D). To correct for vertex distance, first find the far point of the eye. The far point is the point which is conjugate to the fovea when the eye is not accommodating. It indicates where an object would need to be located to create a focused image on the retina. In this case, the correction you have placed indicates a far point 1/(10 D) = 1/10 m or 10 cm in front of the lens. Take this 10 cm and add the 11 mm (1.1 cm) vertex, and you find that the true far point of the eye is 11.1 cm in front of the cornea or 0.111 m. Take the inverse of the far point, 1/(0.111 m) to find that the eye requires a −9.0 D correction at the corneal plane.

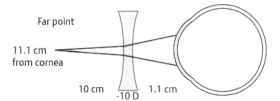

34. Correct: Increasing the lens diameter (A)

Sagittal depth is the elevation of the posterior surface of the contact lens from the edge of the contact lens. Increasing sagittal depth will tend to increase the "tightness" of a contact lens. Increasing the lens diameter will increase the sagittal depth and make a lens fit more tightly. (**B**) Increasing the base curve makes a lens flatter and will decrease sagittal depth. (**C, D**) Adjusting the power of the lens will only change the anterior surface of the lens and will not affect the sagittal depth.

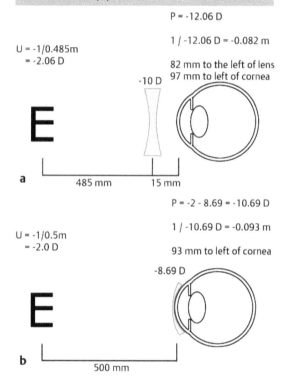

35. Correct: Myopic patients will lose some accommodative range going from glasses to contact lenses (B)

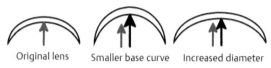

Myopic glasses slightly increase the range of accommodation versus correction at the corneal plane, as encountered with contacts. This occurs because of the vertex distance. Vertex distance refers to a change in effective lens power based on the distance between the lens and the cornea. A near object will have negative vergence, which is made more negative by a myopic correction. The vertex distance will have the effect of reducing this negative vergence closer to that of the eye's distance correction. The result is reduced accommodative demand, or increased accommodative range. Consider an eye with −10.0 spectacle correction at vertex 15 mm viewing a near target at 500 mm. Using the vergence formula, we find that the image of the E will appear to be 82 mm anterior to the lens, which is 97 mm to the left of the cornea. That is the near point the eye must achieve to keep the letter in focus. The second diagram demonstrates the same eye with a vertex-corrected −8.69 contact lens correction in place. The eye needs to focus on a near point of 93 mm in order to keep the letter in focus. This closer near point with the contact lens means that with contact lens correction in place, the eye must accommodate more than it did with glasses. (**B**) Hyperopic glasses will have an opposite effect; they may gain accommodation after switching to contact lenses or postrefractive surgery. The astigmatic correction of the lens (**C, D**) will not affect accommodation, assuming equal spherical equivalents.

36. Correct: Soft toric contact lens (C)

For patients with- or against-the-rule astigmatism of small magnitude, a soft toric lens will be easiest to fit. (**A**) A spherical RGP lens would likely work for this patient but is more difficult to fit than a soft lens. (**B**) A toric RGP lens has adjustments on the back side of the lens to improve fit and is more difficult to fit and adjust. (**D**) A scleral lens is generally more challenging to fit than other types but is useful in very irregular corneas or in severe ocular surface disease.

37. Correct: Scleral lenses may be therapeutic in severe ocular surface disease (A)

Scleral contact lenses form a reservoir of fluid between the lens and the cornea. This can be therapeutic for severe ocular surface disease, such as mucous membrane pemphigoid, ocular graft-versus-host disease, and Stevens–Johnson syndrome. (**B**) Keratoconus patients who failed RGP may benefit from scleral lenses. (**C**) Air bubbles can dry the ocular surface and impair vision (**C**). (**D**) Soft contact lenses can be placed over traditional RGPs in a piggyback configuration but not over scleral lenses.

38. Correct: Increase the base curve of the lens (D)

This diagram shows a tight fit, with central pooling. Remember that the fluorescein will be brighter green where there is more space between the lens and cornea. Increasing the base curve will make the lens less tight. (**A**) This lens should not be ordered in its current state. (**B**) A piggyback lens is useful when the RGP lens moves too much or is uncomfortable, not if a lens is too tight. (**C**) Increasing diameter of the lens would make the lens fit more tightly (**C**).

39. Correct: Keratometry may indicate 44.00 D @ 90, 46.00 D @ 180 (B)

This diagram shows against-the-rule astigmatism. The fluorescein staining at 0 and 180 degrees indicates that the cornea is steeper there (more space between lens and the cornea). The keratometry in (**B**) indicates steepness in the horizontal meridian, which is consistent with the against-the-rule pattern. (**A**) With-the-rule astigmatism tends to cause more staining in an hourglass pattern and vertical rocking. (**C**) The pattern looks regular, so spectacle correction would probably yield good acuity. (**D**) Soft contact lenses tend to be more comfortable than RGP lenses.

40. Correct: None of the above (D)

When the media permits it, optical measurements with devices, such as IOLMaster or Lenstar, are usually the most accurate. (**A**) The density of this posterior polar cataract will probably not allow an optical measurement. Dense cataracts, and particularly posterior subcapsular or posterior polar cataracts, may require ultrasound measurements. Ultrasound measurements can be performed using applanation or immersion. Applanation, like tonometry, has an ultrasound probe directly against the cornea and will indent the cornea, leading to an artificially short axial length measurement. This would cause you to implant a higher power lens, leading to a (**B**) myopic outcome. Immersion ultrasound is preferred. (**C**) Manual keratometry does not measure the posterior corneal curvature directly. It measures the curvature of the anterior cornea and then calculates corneal power using an index of refraction. The index is usually set at 1.3375, halfway between that of cornea and that of tear film. This adjusted index of refraction is designed to account for the posterior cornea, but it is an assumption and not a direct measurement.

41. Correct: Difference in A constant: lower power lens. Sulcus lens placement: lower power lens (A)

Effective lens position changes when placing a lens in the sulcus. Nearly all intraocular lenses are plus power. (**B, D**) Moving a plus power lens anteriorly will cause it to have more effective power. Therefore, you will want to reduce the power of a sulcus lens by 0.5 to 1.0 D, depending on axial length. When thinking about the effects of the A constant of different lenses, think of the Sanders-Retzlaff-Kraff formula: $P = A - 2.5L - 0.9K$, where P is the lens power, A is the A constant, L is axial length, and K is the mean corneal power. In this equation, increasing the A constant would increase the calculated power of the lens. (**C, D**) Going to a lens with a lower A constant would mean you need a lower power lens.

42. Correct: None of the above (D)

Corneal ectasia is a contraindication to multifocal lenses. Multifocal lenses would theoretically allow good vision with rigid gas permeable (RGP) lenses in place. (A) While not wearing RGP lenses, the vision would be diminished by the multifocal lens, so this is not a good choice. (B) Toric lenses can be considered in patients with keratoconus, but only if they do not plan to wear RGP lenses in the future. The sources of astigmatism are cornea and lens. The RGP eliminates nearly all corneal astigmatism. Having a toric lens would increase astigmatism while wearing an RGP lens. (C) Simultaneous penetrating keratoplasty with cataract has unpredictable refractive outcomes, because corneal power is unpredictable following full-thickness transplant. Waiting until the cornea has healed from surgery and performing cataract surgery improves refractive outcomes if circumstances allow for it.

43. Correct: −1.00 +2.00 × 85 (C)

This lens is 15 degrees from its intended axis. As a general rule, every 3 degrees off axis will reduce the astigmatism correction by 10%. Fifteen degrees off axis will result in a loss of half the astigmatic correction. Because the initial astigmatism was 4.00 D, you would expect 2.00 D (A, D) of residual astigmatism. To think of the direction of astigmatism induced, remember that the *manifest refraction indicates the correction which must be applied* to correct the refractive error. Rotating the lens toward 100 would effectively be adding plus cylinder closer to 90 degrees, not 125 degrees. Therefore, the manifest refraction would show plus cylinder closer to 90 degrees (B), not 125.

44. Correct: Formula error (D)

Following myopic corrections, the cornea is made abnormally flat. Standard intraocular lens calculations factor in effective lens position based on the shape of the cornea; a flatter cornea will tend to have a shallower anterior chamber. This discrepancy following refractive surgery is called formula error. (A) Instrument error occurs when corneal measurements do not accurately measure the central cornea. (B) Index of refraction error refers to the difference of anterior and posterior corneal curvature. Keratometers measure curvature, not power, and calculate power by assuming an index of refraction. (C) Capsular error is not a real entity.

45. Correct: Square edges on the lens optic (D)

It is thought that a square lens edge occludes lens epithelial cells from migrating to the central posterior capsule. (A, B) Design of the lens, whether one-piece or three-piece, is not thought to be as critical. (C) A round-edged lens may have some advantages such as decreased incidence of dysphotopsia, but it is thought to lead to more posterior capsular opacification.

46. Correct: Yes, it may reduce the rate of retinal tear or detachment (A)

In addition to helping maintain the structure of the anterior chamber, placing an intraocular lens may reduce the rate of retinal tear or detachment. (B, C) It is not thought to directly affect the rate of endothelial failure or postoperative cystoid macular edema, although this may be confounded by the fact that complicated cataract surgery can lead to aphakia as well as the other complications.

47. Correct: Increase power by 3 to 5 D (C)

Silicone oil has a higher refractive index than vitreous. The silicone oil behind the intraocular lens will effectively act as a minus power lens. The lens power should be increased (A, B) by 3 to 5 D (D) to correct for this.

48. Correct: The total corneal power is less than estimated (B)

The corneal refractive index used to calculate K is artificially lowered to account for the negative power of the posterior cornea. This reduction, about 10%, assumes a typical corneal shape. Since myopic laser correction flattens the anterior corneal surface, keratometry will assume flattening of the posterior corneal surface where no change has occurred. This is called index of refraction error. The posterior corneal power is therefore underestimated (the posterior cornea is more minus than expected). The overestimate of corneal power causes an underestimate of IOL power (A), since cornea and lens together form the total refractive power of the eye. (C) Lens calculations which are not corrected for myopic refractive surgery will tend to suggest a lens, which is less powerful than actually needed, which would cause a hyperopic surprise. Formulas which do not explicitly use anterior-chamber depth make an assumption based on corneal curvature—steeper corneas tend to have deeper chambers. (D) Flattening a cornea with refractive surgery will lead to an assumption that the lens is closer to the cornea than it is in reality (formula error). This can exaggerate a hyperopic surprise.

49. Correct: Apodization of diffractive MFIOL rings may allow for a smoother transition between distance and near images (C)

Apodization refers to decreased height of outer diffractive rings as opposed to inner diffractive rings to lessen the effect of the near component of MFIOL focus in the lens periphery. This may improve the transition between near and far images. Contrast sensitivity is decreased with MFIOLs (A) because of light scatter at the diffractive ring margins that reduce contrast and available image light by 20%. A distant object point is simultaneously imaged by the MFIOL to form an image point and blur circle by the refractive distance and diffractive near components of the MFIOL, respectively. The superposition of an image point and blur circle creates a blur circle that is brightest in the center and lower in periphery (**B**), so it is not uniform. This causes ghosting or halos around objects and lights that is not tolerated by some patients. Similarly, near object points undergo simultaneous focus to form image points and blur circles by the respective near and far components of the MFIOL. Multifocal lenses are very sensitive to corneal astigmatism. As little as 1 D, particularly against-the-rule, can cause significant loss of visual acuity (**D**) and contrast sensitivity. Such a patient may be a candidate for a refractive procedure to reduce astigmatism or a toric multifocal lens.

50. Correct: Light reaches the retina directly, without passing through the IOL (A)

Light from the far temporal side of the eye may pass through the nasal edge of the lens and be refracted towards the central retina. Light from the far temporal side may also have a path around the lens, which is not refracted by the IOL. This results in an arc of peripheral retina which is not illuminated, causing the patient to experience negative dysphotopsia. This is based on ray-tracing studies. It was previously thought that reflections from the edge caused negative dysphotopsia. (**B**) Light reflected from the retina may be reflected back by the anterior lens surface to cause a light spot (**B**) on the retina that is seen as glare. This is a form of positive dysphotopsia. Reflections from the anterior (**C**) and posterior (**D**) surface of the lens (primarily anterior) are thought to play a role in positive dysphotopsia, not negative.

51. Correct: This patient is not a candidate for LASIK (D)

This patient's corneas are too flat to undergo such a myopic treatment. Keratorefractive surgery must flatten the cornea 0.8 D to treat 1.0 D of myopia. In this patient, treating 10.0 D of myopia would require flattening the cornea by 8.0 D. The expected corneal curvature is given by the formula Kpostop = Kpreop + (0.8 × RE). In this case, the expected postoperative curvature is 31.0 D. It is not recommended to leave the cornea flatter than 33.0 D, as it may lead to reduced visual function. A different procedure, such as phakic intraocular lens, could be considered. (**A**) It is generally recommended to treat the manifest refraction when it is similar to the cycloplegic refraction. (**B, C**) There may be a role for adjusting the correction of certain patients, but in this case, it would still result in a cornea which is excessively flat.

52. Correct: Dispense spectacles (A)

This patient currently has a monovision configuration. It's not clear if this was planned, due to regression of LASIK effect, or a myopic shift from an early cataract in the left eye. Some patients with monovision use glasses for certain activities, such as night driving. To differentiate between corneal change and cataract change in this patient, historical refractions can be helpful. Another approach is to perform intraocular lens (IOL) calculations using IOLMaster or Lenstar system; if the myopia in the left eye can be explained by axial length and K values, it is unlikely to be from a myopic shift. (**B**) Treating the left eye with PRK will make this patient, who isn't currently using glasses, dependent on spectacles for near work. You also need to rule out cataract. (**C**) The topographic map is consistent with a slightly decentered ablation, but the patient is seeing well. A rigid contact lens should be considered if the patient is symptomatic despite spectacle correction, but this patient sees well with glasses. (**D**) It is possible that this patient has early cataract with myopic shift, but until he has tried spectacles, surgery is inappropriate

53. Correct: This cornea probably has less spherical aberration than a typical cornea (B)

Spherical aberration is a result of peripheral light rays being refracted more than central rays when passing through a spherical lens. This cornea has a steeper center and flatter periphery (more prolate shape) than a typical cornea, which may be secondary to a hyperopic keratorefractive procedure. This would tend to reduce the amount of spherical aberration in this eye. (**A**) Performing additional laser ablations tends to further increase higher-order aberrations. (**C**) This topography shows asymmetric bow tie configuration with inferior steepening, which is a potential sign of subclinical ectasia when screening patients for refractive surgery. However, this patient already had a refractive procedure. It is not clear whether this was present prior to refractive surgery, or if this is secondary to refractive surgery. It would be prudent to monitor this cornea for ectasia, but this single map does not prove ectasia. (**D**) While there is some irregular astigmatism, the central steepness is still in the normal range (46), so a rigid gas permeable lens may still fit properly.

54. Correct: Reducing the optical zone to 6.0 mm will leave more residual tissue than reducing treatment power to −6.00 (B)

According to the Munnerlyn formula, the thickness (t) required to achieve the necessary refraction correction (**D**) is related by the following formula: t = ({OZ}² × D)/3. Because the optical zone is squared, adjusting it will have a larger effect than adjusting the treatment power. (**A**) LASIK

233

leaves less stromal bed because the flap does not count as stromal bed. (**C**) Wavefront-guided and wavefront-optimized treatments are intended to cause fewer higher-order aberrations, not reduce treatment depth.

55. Correct: A hyperopic LASIK treatment results in a more negative Q factor (D)

Remember that a perfect sphere has a Q factor of zero. This sphere has a high degree of spherical aberration. Healthy corneas have a negative Q factor. Hyperopic LASIK steepens the central cornea further and results in a "hyperprolate" cornea with a more negative Q factor. A more negative Q factor is correlated with a decrease (**A**) in spherical aberration. Healthy corneas tend to have a Q factor of −0.26 (**B**), while an "ideal" cornea has a Q factor of −0.50. Note that it is possible to have negative spherical aberration. The relationship between the Q factor (a dimensionless factor) and the spherical aberration (SA, measured in μm) is not direct. Myopic LASIK flattens the central cornea which results in a more oblate shape and moves the Q factor in a positive direction, increasing positive spherical aberration. Therefore, patients of post-myopic LASIK would still benefit from aspheric intraocular lenses (**C**) that have a negative SA correction (i.e., Tecnis −0.27 μm, Acrysof −0.20 μm). Patients who have undergone hyperopic treatments, on the other hand, might benefit from a spherical intraocular lens (IOL) to avoid inducing negative spherical aberration.

56. Correct: When the corneal apex is decentered from the pupillary axis, significant angle kappa occurs (D)

The pupillary axis is the imaginary line that passes through the midpoint of the pupil and is perpendicular to the cornea. The visual axis connects the point of fixation to the fovea. The difference between the pupillary axis and the visual axis is known as angle kappa, and the corneal apex aligns with the visual axis and not necessarily the midpoint of the pupil. The visual axis, not the center of the cornea (**A**), is the best place to center a treatment. Many excimer lasers used to default to centering the treatment on the midpoint of the pupil (**B**), but this may lead to a "second corneal apex," which can cause visual symptoms such as monocular diplopia. Treatments in patients with large angle kappa should be centered on the visual axis (**C**) to prevent monocular diplopia.

57. Correct: Brimonidine 0.2% may help with postoperative night vision issues (D)

Remember from the Airy disk that a smaller pupil reduces the effects of aberration. With a large pupil, higher-order aberrations become much more noticeable, leading to glare and halos. Brimonidine 0.2% has a mildly miotic effect and may help to reduce night vision issues postoperatively. (**A**) Large pupils are typically defined as greater than 8 mm. The transition zone between ablated and unablated cornea should be 0.5 to 1.0 mm greater (**B**) than the dim pupil size. (**C**) Older generation lasers used both smaller optical zones, and smaller or absent transition zones.

58. Correct: Autorefraction may show a high degree of cylinder (A)

Following refractive surgery, the cornea may have irregular astigmatism. Autorefractors and automated measures of corneal power may read a high degree of astigmatism because they were designed to measure regular astigmatism. (**B**) Because retreatments of residual cylinder may not correct the irregular astigmatism, it is not recommended and may make vision worse. This may change as we get more experience with newer topographic-guided treatments. Regular astigmatism appears as a symmetric bow tie on topography or tomography. (**C**) Irregular astigmatism will have an asymmetric pattern. The axis may be difficult to determine with a cross cylinder (**D**), because it's irregular and has no definite axis.

59. Correct: Horizontal coma (A)

Wavefront aberrations can be described by Zernike's polynomials. The degree of polynomial required to produce the mathematical graph of the wavefront surface is used to label the "order" of the aberration. The lower-order aberrations of clinical significance are all second order: defocus (myopia, hyperopia) and regular astigmatism. Aberrations beyond second order are called higher-order aberrations (HOAs). Coma (vertical and horizontal) and trefoil (vertical and oblique) are the third-order aberrations. Coma tends to be the most visually significant HOA. (**B**) Secondary astigmatism is a fourth-order aberration. (**C**) Spherical aberration is a fourth-order aberration. (**D**) Defocus is a second-order aberration, which encompasses myopia and hyperopia.

60. Correct: PRK treatment centered on the pupillary axis (A)

Although ideally the treatment should be centered on the visual axis, most patients have a small angle kappa, and centering the laser treatment on the pupillary axis will not induce significant irregular astigmatism. Very decentered treatment may induce significant irregular astigmatism and prism. (**B**) Epithelial basement membrane dystrophy, (**C**) flap microstriae, (**D**) and nonuniform hydration more commonly cause irregular astigmatism.

61. Correct: The perceived axial magnification is 2.25 × (B)

The object (the patient's retina) is first acted upon by the 60 D effective power of the patient's eye. Because the eye is emmetropic, this light will be collimated as it leaves the eye (aka zero vergence). The object distance will be the distance to the nodal point of the eye, approximately 17 mm. This light will be "condensed" by the 20 D lens into an image at the secondary focal point of the lens: $1/(20\ D) = 0.05\ m = 50\ mm$ toward the indirect ophthalmoscope. This is where the clinician views the retina, floating 5 cm in front of the condensing lens. Using the formula for transverse magnification, we can calculate (image distance)/(object distance) = $(50/17\ mm) = \sim3 \times$ transverse magnification. See the diagram below. For indirect ophthalmoscopy, the transverse magnification simplifies to $-(P_{eye}/P_{lens})$, where the P variables correspond to the refractive power of the eye and lens. $-60/20\ D = -3 \times$ transverse magnification. To calculate axial magnification, you need to square the transverse magnification, so $3^2 = 9 \times$. However, because the mirrors of the ophthalmoscope reduce the pupillary distance by a factor of 4, the axial magnification will also be reduced by a factor of 4, which results in $9/4 = 2.25 \times$ axial magnification. (**A**) The image produced is real and inverted. (**C**) The retinal image is between the condensing lens and the clinician, not between the condensing lens and the patient. (**D**) For *direct* ophthalmoscopy, the patient's eye acts as a simple magnifier. The equation for a simple magnifier is $D/4$, which would result in $60/4$ or $15 \times$ transverse magnification. This question asked about an *indirect* ophthalmoscope.

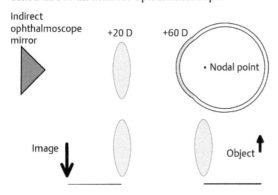

62. Correct: The image size is 2 × 4 cm (C)

Start with the vergence formula: $U + P = V$. The object vergence is $U = -1/(0.5\ m) = -2$, adding the lens gives us $-2 + 3 = 1$, and so image vergence $V = +1$. You can use U/V to calculate magnification. For this question, transverse magnification = $(-2/+1) = -2 \times$. Transverse magnification of -2 means that each linear dimension is doubled in size. This yields an image size of 2 × 4 cm. The sign of the magnification determines whether the image is upright (+) or inverted (−). (**A**) The negative sign indicates that image is inverted. (**B, D**) The magnification of −2 means that the image is larger, not minified.

63. Correct: 12 D (D)

To focus an emmetropic eye on 33 cm would require $1/(0.33\ m) = +3\ D$ of accommodation. The formula for accommodation through a telescope is normal accommodation required × (power of telescope)². In this case, it is $(3\ D) \times (2)^2 = 12\ D$. This is the same optical principle that reduces depth of field under an operating microscope. Tying sutures is easiest with lower magnification, because more accommodation is possible and depth of field is greater. Calibrating the focus between the primary and assistant eyepieces of the microscope is best performed at high magnification, since it is much harder for either surgeon to accommodate.

64. Correct: Field of view–the range of object space visible in the image plane (C)

These terms can be confusing. Here are the definitions: *Field of view*–visible extent of object space in the image plane. *Aperture stop*–(**A**) the opening (i.e., rim of lens, or edge of pupil) that limits the light rays to pass through the system. *Entrance pupil*–(**B**) image of the eye's aperture stop when viewed through the optical elements preceding it (the eye's aperture stop is the physical pupil of the eye, not the image of it). *Depth of field*–the distance an object can be moved without significant blurring of the image. *Depth of focus*–(**D**) range over which the image can be seen without significant blurring (i.e., how far you can move a screen toward or away from a focused projector).

65. Correct: 12 × (B)

When viewing an emmetropic patient's eye, the approximately 60 D of eye power acts as a simple magnifier creating a magnification of $D/4$ or about $15 \times$. Conversely then, a $+12\ D$ hyperopic eye as in this case would have only about 48 D of power giving $48/4 = 12 \times$ simple magnification. In reality, it's a little more complex because the lack of eye power creates divergent light leaving the eye which has to be neutralized by some (+) power in the direct ophthalmoscope. This creates the effect of looking through a reverse Galilean telescope, which results in some minimization of the image compared to an emmetropic eye.

66. Correct: Specular reflection (C)

Specular reflection means that the reflected light has a specific direction, such as the reflection from a mirror or the surface of water. Partial specular reflection at the cornea–aqueous interface allows visualization of the corneal endothelial cell pattern. To perform this, make a narrow, oblique bright beam focused on the posterior cornea. Sweep the beam until you get a specular reflection from Descemet's membrane and increase the magnification. See the two images below, which demonstrate guttae in Fuchs' endothelial dystrophy and pseudoguttae in chronic uveitis. The honeycomb pattern in the Fuchs patient is barely visible. (**A**) In direct illumination, light is reflected directly from the object to the observer. This is the most common way to examine the anterior segment, but it does not allow detailed visualization of endothelium. (**B**) In retroillumination, light bouncing back off structures silhouettes features. Retroillumination from the retina is particularly useful in visualizing posterior subcapsular cataracts, posterior capsular opacification, and iris transillumination defects. It is possible to see endothelial changes using this method, but typically only if there is advanced pathology. (**D**) Sclerotic scatter involves shining the slit beam at the limbus and examining the central cornea with the internally reflected light. This can be used to determine the presence of endothelial changes such as guttae, but it is not ideal for determining cell pattern.

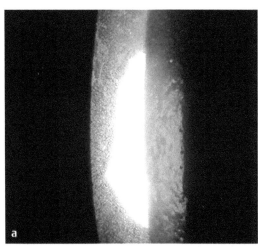

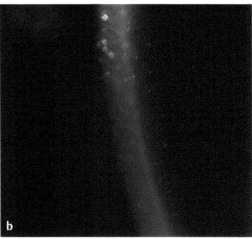

67. Correct: The patient is hyperopic (B)

A hyperopic patient would have the images focused behind the retina. This means the image from the upper pinhole falls on the superior retina, which is interpreted as the lower light being extinguished. (**A**) If the patient is emmetropic, both pinhole images would be focused approximately to a single point. (**C**) If the patient is myopic, the images would have crossed before the retina and the spot on the lower retina would disappear. (**D**) Changing which pinhole is illuminated would yield the same information.

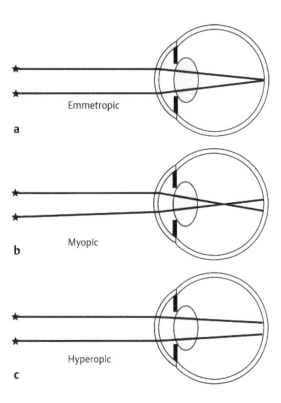

68. Correct: It relies on the cornea's reflective power (C)

Manual keratometry uses reflections from the anterior cornea to measure corneal steepness. The cornea acts as a convex mirror, and the curvature of the mirror displaces mires seen by the operator. By adjusting the position of these mires until they touch, a measurement of anterior corneal curvature can be obtained. (**A**) It measures reflective, not refractive, power. Conversion to refractive power is made by an index of refraction assumption of 1.3375, which is reduced to take into account the negative power of a typical posterior cornea. (**B**) Keratometry measures at a 3-mm diameter, not 2 mm. (**D**) It is not be as reliable in cases of irregular astigmatism, where topography or tomography may be more informative.

69. Correct: A +4 D hand magnifier can have 2 × magnification (A)

When compared to the standard "reference" distance of 25 cm for reading, the relative angular size of the image compared to the object is called the "power" or "magnification factor." It is equal to the power of the lens in diopters divided by 4 (D/4). This magnification occurs when the print is held at the anterior focal point of the lens. If a 4 D lens is used this way, its magnification factor would be 1 ×. However, holding the print at 12.5 cm (half of the focal length) produces a virtual, erect image with transverse magnification of 2 ×. (B) A patient with a tremor would not be able to hold a handheld magnifier, especially a high-power one, steadily enough to use it effectively. Patients with arthritis, tremors, paralysis, or poor hand–eye coordination would do better with a stand magnifier. (C) The common range for hand magnifiers is +5 to +20 D. (D) Low- or medium-power magnifiers provide a larger field of view and are better for continuous print reading.

70. Correct: Bioptic spectacle-mounted telescopes are allowed for driving in certain regions (C)

Bioptic telescopes are mounted in the upper portion of spectacles. The low-vision patient uses the bioptic telescopes to read signs, but otherwise looks through the normal portion of the spectacles. They require a prescription, and driver training, but are permitted in certain states. (A) Near vision loupes give magnification at a useful working distance, but suffer from narrow field of view and narrow depth of field. (B) Distance telescopic aids can be helpful but have the same shortcomings as near loupes, along with reduced contrast, as the magnification is at the expense of luminance. (D) Simple plastic dual optic distance telescopic lenses are available relatively inexpensively and without a casing.

71. Correct: +6.00 laptop computer reading glasses with 8 prism diopter (PD) base-in OU (D)

Kestenbaum's rule estimates the reading add required to read 1M print as the inverse of the visual acuity fraction. For this patient's vision, the inverse of 20/120 gives 120/20 = 6, so a +6.00 reading add would be required. High plus power near glasses require base-in prism to aid in convergence. The general rule is to take the plus power correction, add 2, and put that much base-in prism in each eye. Computer glasses with +6.00 would require 8 prism diopters of base-in prism in each eye. These glasses would act as an intermediate add (+4.00 accounting for the patient's

hyperopia) and would probably allow the patient to use a computer at a shorter-than-normal working distance. (A) Bifocal adds beyond +4.50 are generally not tolerated. (B) +8.00 reading glasses would allow for good reading acuity, but without 8 PD of base-in prism, would likely cause diplopia. (C) A +12.00 monocular reading would not be the most suitable, because it only allows monocular vision, and is much more power than we expect this patient needs, which decreases working distance and would slow reading unnecessarily.

72. Correct: Video magnifiers (A)

Once visual loss is "profound," video magnifiers are unlikely to be very useful. (B–D) The other choices listed are all very useful and fall in the category of "nonvisual assistance" or "visual substitution skills."

73. Correct: Observer and patient pupils are conjugate (A)

The light source, which is in the same plane as the observer's pupil, must be conjugate with the patient's pupil so that an image of the light source is formed in the pupil plane. It is as if the light is reduced in size so that it fits within the pupil and illuminates the retina widely. Otherwise, only some of the light gets through, and this light will illuminate only a small area of retina behind the pupil. You can see this for yourself by moving the condensing lens closer or farther from a patient's eye during indirect ophthalmoscopy. If the lens is not positioned properly, you will not have a full image of the retina. If the observer pupil and patient retina were conjugate (B), then the retina would not be in focus for the observer. Instead, the observer and patient's retina must be conjugate. The patient's far point being in front of the observer (C) is irrelevant, as the condensing lens will still create a real image in front of the observer.

74. Correct: The effect of a telescope (B)

Any variation from emmetropia (i.e., ametropia) requires additional lens power in the ophthalmoscope. In the setting of myopia, the direct ophthalmoscope will be set to a minus power lens. This acts like a Galilean telescope, with the direct ophthalmoscope acting as an eyepiece. This magnification is multiplied by other forms of magnification in play. The direct ophthalmoscope provides the magnification of a simple magnifier when viewing a fundus, but in this case, the additional magnification from the telescope will make the fundus appear larger (A) than an emmetropic eye. (C) Pincushion distortion is a result of a high plus power lens, which is not used to examine a myopic fundus with a direct ophthalmoscope.

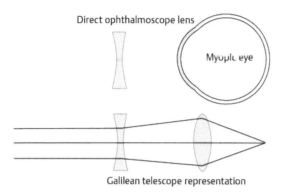

Direct ophthalmoscope lens

Myopic eye

Galilean telescope representation

75.   Correct: Diffraction and aberration play an equal role (D)

The PSF is a measure by which an object point of light is formed into an image by an optical system. An ideal PSF would be a single dot, however, any optical system leads to an imperfect PSF and an imperfect image. When the pupil size is intermediate at 2.3 to 2.4 mm, the effects of diffraction and aberration are balanced and give the smallest overall PSF. This is considered the "optimal pupil size." (**A**) The PSF is larger when the pupil is small and light undergoes significant diffraction, so this is not the optimal pupil size. (**B**) Similarly, the PSF is large when the pupil is large and light undergoes more aberration. (**C**) The PSF is always affected to some degree by diffraction and aberration.

76.   Correct: Interference (C)

This is an antireflective coating. A coating is deposited at a thickness of one-fourth of the desired wavelength of light. Light striking the coating will be reflected by the front and back surface of the coating. Light reflecting from the back coating will be 2 × 1/4 = 1/2 wavelength out of phase with light reflecting from the front surface. This results in destructive interference, so that any light that would be reflected interferes, and therefore cannot be reflected. Because the coating only prevents certain wavelengths from reflecting, some wavelengths are reflected, resulting in the green color in this case. (**A**) Diffraction is the bending of light around the edge of an aperture. (**B**) Dispersion is the varying refraction of light of different wavelengths by a lens material, such as chromatic aberration. (**D**) Refraction is the transmission of light at an interface rather than reflection.

77.   Correct: They reduce reflected light (B)

Polarized lenses block reflected light from horizontal surfaces that is linearly polarized parallel to these surfaces. The maximum polarization of light by such surfaces occurs at the Brewster angle of incidence. The reflection of such light from water or road surfaces that causes glare is thus removed. Although they diminish light like all sunglasses, polarizing lenses have additional specific features (**A**), so this is

not the best answer. (**C, D**) Refracted light is transmitted light, and not all transmitted light is polarized. In any case, glare from surfaces is caused by reflections and not refraction.

78.   Correct: Dispersion (A)

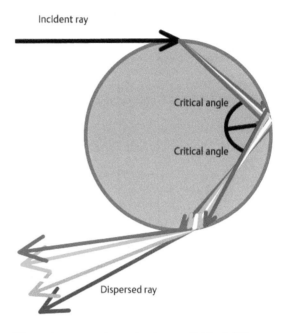

Incident ray

Critical angle

Critical angle

Dispersed ray

Dispersion separates out colors as light of different wavelengths undergo different degrees of refraction at interfaces. In the case of a rainbow, water droplets cause multiple total internal reflections within the droplet. Some of the light will escape the droplet after being reflected, and at this transition, the magnitude of refraction is wavelength dependent (as it is with chromatic aberration). Usually, the sun is behind the observer, and the water droplets in front redirect the light back toward the observer (see diagram). (**B**) Diffraction is bending of light waves around edges or boundaries. (**C**) Scatter is redirection of light in many directions other than that of the original incident light by particles. (**D**) Absorption is the transfer of energy from a photon to an electron. When an electron absorbs a photon, it moves to a higher potential energy level.

79.   Correct: Diffraction (B)

Diffraction is bending of light around edges. A scratch on the surface forms a diffracting edge that bends a light wave outward in a direction at right angles to the scratch line, analogous to Airy's disk that is formed by a round aperture. (**A**) Refraction is the redirection of light travel by an interface where refractive index changes. (**C**) Reflection is the redirection of light to the same side of an interface where refractive index changes so that angle of reflection equals the angle of incidence. (**D**) Prismatic deviation is the refraction of light by an angled interface where refractive index changes. If the interface is flat, then the direction of light travel is changed, but the vergence is unchanged. However, if the surface is curved, then both direction of light and vergence of the light changes across the interface.

80. Correct: Short-wavelength light scatter between subject and object is screened out (A)

As stated in Rayleigh's formula, blue light is scattered by air more than longer wavelengths. This is why the sky appears blue. (**B, D**) Orange tint is effectively a filter which blocks blue light (short wavelength). (**C, D**) The scatter occurs throughout the air between the subject and object.

81. Correct: Diffraction (C)

A healthy cornea is clear because the well-organized bands of collagen are evenly spaced so that any scattered or diffracted light will be lost to destructive interference, similar to the function of antireflective coating. An edematous cornea becomes disorganized, and light can be scattered and diffracted. Point-like light sources will appear more diffuse, like a halo. Diffraction from the edges of each collagen fibril can act as a diffraction grating, causing colored halos. (**A**) Total internal reflection is when light cannot travel from a material of high index of refraction into a lower index of refraction. Total internal reflection is what necessitates a gonio lens to visualize the angle, and what allows fiber optic cables to function. (**B**) Absorption causes the selective removal of some wavelengths of light by pigments such as blue-blocking lenses absorbing blue light and making images appear yellow. (**D**) Refraction is the redirection of light waves by an interface where the index of refraction changes.

82. Correct: Absorption (D)

The shorter wavelengths of incident white light are absorbed by the retinal pigment epithelium, choroid pigment, and blood of the choroidal vasculature. What remains is longer wavelength orange and red light. (**A**) Dispersion is variable refraction based on wavelength and is responsible for chromatic aberration and rainbows. (**B**) When you examine a retina, you are viewing light reflected from the retina, but the reflection is red because colors other than red are absorbed.

83. Correct: 1.4 mm (D)

For chromatic aberration, the smaller the pupil, the better. If the image of an object point is larger than a point (such as a blur circle, coma, or other shape), then the size of that image is reduced by the smaller aperture and approximates a point. This reduces the effect of lens aberration. Diffraction, on the other

hand, increases in magnitude at smaller apertures. Note that 2.4 mm (**B**) is best overall to balance aberration and diffraction (Airy's disk), because it is midway between a large and small pupil. However, the question asked only about minimizing aberration.

84. Correct: 2.4 mm (B)

Airy's disk lets us know that a 2.4-mm pupil will tend to balance diffractions and aberrations to give the best possible resolution. At a pupil smaller than 2.4 mm (**A**), diffraction limits resolution. At pupils larger than 2.4 mm (**C, D**), aberration limits resolution.

85. Correct: Long-wavelength light penetrates lower in the atmosphere and is scattered by dust particles (D)

Small particles (such as air in the atmosphere) scatter short-wavelength (blue) light more than other wavelengths. Larger particles, such as dust, scatter all wavelengths. In this situation, the short-wavelength light has already been scattered away by the upper atmosphere by the time it reaches the lower levels. The longer (red) wavelengths that reach the lower levels are scattered in all directions by the dust particles. Normally, we would see scattered blue in the air in any direction other than the sun, and a yellow sun that has had some blue scattered away. Here, we see mainly red scattered in all directions. Short-wavelength light is scattered more (**A, C**) by the small particles in the atmosphere and therefore doesn't penetrate as well. (**B**) Short-wavelength light and long-wavelength light are scattered equally by large particles such as dust.

86. Correct: −5.00 +2.00 × 90 (C)

Contact lenses are usually prescribed in minus cylinder. To convert between these two, you can use a power cross to avoid making mistakes. The diagram demonstrates these two refractions in a power cross. The resultant refraction is −5.00 +2.00 × 90, or in minus cylinder, −3.00 −2.00 × 180.

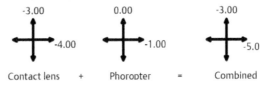

| Contact lens | + | Phoropter | = | Combined |

87. Correct: Blue light creating images in fluorescein angiography (B)

Light has a wave-particle duality. Fluorescence is an example of the particle nature of light, in the form of a photon. Shorter-wavelength (higher-frequency) light means each individual photon has higher energy. In the case of fluorescence, a photon is absorbed by an electron in the fluorescent pigment. This electron elevates to a higher-energy level and then rapidly decays back to a lower-energy state. Each time the electron drops to a lower-energy level, it emits a secondary, lower-energy photon. In the case of fluorescein, most energy is emitted as a green photon, which is imaged by the camera. Interference patterns (**A**), polarization (**C**), and antireflective coating (**D**) (an example of destructive interference) are all examples of the wave properties of light.

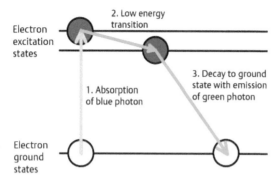

88. Correct: The ciliary muscle contracts, which loosens the zonular fibers (A)

Zonular fibers exert baseline tension on the lens. When accommodation is relaxed, the tension from the zonular fibers is at its maximum, which tends to flatten the lens slightly. The ciliary muscle forms a ring around the zonular insertions. When the ciliary muscle contracts, it decreases the diameter of the ring. This causes the zonular fibers to become looser. This decreased tension on the lens causes the lens to become slightly steeper, which increases lens power. The other answer choices have part of this relationship backward (**B–D**).

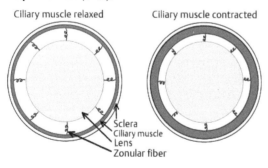

89. Correct: "x" represents the direction of travel of the wavefront (B)

The rays serve to indicate the direction of travel of various parts of the wavefront. The wavefront moves outward in a spherical manner from the starting point. Rays of light in a diagram are just markers of direction of travel of various parts of a wavefront. There are infinite number of "rays" emanating from the object point corresponding to all parts of the wavefront, but only a few are shown. Textbook diagrams often dispense with the wavefront drawing, but keep the rays, because they can be used to create geometric diagrams for calculation of vergence and refraction. "w" represents the object point, because light is shown by the arrows to be leaving the point rather than arriving to it as expected for an image point (**A**). "y" is a measure of crest-to-crest distance, which is the wavelength of the light shown. Frequency is equal to speed of light divided by the wavelength (**C**). "z" represents a wavefront of light, not a ray (**D**).

90. Correct: The lens material must have higher refractive index than the surrounding medium (B)

The lens must have plus power since it takes nonvergent entering light and converts it to convergent light. Since the lens is convex, it must have a higher index of refraction to cause positive vergence. If the convex lens refractive index were lower than the surrounding medium, then the power would negative (as seen with an air bubble in the eye during surgery). The planar wavefront may have originated far away but may also have originated due to another lens system (**A**), such as originating from the focal point of a converging lens. Light with no vergence that enters a convergent lens will be focused to the focal point of the lens. The vergence of light at this point approaches infinity, not zero (**C**). The vergence of light on the left is uniform and of zero vergence, while that on the right it is increasing steadily toward the image point where it has infinite vergence. Calculating any lens configuration using the vergence formula will demonstrate different vergences (**D**) at different distances from the lens.

91. Correct: The lens induces base-down prism in the upper half of the lens (D)

Lenses act as a prism for light which does not pass through the optical center of the lens. To remember the direction of the prism, think of the shape of a convex and concave lens as stacked prisms (see diagram). For a convex (plus power) lens, the shape of the lens is with a base-down prism in the top half and a base-up prism in the bottom half. Note that this also applies in the horizontal plane: the base of the prism will be at the center of the lens. Prentice's rule allows us to calculate the magnitude of induced prism. Multiply the lens power (in diopters) by the distance from the optical center (in centimeter) to calculate induced prism. In this case, point x would be 5 D × 1 cm = 5 prism diopters. From our diagram, we see that it should be base up (**A**), not base down. You can use the distance formula to determine that point z is $\sqrt{2}$ cm from the optical center, so it would induce $5\sqrt{2}$ prism (**B**) with the base toward the center of the lens. Point y would be 5 prism diopters base in (**C**), not base down.

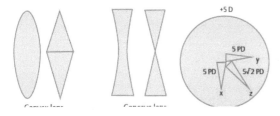

92. Correct: −4 (D)

Transverse magnification can be calculated by M = (image height)/(object height) or by M = (image distance)/(object distance). It can also be calculated by M = (object vergence)/(image vergence). For this problem, the calculation with vergences makes the answer much simpler. Object vergence is −4. Image vergence can be calculated using the vergence formula, U + P = V, or −4 + 5 = 1. The magnification is then (−4)/(1) = −4. If you cannot remember this formula, this can still be solved using (image distance)/(object distance). To solve it this way, you need to calculate that light with vergence −4 could have originated from an object at distance of (−1)/(4) = −1/4 m or −0.25 m. The image distance is 1/1 = 1 m. M = (1 m)/(−0.25 m) = −4. Diagram: Vergence calculation with 5-D lens.

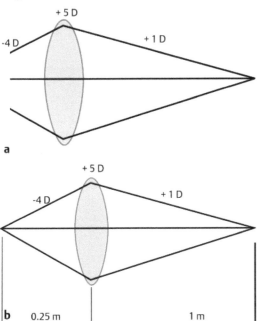

93. Correct: −1.00 +2.00 × 135 OD −1.00 +2.00 × 045 OS (C)

Oblique astigmatism correction can cause symptomatic distortion. Under monocular conditions, the oblique correction would cause a minor (< 1 degree) of image tilt. With both eyes opened, the discrepancy in stereopsis can cause this image tilt to be perceived as more than 30 degrees of image tilt. The other corrections can cause distortion, but the distortion caused by vertical or horizontal astigmatism is much less symptomatic (**A, B, and D**). If you have a patient complaining of image tilt with new glasses, you can try adjusting the axis closer to 90 or 180 or undercorrecting the cylinder.

94. Correct: Real images are always formed by converging rays (A)

Real images occur any time the rays creating it are converging or have positive vergence. If the image created is due to a diverging ray, the image is virtual. This most commonly occurs in a compound optical system, such as the example below. Two converging lenses together create a real intermediate image, which then creates a virtual image which is inverted. Virtual images are always formed by diverging rays (**B**). Virtual images are often upright, but not always (**C**). Real images are often inverted, but not always (**D**).

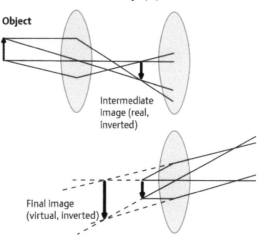

95. Correct: 1.25 × (C)

Sunlight entering this unknown lens has zero vergence and is focused 20 cm beyond the lens. That is the definition of a secondary focal point, so this lens has a focal length of 20 cm. Therefore, this lens has a power of 1/(0.2 m) = 5 D. Simple magnifiers are compared to a reference distance of 25 cm. You can calculate the magnification of simple magnifiers with the formula (D/4), in this case 5/4 = 1.25 ×.

96. Correct: The conjugate plane to the fovea in a cyclopleged eye is at the far point of the eye (A)

If two planes are conjugate, it means that an object in one plane will correspond to an image in the other. It also means that the directions of rays can be reversed; the image can act as an object and project an image to the original object. As an example, a corrected eye will have its fovea conjugate to what it is viewing. This means that an "E" on an eye chart creates an image of an "E" on the fovea. It also means that there is an image of the fovea created on the "E!" Anywhere you look, you are projecting a very faint image of your fovea. This is how a fundus camera is able to function. For a lens, every plane in the optical axis will have a corresponding conjugate plane. There are infinite conjugate planes (**B**), not two. This is what you are solving for in most geometric optics questions. The focal points of a lens are by definition not conjugate (**C**); if you placed an object at the anterior focal point of a plus lens, the image will be created at infinity, not at the other focal point. Nodal points are unique to each lens system. Rays from an object that pass through the anterior nodal point (**D**) will appear to come out of the posterior nodal point toward the conjugate image. They are important to working with conjugate planes

97. Correct: None of the above (D)

Pinhole occluders typically have holes which are 1 to 1.2 mm in diameter, which is less than the Airy disk. To understand the reason, you need to think about why we use pinhole occluders as a quick way to reduce aberrations. The vision through a 1.2-mm pinhole will be limited somewhat by diffraction, but it does a much better job at correcting refractive error. Diffraction will be less for a 2.4-mm pinhole and in an emmetropic eye, this may improve acuity. However, we don't need pinhole occluders for emmetropic eyes (**A**). The larger pinhole will allow aberration, including refractive error, to have a larger detrimental effect (**B**) on vision. The larger pinhole means less diffraction (**C**), not more.

98. Correct: Infinity (B)

This optical system in this question is a Keplerian or astronomical telescope, which is an afocal optical system. In this case, the image is created at infinity (to the right in our diagram). To see why, we can use the vergence formula and solve it in steps. The object vergence entering the first lens is $-1/(5 \text{ m})$ = -0.2. Adding the vergence of the lens, we get the intermediate image vergence of $-0.2 + 5.2 = 5$ D. This means the intermediate image is created $1/(5)$ = 0.2 m to the right of the first lens. We then use this image as our object for the second lens. Light from this object will travel 10 cm to the right toward the

+10 D lens. The object vergence is $-1/(0.1) = -10$ D. Adding the vergence of the lens, we get an image vergence of 0 D. Because these rays continue to travel to the right, the object will be at an infinite distance to the right of the lenses. By convention, this is positive infinity. If it were to the left, it would be (**A**) negative infinity.

99. Correct: 10 PD base in both eyes (D)

To answer this correctly, you must remember two important facts about prisms. First, the image in a prism is displaced toward the apex of the prism. Second, 1 prism diopter is defined as deviating an image 1 cm at a distance of 100 cm. In this question, she reports that the right eye image is too far to the left. This would require a prism with apex to the right over the right eye, which is the same as base in. Since the image is displaced 10 cm at a distance of 50 cm, you must convert this to a distance of 100 cm. By similar triangles, the image would be displaced 20 cm at a distance of 100 cm, so the total prism must be 20 prism diopters base in (equivalent to 10 prism diopters base in OU). Base-out prism (**A, B**) would worsen the deviation. Not adjusting the distance to 100 cm would result in undertreating (**A, C**) the deviation.

100. Correct: Red: less absorption by hemoglobin (B)

It seems counterintuitive, but pigments are colored because they absorb everything other than their color. For instance, plants are green because chlorophyll absorbs all colors but green. Hemoglobin is red because it absorbs all colors but red. A dispersed vitreous hemorrhage acts as a red filter. As a result, red light (such as from a Xenon laser) would have better penetration through hemorrhage. Similarly, a yellow laser has better penetration through a brunescent cataract. (**A**) Blue does have higher energy per photon, but it will be absorbed by the hemorrhage and not reach the retina. (**C**) Green will be absorbed by hemoglobin and can be scattered by small particles. The melanin in retinal pigment epithelium (RPE) cells absorbs all colors of visible light. (**D**) Yellow light for retinopexy is absorbed more by hemoglobin than by melanin.

Chapter 8

Retina and Ocular Oncology

Syed A. Hussnain, Norimitsu Ban, Aliaa H. Abdelhakim, Spencer Langevin, Tarun Sharma, Brian P. Marr,
Tongalp H. Tezel

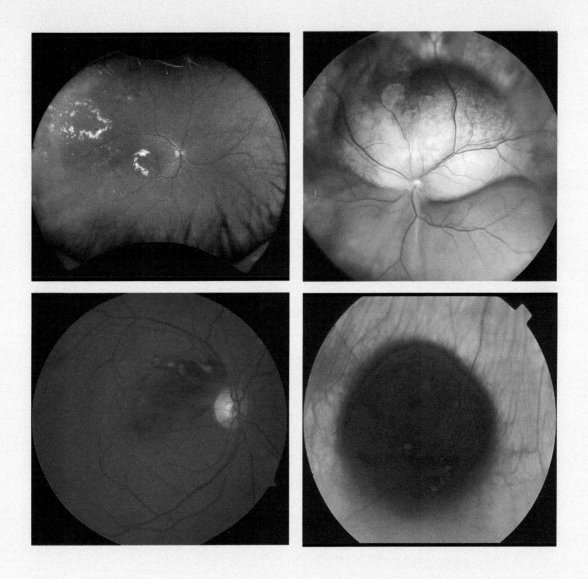

8.1 Questions

Easy | Medium | Hard

1. A 48-year-old woman with diabetes presents to your office for examination. You order a high-definition swept-source optical coherence tomography (OCT) to assess for diabetic macular edema. What is the space in front of the optic nerve on her OCT called?

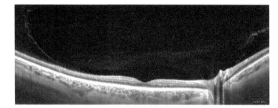

A. Weigert's ligament

B. Vitreous base

C. Area of Martegiani

D. Cloquet's canal

2. You have just finished performing an optical coherence tomography (OCT) of the macula on a new patient. The patient asks you to describe the macula. Which one of the following best describes the anatomical macula?

A. An area composed of only cones photoreceptors.

B. An area where there are no capillaries.

C. An area ~5.5 mm in diameter bordered by the disc and temporal vascular arcades.

D. An area 3.0 mm temporal and 0.8 mm superior to the center of the optic disc.

3. A 29-year-old woman with systemic lupus erythematosus presents for eye examination after her rheumatologist recently started her on hydroxychloroquine (HCQ). In HCQ toxicity, what retinal layer is initially affected?

A. Retinal pigment epithelium (RPE)

B. Choroid

C. Outer plexiform layer

D. Photoreceptor layer

4. A 68-year-old man with diabetes and hypertension presents with blurry vision in his right eye and is found to have the dilated fundus as shown in figure. In patients with this entity, what imaging modality is most predictive of the likelihood of visual acuity recovery?

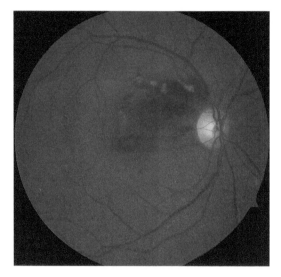

A. Autofluorescence

B. Optical coherence tomography (OCT)

C. Fluorescein angiography (FA)

D. Indocyanine green (ICG) angiography

5. You decide to obtain fluorescein angiography on a patient with a branch retinal vein occlusion. What is the most common side effect of fluorescein angiography?

A. Photosensitivity

B. Hives

C. Anaphylaxis

D. Nausea

6. A 30-year-old pregnant woman with a history of proliferative diabetic retinopathy presents with new onset blurry vision in her left eye and is found to have mild vitreous hemorrhage. An area suspicious for neovascularization is noted along the superotemporal arcade. What is the best way to confirm the presence of retinal neovascularization in this patient?

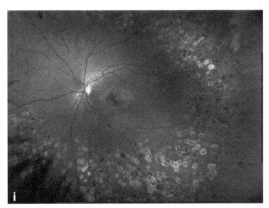

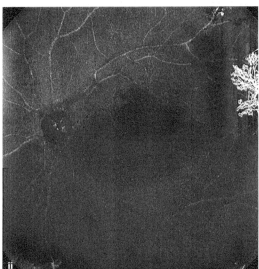

A. Optical coherence tomography (OCT)
B. OCT angiography
C. Fluorescein angiography
D. Indocyanine green (ICG) angiography

7. A 72-year-old White woman with age-related macular degeneration presents for her routine follow-up. You obtain the following image to monitor progression. What layer of the retina does this imaging modality measure?

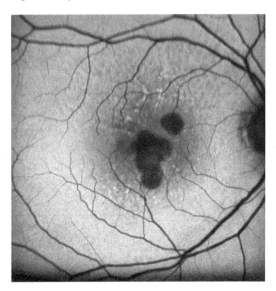

A. Nerve fiber layer
B. Inner nuclear layer
C. Outer nuclear layer
D. Retinal pigment epithelium (RPE) layer

8. You order fluorescein angiography (FA) and indocyanine green (ICG) angiography on a patient with central serous chorioretinopathy. When comparing fluorescein to indocyanine green:

A. Fluorescein optimally fluoresces at a shorter wavelength than ICG.
B. ICG fluoresces brighter than fluorescein.
C. Fluorescein is more protein-bound than ICG in the bloodstream.
D. Fluorescein optimally fluoresces at a longer wavelength than ICG.

9. An 80-year-old woman in your retina clinic asks how do you know that she does not have exudative age-related macular degeneration (AMD). Which of the following does she not demonstrate?

A. Retinal pigment epithelium (RPE) pigmentary changes
B. Drusenoid pigment epithelial detachments (PEDs)
C. Thickening of Bruch's membrane
D. PED that exhibits leakage on fluorescein angiography

10. Which of the following patients has been determined to benefit from Age-Related Eye Disease Study (AREDS) vitamin supplementation?

A. 40-year-old man with numerous large drusen

B. 14-year-old girl with Stargardt disease

C. 62-year-old man with geographic atrophy in one eye

D. 78-year-old patient with previous bilateral choroidal neovascularization

11. A 90-year-old woman comes to your office for a routine eye exam. Normal retinal changes with age include all factors except:

A. Photoreceptors are reduced in density.

B. Lipofuscin accumulates in the retinal pigment epithelium (RPE).

C. Deposits accumulate between Bruch's membrane and the choriocapillaris.

D. Involutional changes occur in the choriocapillaris.

12. A 75-year-old woman presents to your clinic for evaluation of age-related macular degeneration (AMD). You obtain an optical coherence tomography (OCT) that shows the following findings shown in the figure. Which of the following findings are not part of the spectrum of disease in nonexudative AMD?

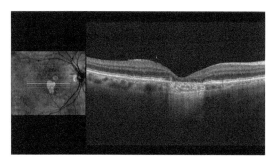

A. Subretinal fluid

B. Geographic retinal pigment epithelial atrophy

C. Hard drusen

D. Retinal pigment epithelium (RPE) pigmentary changes

13. While examining a 77-year-old woman, you notice the presence of many intermediate, soft drusen. Which drusen carry the worst prognosis for visual loss from macular neovascular complications?

A. Cuticular

B. Hard

C. Small

D. Soft

14. You have been asked to examine a patient known to have age-related macular degeneration (AMD). What aspect of evaluation is of primary importance?

A. A complete fundus examination

B. Fluorescein angiography

C. Optical coherence tomography (OCT)

D. Fundus photography

15. An 82-year-old man with cardiovascular disease presents with an acute change in his vision. In the disease pictured, what is the material causing the pathology?

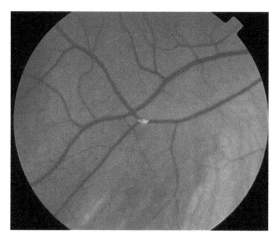

A. Fibrin

B. Cholesterol

C. Calcium

D. Parasite

16. A 75-year-old man with a history of cardiovascular disease presents with 20/40 vision in the same eye as findings consistent with central retinal artery occlusion (CRAO). What is the most likely explanation?

A. This is a nonischemic CRAO and so he has good central vision.

B. The long anterior ciliary arteries maintain redundant circulation, thus there is good central vision.

C. The cilioretinal arteries provide circulation to the fovea and are not affected.

D. The occlusion has been detected early enough and with anti-VEGF therapy, he can maintain good vision.

17. An 80-year-old woman had a central retinal artery occlusion (CRAO) in her left eye 4 days ago and now presents with sudden total loss of vision in her right eye. Which of the following tests should be considered immediately?

A. Carotid ultrasound

B. MRI of the brain

C. CT of the orbits

D. Erythrocyte sedimentation rate (ESR)/C-reactive protein (CRP)

18. While examining a 68-year-old man with a history of stroke, you notice narrowed retinal arteries, dilated retinal veins, midperipheral intraretinal hemorrhages, and neovascularization of the iris in his right eye. The left eye fundus exam is unremarkable. What is the most important next step in the management of this patient?

A. Panretinal photocoagulation

B. Intravitreal anti-VEGF therapy

C. Carotid ultrasound and referral to vascular surgery

D. Cardiac stents

19. You are examining a 2nd-year medical student who mentions to you that all pigmented structures in the body are derived from neural crest cells. You show him a swept-source optical coherence tomography (OCT) of his right eye. What is the origin of the cells that are part of the the bottom most hyperreflective layer on the OCT?

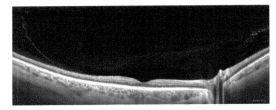

A. Surface ectoderm

B. Neural crest cells

C. Mesoderm

D. Neuroectoderm

20. Your 60-year-old with severe nonproliferative diabetic retinopathy (NPDR) asks you if it is OK for him to take aspirin recommended by his cardiologist. Based on Early Treatment Diabetic Retinopathy Study (ETDRS) reports, which of the following statements regarding the use of aspirin is FALSE?

A. It has no effect on progression of retinopathy.

B. It has no effect on rates of progression to high-risk PDR.

C. It has no effect on rates of vitreous hemorrhage.

D. It significantly increases the rate of vitrectomy for nonclearing vitreous hemorrhage.

21. After examining a diabetic patient with you, a rotating medical student asks you if the patient has clinically significant macular edema (CSME). According to the Early Treatment Diabetic Retinopathy Study (ETDRS), which of the following is defined as CSME?

A. Retinal thickening anywhere within temporal arcades

B. Hard exudate with 7500 μm of the center of the macula with adjacent thickening of the retina

C. Extensive foveal and parafoveal nonperfusion on fluorescein angiography

D. An area of retinal thickening <= one disc area, any part of which lies within one disc diameter of the center of the macula

22. Which of the following statements regarding the Early Treatment Diabetic Retinopathy Study (ETDRS) is false?

A. The ETDRS concluded that panretinal photocoagulation (PRP) reduces the risk of severe visual loss in patients with high-risk proliferative diabetic retinopathy (PDR).

B. The ETDRS identified the risk factors for development of PDR.

C. The ETDRS defined clinically significant macular edema (CSME).

D. The ETDRS showed that aspirin does not affect disease progression.

23. One of your patients with no significant ocular history was recently diagnosed with gestational diabetes and calls you to inquire when during her pregnancy should you screen her for diabetic retinopathy. Pregnant women with gestational diabetes mellitus should be examined:

A. Only if symptomatic

B. Every trimester

C. Once during pregnancy

D. During first trimester and after delivery

24. A 23-year-old man presents to your office with blurry vision. His fundus findings are shown below in the ultrawide-field imaging. What is the genetic inheritance pattern of this disease?

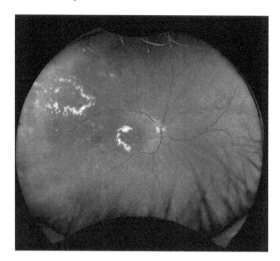

A. Autosomal recessive

B. Autosomal dominant

C. X-linked recessive

D. None of the above

25. A 68-year-old man with diabetes and hypertension presents with blurry vision in his right eye and is found to have an abnormal dilated fundus exam as shown in the color photograph below. Which one of the following is NOT a risk factor for this entity?

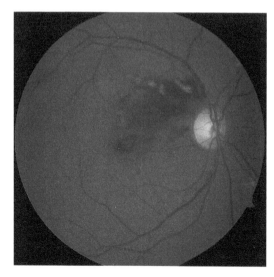

A. Diabetes mellitus

B. Hypertension

C. Increased body mass index (BMI) at an age of 20

D. Hyperlipidemia

26. A 17-year-old girl with sickle cell SS disease presents for retinal evaluation and is found to have the following findings. Which proliferative sickle cell retinopathy feature is depicted in the color and fluorescein angiography images below?

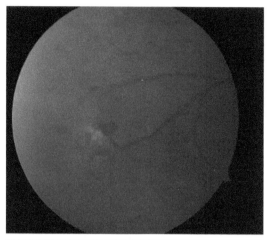

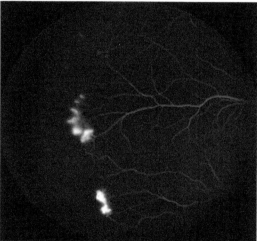

A. Iridescent spots

B. Salmon patch

C. Black sunburst lesions

D. Sea fan

27. A sickle cell patient is lost to follow-up and presents 2 years later with a retinal detachment. Which one the following cannot be listed as a reasonable precautionary action while planning retina detachment repair in a patient with SS disease?

A. Avoiding sclera buckle

B. Avoiding epinephrine in the local anesthetics

C. Not removing extraocular muscles

D. Applying cryopexy around the peripheral retina

28. A 68-year-old man with diabetes and hypertension presents with blurry vision in his right eye and is found to have a branch retinal vein occlusion (BRVO). Which one of the following is an indication for laser photocoagulation in the setting of BRVO?

A. Macular edema with central thickness more than 500 μm

B. Macular edema for 3 months with vision 20/40

C. Macular edema with vision 20/200 and central thickness more than 300 μm

D. Patients with more than five disc areas of capillary drop out in fluorescein angiography

29. A 41-year-old patient with "plucked chicken-skin" appearance presents with fundus and optical coherence tomography (OCT) findings shown below. Subretinal hemorrhages in this entity:

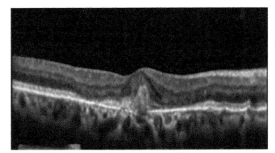

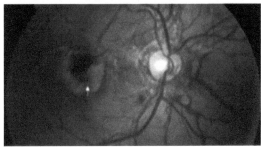

A. May resolve spontaneously without evidence of choroidal neovascularization (CNV)

B. Requires intravitreal dexamethasone

C. Can be managed with photodynamic therapy if extrafoveal

D. Can be managed with thermal laser if peripapillary

30. A 45-year-old man presents with blurry vision in his right eye and is found to have the following finding on his fundus examination. Which one of the following clinical characteristics is typical of this finding?

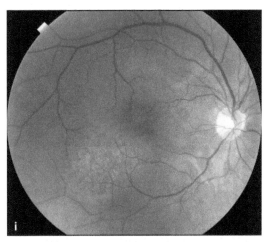

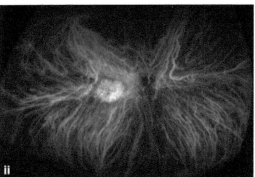

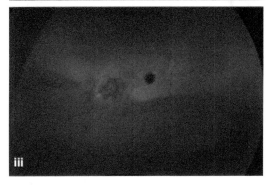

A. Serous detachment of the retinal pigment epithelium (RPE)

B. Myopia

C. Low internal reflectivity on A-scan

D. Wash-out pattern on indocyanine green (ICG) angiography

31. You notice the following finding while performing a dilated fundus examination on your patient. What is a potential complication of the condition shown below?

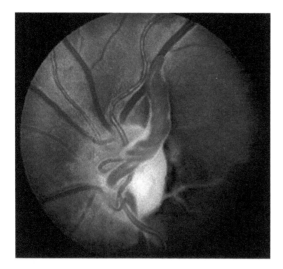

A. Vitreous hemorrhage

B. Branch retinal artery occlusion

C. Branch retinal vein occlusion

D. All of the above

32. A 63-year-old woman presents to your office with acute onset of flashes and floaters. What is the chance of finding a retinal tear in a patient who has a symptomatic posterior vitreous detachment?

A. > 1%

B. 3 to 5%

C. 8 to 15%

D. 20 to 25%

33. During your routine dilated exam on a patient with age-related macular degeneration, you find a peripheral retinal break. The patient does not report any symptoms of flashes or floaters. Which of these may increase the risk of retinal detachment in a patient with an asymptomatic break?

A. Family history

B. Aphakia, pseudophakia

C. History of retinal detachment (RD) in the fellow eye

D. All of the above

34. What is the correct order of the name of the pathologies shown below?

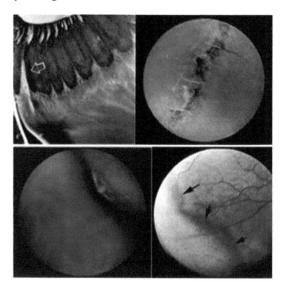

A. Slit tear, lattice degeneration, peripheral retinal excavation, retinoschisis

B. Meridional fold, lattice degeneration, cystic tuft with peripheral retinal excavation, white-without-pressure

C. Dentate process, paving-stone, lattice degeneration, white-with-pressure

D. Peripheral retinal excavation, lattice degeneration, cystic tuft with peripheral retinal excavation, reticular degeneration

35. A 38-year-old investment banker under high stress presents to your office with blurry vision in his right eye. You obtain the imaging shown. What fluorescence patterns are demonstrated in the angiogram?

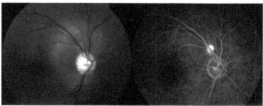

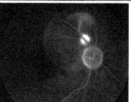

A. Window defect

B. Leakage

C. Pooling

D. B and C

36. You obtain an optical coherence tomography (OCT) of the macula in a patient with decreased vision in the left eye. Which layer is affected in the OCT scan shown?

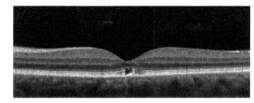

A. Ganglion cell layer
B. Inner nuclear layer
C. Ellipsoid layer/interdigitation zone
D. Outer plexiform layer

37. You observe the optic nerve to be raised with edematous appearance in a young, asymptomatic woman. What kind of an imaging technique has been employed to obtain the fundus picture below and what is depicted in the image?

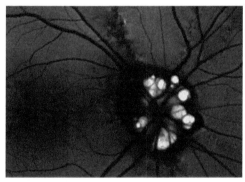

A. Fluorescein angiography (FA): Neovascularization on or within one-disc diameter of the optic nerve head (NVD)
B. FAF: Optic nerve drusen
C. Near infrared: choroidal neovascularization (CNV)
D. Indocyanine green (ICG) angiography: polypoidal choroidal vasculopathy

38. A 70-year-old man presents with distorted vision in his left eye. An optical coherence tomography (OCT) of the macula is obtained. What condition is depicted in the OCT scan below?

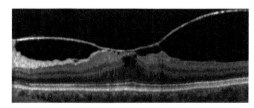

A. Vitreomacular traction (VMT)
B. Wet age-related macular degeneration
C. Acute posterior vitreous detachment
D. Diabetic macular edema

39. An 80-year-old Caucasian woman presents with acute decline in vision in her right eye and is found to have subretinal fluid in the macula. The differential diagnosis for neovascular age-related macular degeneration (AMD) includes which of the following pathologies?

A. Idiopathic polypoidal choroidal vasculopathy (IPCV)
B. Retinal arterial macroaneurysm
C. Vogt–Koyanagi–Harada (VKH) disease
D. All of the above

40. A 70-year-old man with a history of stroke has narrowed retinal arteries, dilated retinal veins, mid-peripheral intraretinal hemorrhages, and neovascularization of the iris in his right eye suggestive of ocular ischemic syndrome. Which one the following fluorescein angiography pattern IS NOT typical for ocular ischemic syndrome?

A. Delayed choroidal filling
B. Increased transit time
C. Vascular staining
D. Pooling of dye under the retinal pigment epithelium (RPE)

41. You diagnose a patient with ocular ischemic syndrome. Which statement is correct regarding ocular ischemic syndrome?

A. Two-third of the eyes develop neovascularization of the iris (NVI)
B. One-fifth of the eyes have flare and cells
C. Half of the eyes develop neovascular glaucoma (NVG)
D. All of the above

42. A 76-year-old woman presents with a headache and acute vision loss in the left eye and is found to have a central retinal artery occlusion (CRAO) on dilated fundus exam in the emergency room. What test would you not consider?

A. Erythrocyte sedimentation rate (ESR)
B. C-reactive protein (CRP)
C. Platelet count
D. Interleukin 6 (IL-6)

43. A 20-year-old patient who recently had brain surgery presents to you for a routine eye exam and is found to have the lesion shown below in his right eye. The left eye shows a similar but smaller lesion. What is the most common cause of death in these patients?

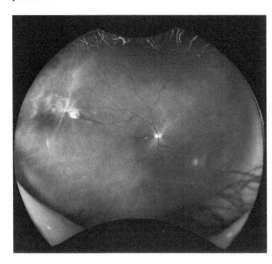

A. Pheochromocytoma and cerebellar hemangioblastoma

B. Cerebellar hemangioblastoma and renal cell carcinoma

C. Liver cysts and meningiomas

D. Spinal cord tumors and pheochromocytomas

44. You see a patient in clinic who has cystoid macular edema. What structure comprises the inner blood–retinal barrier that is compromised in this condition?

A. Inner nuclear layer–ganglion cell layer junction

B. Tight junctional girdles of retinal pigment epithelium (RPE)

C. External limiting membrane

D. Endothelial cell tight junctions

45. You order a fluorescein angiogram on a patient with diabetes. What are the excitation and emission wavelengths for sodium fluorescein, respectively?

A. 530 nm, 700 nm

B. 465 nm, 530 nm

C. 830 nm, 1000 nm

D. 700 nm, 530 nm

46. While performing a dilated fundus exam on an asymptomatic patient, you notice a cystic retinal tuft in the right eye. Which of the following contributes the highest risk for a retinal tear?

A. Noncystic retinal tufts

B. Cystic retinal tufts

C. Anteriorly located zonular traction tufts

D. Posteriorly located zonular traction tufts

47. A 65-year-old woman presents with acute flashes and floaters in her left eye and is diagnosed with a posterior vitreous detachment. Which one of the following is defined as the liquefaction of the vitreous?

A. Syneresis

B. Synchysis

C. Posterior vitreous detachment

D. Synchysis scintillans

48. During your busy retina clinic, you diagnose four different patients with a giant retinal tear, horse-shoe tear, dialysis, and slit-tear in a single day. Which one may not result in an immediate retinal detachment?

A. Giant tear in a 60-year-old

B. Horse-shoe tear in a 25-year-old myopic patient

C. Traumatic dialysis in a 35-year-old

D. Slit-tear in a 50-year-old pseudophakic patient

49. A 74-year-old man presents with acute vision loss and is found to have choroidal infarction on fluorescein angiography. Which one of the following symptoms/findings may give a hint as to the etiology of choroidal occlusion?

A. Temporal scalp tenderness

B. Glomerulonephritis

C. History of YAG capsulotomy

D. A and B

50. You are seeing a 26-year-old man with blurry vision. His optical coherence tomography is shown below. You perform a fluorescein angiography (FA) that does not show any leakage. Which of the conditions below are these imaging findings most consistent with?

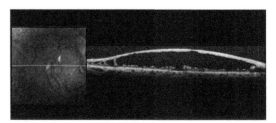

A. Goldmann–Favre disease

B. Irvine–Gass syndrome

C. Choroidal hemangioma

D. Cryopexy

51. An 80-year-old male patient with headaches and sudden vision loss in the right eye presents with the fundus appearance as shown. Recently he had carotid Doppler ultrasonography which revealed > 20% stenosis. His recent erythrocyte sedimentation rate (ESR) was 20 mm. What is the next best step in management?

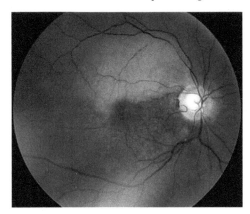

A. Anterior chamber paracentesis

B. IV bolus steroids

C. Temporal artery biopsy

D. Carotid endarterectomy

52. A 42-year-old woman was recently diagnosed with non-insulin-dependent diabetes. Which statement is most correct?

A. Immediate focal laser photocoagulation should be performed if she has clinically significant macular edema (CSME) and her vision is 20/20.

B. According to the DCCT, tight control of the patient's blood sugar would decrease her risk of developing diabetic retinopathy.

C. Immediate scatter photocoagulation should be applied if neovascularization of the disc and vitreous hemorrhage are present.

D. Focal laser photocoagulation should be performed if fluorescein leakage is present in the center of the fovea, even if the clinical examination does not show retinal thickening.

53. Which of the following statements is most correct?

A. In the Wisconsin Epidemiologic Study of Diabetic Retinopathy (WESDR) after 20 years of type 1 diabetes mellitus, half of patients had retinopathy.

B. In the National Health and Nutrition Survey III among type 2 diabetics, non-Hispanic Caucasians had a higher frequency of retinopathy than those of African descent.

C. In the WESDR, older onset diabetics after 20 years of DM were twice as likely to be legally blind than their counterparts who were >= 30 years old at DM onset.

D. In the WESDR, 60% of patients had diabetic retinopathy after 20 years of type 2 diabetes.

54. Which is false regarding peau d'orange?

A. Represents stippled appearance at the interface between abnormal light colored and normal darker colored fundus.

B. May be found along with optic nerve drusen and peripheral atrophic spots.

C. Associated with ABCC6 mutations.

D. Noted as orange color of skin after intravenous injection of fluorescein dye.

55. Which one of these is true?

A. SCORE study shows intravitreal steroids are five times more effective than sham in branch retinal vein occlusion (BRVO).

B. GENEVA study shows steroids are less effective than laser photocoagulation in BRVO and central retinal vein occlusion (CRVO).

C. SCORE study shows laser photocoagulation is better than intravitreal steroids for BRVO.

D. BRAVO study showed similar efficacy of ranibizumab and laser photocoagulation in BRVO.

56. Which one of these statements is incorrect?

A. Grid laser treatment does not improve vision in patients with cystoid macular edema secondary to central retinal vein occlusion (CRVO).

B. Grid laser treatment decreases angiographic macular edema in CRVO.

C. Grid laser treatment may improve vision in younger individuals in CRVO.

D. Panretinal photocoagulation (PRP) in CRVO should be done in patients with widespread ischemia.

57. Which one of these medications can cause this condition?

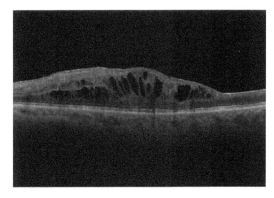

A. Latanoprost

B. Niacin

C. Rosiglitazone

D. All of the above

58. A 25-year-old male patient with renal hypertension is referred by the internist. Dilated fundus exam showed some hypertensive changes. What is the name of linear hyperpigmentations suggestive of hypertension?

A. Focal intraretinal periarteriolar transudates

B. Elschnig spots

C. Vogt's striae

D. Siegrist streaks

59. A 50-year-old male patient with no past medical history noticed sudden vision change in the left eye. Dilated fundus exam showed intraretinal hemorrhage and dilated tortuous retinal vasculature inferotemporally. Which one of the following indicates an inflammatory condition as the cause of this condition?

A. Volcano-style macular edema

B. Extensive hemorrhages

C. Occlusion at a non-arteriovenous (AV) crossing site

D. Presence of hard exudates

60. A 77-year-old female patient with hypertension and hyperlipidemia noticed sudden vision loss in the right eye. There is an afferent pupillary defect. Dilated fundus exam showed dilation and tortuosity of all branches of the central retinal vein with cotton wool spots. Which one the following is the most important risk factor for prediction of iris neovascularization after this condition?

A. Decreased electroretinogram bright flash/dark adapted b-wave

B. Four quadrants of hemorrhage

C. Prolonged retinovascular circulation times

D. Poor visual acuity

61. Which one the statements describe the genetic basis of the majority of the neuronal ceroid lipofuscinoses (NCLs)?

A. They are a group of neurodegenerative disorders with autosomal recessive inheritance.

B. They are a group of neurodegenerative disorders with autosomal dominant inheritance.

C. They are a group of neurodegenerative disorders with X-linked inheritance.

D. They are a group of sporadic neurodegenerative disorders.

62. Which of the following statements for Fabry's disease is correct?

A. It is an autosomal dominant disorder.

B. It is caused by a mutation in the gene encoding alpha-galactosidase A.

C. It is associated with accumulation of ceramide trihexoside in joints.

D. It is associated with whorls in the skin.

63. What percent of the patients with type A Niemann–Pick disease manifest with a cherry-red spot in the fundus?

A. 100%

B. 75%

C. 50%

D. 25%

64. A 26-year-old male patient presents with decreased and distorted vision of his left eye and on examination shows the following image. Which of the following is not consistent with his diagnosis?

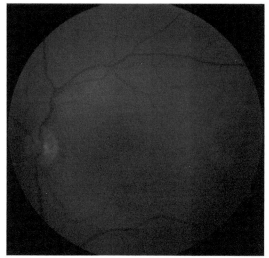

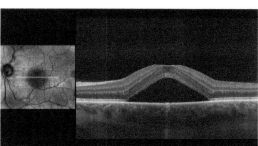

A. Visual prognosis may not be good for chronic, recurrent, and bullous cases.

B. 80–90% of the subretinal fluid undergoes spontaneous resorption in 6 weeks.

C. Functional recovery follows anatomical recovery but can take up to 1 year.

D. Contrast sensitivity and color vision defects may persist despite anatomical recovery.

65. A 51-year-old male patient with uncontrolled diabetes has cataract in the right eye. Dilated fundus exam shows one-fourth area of NVD but not vitreous hemorrhage. You wish to plan cataract surgery. Which of the following is the most appropriate statement?

A. Avoid cataract surgery.

B. Ideally have scatter laser immediately after planned cataract extraction.

C. Ideally have scatter laser 1 to 2 months before planned cataract extraction.

D. Ideally have scatter laser immediately before planned cataract extraction.

66. A 65-year-old male smoker with a history of hyperopia presents with drusen of both eyes. He is worried because his mother became blind from her age-related macular degeneration (AMD). Which of the following does not increase his risk of progressive vision

loss from AMD?

A. Hyperopia

B. Smoking

C. Male sex

D. Family history of vision loss from AMD

67. A 70-year-old male patient with gradual decrease in vision over 5 years in the left eye presents with the fundus appearance as shown in figure. The most common form of this lesion develops from which of the following?

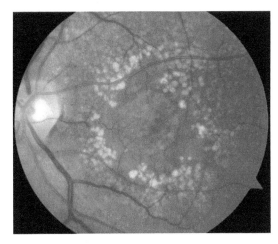

A. Choroidal neovascular membrane

B. Retinal pigment epithelium (RPE) mottling

C. Atrophic drusen

D. RPE detachment

68. A 35-year-old female patient presents with blurred vision and metamorphopsia in the left eye. Fundus exam shows small, round, discrete, and yellow-white spots in macula. Which of the following makes the diagnosis of multifocal choroiditis more likely than histoplasmosis?

A. Punched out chorioretinal lesions

B. Choroidal neovascularization (CNV)

C. Vitritis

D. Peripapillary pigmentary changes

69. "Full panretinal photocoagulation (PRP)" as defined by the Diabetic Retinopathy Study (DRS) and Early Treatment Diabetic Retinopathy Study (ETDRS) includes at minimum

A. 800 laser burns

B. 1000 laser burns

C. 1200 laser burns

D. 1500 laser burns

70. A 37-year-old male patient with sudden vision decrease in the left eye presents with fluorescein angiography (FA) as shown. Detachment of which one of the following structures can occur in this patient?

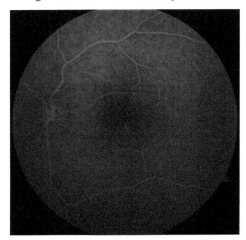

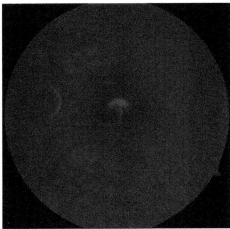

A. Sensory retina

B. Choroid

C. Retinal pigment epithelium

D. A and C

71. Which of the conditions below may result in the changes demonstrated?

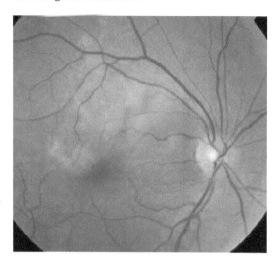

A. Disseminated intravascular coagulation (DIC)
B. Thrombotic thrombocytopenic purpura (TTP)
C. Giant cell arteritis (GCA)
D. All of the above

72. A 77-year-old female inpatient hospitalized for a new diagnosis of ovarian cancer complains of severe loss of vision bilaterally over the past few weeks. On fundus exam, you notice large nevus-like regions of increased pigmentation and thickening of the choroid. Which of the following is correct regarding her most likely diagnosis?

A. It is a benign condition.
B. The associated gene is located on chromosome 4.
C. It does not affect retina.
D. Fifty percent of cases have a known malignancy at the time of diagnosis.

73. A 10-year-old male patient followed by neurology for a diagnosis of Refsum disease is sent for consultation regarding visual prognosis. Which of the following clinical features is associated with his condition?

A. Pigmentary retinopathy with decreased electroretinogram (ERG) signals
B. Cataracts
C. Enlarged corneal nerves
D. All of the above

74. A 74-year-old female patient previously diagnosed as neovascular age-related macular degeneration with monthly intravitreal anti-VEGF injection comes back to your clinic. What is featured in this optical coherence tomography (OCT) image?

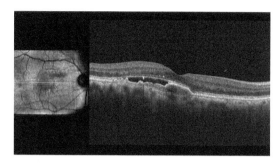

A. Subretinal fluid
B. Pigment epithelial detachment
C. Epiretinal membrane
D. A and B

75. The differential diagnosis for dry age-related macular degeneration (AMD) includes which of the following conditions?

A. Late onset Stargardt disease
B. Plaquenil or chloroquine toxicity
C. Old central serous chorioretinopathy
D. All of the above may be included

76. A 54-year-old Caucasian male presents to your clinic with the finding shown after seeing flashes of light and floaters. Which genetic mutation is associated with the worst prognosis for this condition?

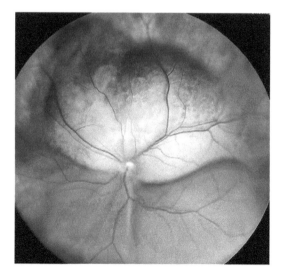

A. Trisomy 21
B. Monosomy 6
C. Disomy 8
D. Monosomy 3

77. A 70-year-old African American female presents to your clinic with multifocal white creamy subretinal lesions in the macula of both eyes. Which is the most likely history associated with this finding?

A. History of rheumatoid arthritis

B. History of breast cancer in remission, treated 5 years ago with combination of chemotherapy and radiation

C. History of ovarian cancer in sister

D. Von Hippel's disease

78. A 55-year-old Asian female presents to your clinic after being treated for "chronic" vitritis for many months. She has been on topical steroids for several months with courses of both oral and sub-tenons steroids as well. She responds initially to treatment but then worsens each time her steroids are decreased. What is the next best step in management?

A. Injection of intravitreal dexamethasone implant

B. Vitreous biopsy with intravitreal injection of antibiotics

C. Vitreous biopsy with culture and cytology

D. Referral to rheumatologist for systemic evaluation

79. A 90-year-old male is referred to your office due to uncontrolled glaucoma from his primary care physician. Anterior segment examination is shown in figure. What is the most likely primary malignancy in this patient?

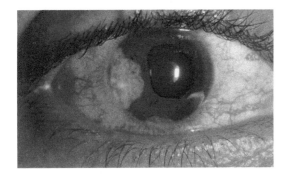

A. Prostate

B. Lung

C. Skin melanoma

D. Brain

80. Patient presents to your clinic with the finding shown in figure. What neurocutaneous disorder is this mass most commonly associated with?

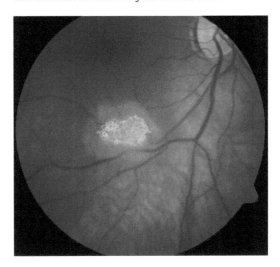

A. Bourneville's disease

B. Encephalotrigeminal angiomatosis

C. Von Recklinghausen's disease

D. Wyburn-Mason syndrome

81. A 6-year-old male comes to your clinic and has the following multiple fundus finding (capillary hemangioma hemangioblastoma). The causal gene is associated with which chromosome?

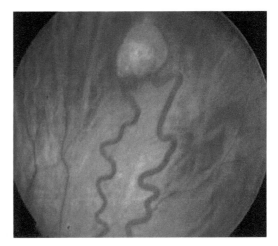

A. 17

B. 9

C. 22

D. 3

82. Fundoscopy of a 15-year-old male revealed few pigmented lesions along the equator of the eye. Each of the lesions are flat, sharply demarcated, hyperpigmented, and have a surrounding halo and tail of depigmentation that is directed at the optic nerve. What is the most appropriate next step?

A. External beam radiation

B. Referral for colonoscopy

C. Laser photocoagulation

D. Serial photographs to assess for malignant change

83. Parents bring their 2-year-old to your office after noticing that their child has a white pupil in one eye during their last family photograph. On examination, white creamy lesions are noted in the fundus with a dense nodular vitreous debris. Which chromosome carries the mutation leading to this condition?

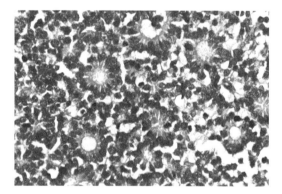

A. Chromosome 17

B. Chromosome 13

C. Chromosome 5

D. Chromosome 3

84. The parents of a 3-year-old successfully treated for retinoblastoma ask whether their child is at risk for any other malignancy. What is the most common secondary tumor in these patients after successful treatment of the primary tumor?

A. Lymphoma

B. Osteosarcoma

C. Ewing's sarcoma

D. Lung

85. A 70-year-old male is diagnosed with uveal melanoma. When ordering the imaging to evaluate for metastasis, where should you direct the radiologist to pay special attention?

A. Brain

B. Skin

C. Liver

D. Bone

86. A 1-year-old is brought to your clinic for evaluation of strabismus. During exam, you notice a white pupil in the left eye and ultimately diagnose the child with retinoblastoma. The patient unfortunately has a germline mutation and is diagnosed with trilateral retinoblastoma. Which structure is involved in this rare condition?

A. Sclera

B. Long bones

C. Frontal lobe

D. Pineal gland

87. A patient is referred to your office to rule out malignant melanoma of the right eye. The fundus photograph is shown in the given figure. What is the diagnosis?

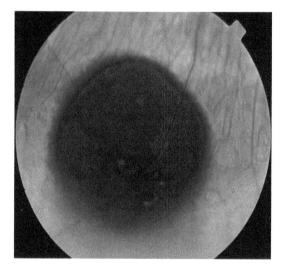

A. Choroidal melanoma

B. Congenital hypertrophy of the retinal pigment epithelium

C. Choroidal nevus

D. Circumscribed choroidal hemangioma

88. The Collaborative Ocular Melanoma Study (COMS) medium choroidal melanoma trial evaluated survival of standard enucleation versus I-125 brachytherapy. The study concluded which of the following?

A. Survival rates were equivalent for both 5 and 10 years.

B. Plaque brachytherapy was associated with better survival outcomes at both 5 and 10 years.

C. Enucleation was associated with better survival outcomes at 5 and 10 years.

D. Survival rate at 5 years was equivalent, but was better with enucleation at 10 years.

89. A 48-year-old male is diagnosed with a small choroidal melanoma 2 mm from the optic nerve. Which of the following is not an accepted treatment for this condition?

A. Transpupillary thermotherapy

B. External beam radiotherapy

C. Transscleral thermotherapy

D. Observeration

90. An 18-year-old male presents for routine examination. He has a diffusely red fundus of the right eye with normal fundus pigmentation of the left eye. He also has an associated port-wine stain of the right side of his face. Which inherited chromosome is this abnormality associated with?

A. 17

B. 9

C. 22

D. No genetic inheritance is associated with this condition

91. A 3-year-old male is diagnosed with endophytic retinoblastoma with vitreous seeding. In addition to intra-arterial chemotherapy, what other treatment is the best option for this patient?

A. Intravitreal melphalan

B. External beam radiation

C. Intravenous chemotherapy

D. Observation

92. A patient is referred to your office for serous detachment of the right retina recalcitrant to repeated intravitreal anti-vascular endothelial growth factor injections. His vision is 20/80 in the right eye and 20/20 in the left eye without correction. Anterior segment examination reveals no abnormalities. You decide to perform ultrasonography and discover a subretinal mass that shows high internal reflectivity with focal diffuse choroidal thickening. The patient is asking you to please provide him with treatment as his vision is greatly affected. What is the best treatment for this patient's condition?

A. Laser photocoagulation

B. Oral diamox

C. Photodynamic therapy

D. Intravitreal dexamethasone depot injection

93. A patient is referred to your office by her primary ophthalmologist for a white, slightly elevated subretinal mass without overlying fluid in the left eye. She denies visual symptoms and vision is 20/20 on Snellen testing in both eyes. B-scan ultrasonography is performed and reveals a highly reflective mass replacing the normal choroid. A computed tomography (CT) scan shows calcification in the area of the lesion. What is best treatment?

A. Biopsy of the lesion

B. Observation

C. Intravitreal injections of anti-vascular endothelial growth factor

D. Thermal laser

94. A 40-year-old female comes to you complaining of decreased vision and severe floaters in both eyes. Dilated fundus examination reveals creamy subretinal infiltrates, subellipsoid zone thickening in both eyes, and dense vitritis. Vitreous shows primary vitreoretinal lymphoma (VRL). Which is the most common subtype associated with this condition?

A. Marginal zone lymphoma

B. Mantle cell lymphoma

C. T cell lymphoma

D. Large B cell lymphoma

95. A 70-year-old patient presents to your office with a pigmented lesion in the fundus of the right eye. Which of the following findings is associated with increased risk of malignant transformation?

A. Orange pigment present on the tumor surface

B. Tumor thickness of > 2 mm on ultrasonography

C. Presence of drusen on the tumor surface

D. Distance < 3 mm from optic nerve

96. A 65-year-old male presents to your office complaining of decreased vision in his left eye. On slit lamp examination, you notice nuclear sclerosis of both lenses. However, upon careful examination you notice that a portion of the left cataract is more opaque than the rest of the lens. What is the next best step in management of this patient?

A. Removal of cataract

B. Visual field examination

C. Ultrasound biomicroscopy

D. Peripheral iridotomy over region of dense cataract

97. What was the primary outcome of the Collaborative Ocular Melanoma Study (COMS) large choroidal melanoma trial?

A. Standard enucleation and brachytherapy had equal survival outcomes.

B. Pre-enucleation radiotherapy did not improve overall survival compared to primary enucleation alone.

C. Brachytherapy should not be considered for large tumors.

D. Melanoma specific mortality was 1% at 5 years.

98. An 80-year-old male who recently died underwent autopsy and a glistening, white solid tumor was noted in the area of the ciliary body. What is the most likely lesion in this patient?

A. Iris pigment epithelial cyst

B. Ciliary body melanoma

C. Fuch's adenoma

D. Pars plana cyst

99. An 8-month-old male was referred to your office by his pediatrician after noticing a white pupil during well-child visit. Which of the following is not in the differential diagnosis for this child?

A. Retinal capillary hemangioblastoma

B. Coat's disease

C. Retinoblastoma

D. Persistent fetal vasculature

100. Patient undergoes computed tomography (CT) scan of the head after complaining of headache following vehicle collision. What is the incidental finding noted in the given image?

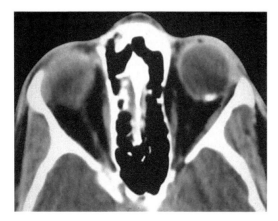

A. Vitreous hemorrhage

B. Disciform scar

C. Choroidal osteoma

D. Choroidal melanoma

101. A 25-year-old male presents to your clinic with decreased vision in the right eye. He has a serous retinal detachment causing diminished visual acuity and visual distortion. He undergoes significant investigation and is diagnosed with a circumscribed choroidal hemangioma. What is the single best test to diagnose this lesion?

A. Indirect ophthalmoscopy

B. Indocyanine green angiography

C. B-scan ultrasonography

D. Fluorescein angiography

102. You are seeing a patient referred to you with a retinal detachment in the right eye. As you finish examining him, the patient asks if he is a candidate for a "bubble" procedure. Which of the following is a contraindication for the procedure to which the patient is referring?

A. A single break at 12 o'clock with PVR grade B

B. Two breaks at 2:30 and 3:30 clock hours with mild nuclear sclerosis

C. Pseudophakic patient with three breaks between 9:30 and 10:30 clock hours

D. Single break at 12 o'clock with severe vitreous hemorrhage

103. A 32-year-old man presents 6 months after sustaining a firecracker injury to his eye. Immediately after the injury, he was noted to have hyphema that later resolved. Which of the following retinal defects is *least* likely to be associated with the blunt traumatic injury?

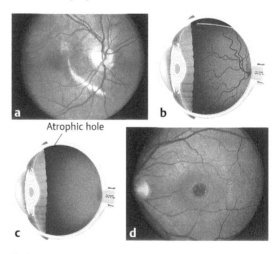

A. Image a

B. Image b

C. Image c

D. Image d

104. A 32-year-old male with a firecracker injury to his eye is wondering what his odds would have been for needing a retinal detachment surgery if a retinal issue were found. You tell him that retinal detachment surgery is most commonly necessary with:

A. Penetrating scleral injury

B. Retinal sclopetaria

C. Choroidal rupture

D. Traumatic macular hole

105. A 30-year-old construction worker presents to your clinic for follow-up after being seen in the emergency department for an intraocular foreign body. When a coworker was using a jackhammer, a large, oddly shaped iron shard had penetrated through his safety glasses and globe into the vitreous cavity. Computed tomography (CT) of orbits was consistent with this history. Despite the recommendation for vitrectomy with foreign body removal, surgical repair was not elected by the patient, who instead opted for observation. Which of the following is best for long-term monitoring in this patient?

A. CT scan

B. Color plates

C. Electroretinogram (ERG)

D. Magnetic resonance imaging (MRI) scan

106. A 30-year-old man with an intraocular foreign body is wondering about the chances of endophthalmitis with injuries like the one he sustained. Which one is correct regarding endophthalmitis after penetrating scleral trauma?

A. Endophthalmitis occurs in about 25% of cases of penetrating scleral trauma.

B. *Bacillus cereus* is the causative organisms 2 to 7% of the time.

C. A rural location for the trauma is relatively protective.

D. Loss of the eye is common with *B. cereus* endophthalmitis

107. You are seeing a patient every 3 months for a condition, and he tells you that he is religious about using the "chart with the straight lines and black dot in the center" every day. The patient most likely has which of the following conditions?

A. Scleral rupture

B. Solar retinopathy

C. Choroidal rupture

D. Posttraumatic endophthalmitis

108. A 37-year-old woman presents to your office for a "screening eye exam" after being referred by her primary care physician. The patient is not sure why she was specifically referred, does not endorse any visual complaints, and does not have any records with her or recall the names of the medications that she takes. On exam, you notice pigmentary changes in the macula and mid-periphery. Which drug is she most likely taking?

A. Docetaxel

B. Paclitaxel

C. Niacin

D. Thioridazine

109. Intake of which compound can cause the following on spectral-domain optical coherence tomography imaging?

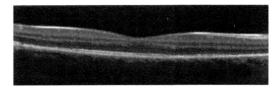

A. Alkyl nitrate ("poppers") inhalation

B. Nitrofurantoin therapy

C. Canthaxanthin ingestion

D. Talc injection

110. A 60-year-old patient with long-standing lupus nephritis presents for her regular eye examination. On medication review, she says that her rheumatologist finds that high-dose Plaquenil works best for her condition and she's been well controlled. Which of the following would be most expected on spectral-domain optical coherence tomography (SD-OCT) imaging?

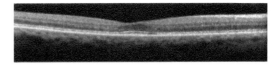

A. Figure

B. Inner segment ellipsoid loss in a parafoveal location

C. Thick choroid

D. A and B

111. A 36-year-old woman is new to your clinic and arrives for a retinal consultation. You notice yellow-orange crystalline macular deposits and ask the patient whether she might have been exposed to canthaxanthin. What is canthaxanthin used for?

A. Tanning

B. Antibiotics

C. Anesthesia

D. Breast cancer

112. A 40-year-old man presents for an ophthalmologic evaluation at the county hospital. He is actively being treated for tuberculosis, but does not know his current medications. Your concern for rifabutin-related toxicity is increased given the presence of which finding?

A. Choroidal folds

B. Anterior and posterior uveitis with hypopyon

C. Retinal pigment epithelium (RPE) loss

D. Cataract

113. You are examining a patient who asks you about possible effects to the eyes from exposure to different metals. He has been a metalworker for about 20 years. What can ocular argyrosis include?

A. Gray or blue coloring of skin

B. Black tears

C. Dark choroid

D. All of the above

114. You are consulted in the emergency room for a 78-year-old man who noticed sudden yellowing of his vision since he started taking a medication newly prescribed by his primary care physician. He has dementia and cannot recall the name of the drug. Which of the following is the most likely culprit?

A. Sildenafil

B. Digitalis

C. Topamax

D. Nitrofurantoin

115. A 57-year-old woman is referred to you from a local optometrist due to new floaters and flashes of light, followed by a shadow over her vision. On examination, you notice a break with subretinal fluid extending into the macula consistent with macula-off retinal detachment, and decide to take her to the operating room for a primary, segmental, radial buckle with cryotherapy and no drainage the next day. Ultrasound from her postoperative day 1 visit is given in the figure, confirming support of the break by the buckle with resolving subretinal fluid. Which statement is *correct* regarding peripheral retinal lesions leading to retinal detachment?

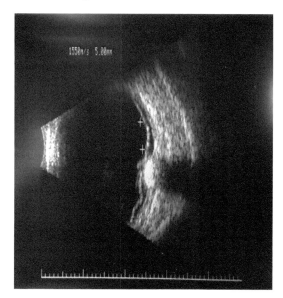

A. A hole is not a full-thickness break.

B. A tear occurs due to atrophy of the inner retina.

C. A horse-shoe retinal tear occurs if retina is pulled anteriorly.

D. A tear covering 2 clock hours is termed as giant tear.

116. A 30-year-old man at the county hospital emergency room was "minding his own business" when he was "jumped out of nowhere" and punched in his right eye. He has symptoms concerning for a retinal tear or detachment. At which locations should you have greatest suspicion for a traumatic retinal break?

A. Inferotemporal and superonasal quadrants

B. Superotemporal and superonasal quadrants

C. Inferonasal and superonasal quadrants

D. Superotemporal and inferonasal quadrants

117. What is the definition of a "giant retinal tear"?

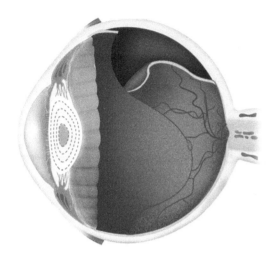

A. A tear anterior to the base of the vitreous

B. A tear that extends circumferentially more than 3 clock hours

C. A large horse-shoe tear with a bridging blood vessel

D. A tear that extends radially toward arcades or posterior pole

118. You are seeing a patient on a Sunday night at 8 pm for new flashes and floaters, and notice a posterior vitreous detachment (PVD) on exam, but no retinal breaks. Which statement related to PVD is *incorrect*?

A. During PVD vitreous gel starts separating 3 mm away from the ora serrata.

B. Release of vitreous from the area of Martegiani causes a Weiss ring.

C. Prevalence of PVD is higher among myopes.

D. Syneresis is the collapse of the vitreous gel.

119. It is 9 pm on Sunday night, and a patient calls with "tons of red spots" in her vision. On her exam, you notice not only a posterior vitreous detachment (PVD), but vitreous hemorrhage also. You then begin the scleral-depressed portion of the exam. What is the chance of finding a tear in a patient like this with vitreous hemorrhage and PVD?

A. 10%

B. 25%

C. 40%

D. 60%

120. Which lesion, as per the given figure, requires immediate retinopexy to prevent retinal detachment in a symptomatic patient?

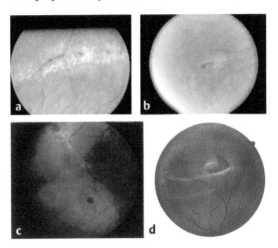

A. Image a

B. Image b

C. Image c

D. Image d

121. Which statement is INCORRECT?

A. Flap tears in fellow eyes of eyes with retinal detachment must be prophylactically treated.

B. Laser retinopexy of the fellow eyes of retinal detachment with lattice degeneration can decrease retinal detachment rate.

C. Lattice degeneration with a retinal hole does not require treatment unless there is a risk factor.

D. Patients with demarcation line should be considered risk-free of further progression of a subclinical retinal detachment.

122. If a patient presents with a left inferior retinal detachment extending between 3 and 11 o'clock, where is the most likely place you will find a retinal tear?

A. 3 o'clock

B. 4 o'clock

C. 5 o'clock

D. 10 o'clock

123. A 65-year-old patient needs urgent surgery for a retinal detachment. He asks about his prognosis. Which statement about the functional and anatomical outcomes of retina reattachment surgery is incorrect?

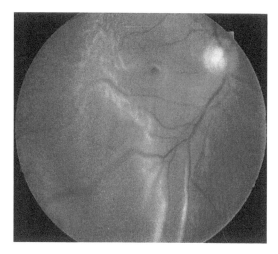

A. Success rate of retinal reattachment surgery is 80 to 90%.

B. Eighty-seven percent of the eyes with macula-on retinal detachments recover vision equal to or better than 20/50.

C. 33 to 50% of the macula-off detachments can see equal to or better than 20/50.

D. Delay in repair of macula-off detachments does not affect the functional outcome.

124. Which of the findings indicates the exudative nature of a retinal detachment?

A. Shifting subretinal fluid

B. Smooth retinal surface

C. Lack of intravitreal pigment

D. All of the above

125. What is the cleavage plane in typical retinoschisis?

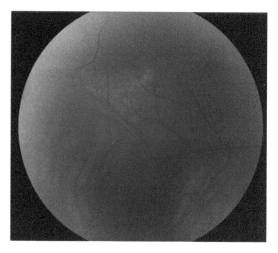

A. Nerve fiber layer

B. Inner plexiform layer

C. Inner nuclear layer

D. Outer plexiform layer

126. A patient with + 3.00 hyperopic correction presents as a referral from another retina surgeon given concern for retinoschisis and possible retinal detachment. You notice a thin, transparent elevation involving the retina inferotemporally, but also the presence of demarcation line. Along with retinoschisis, what else do you suspect is present?

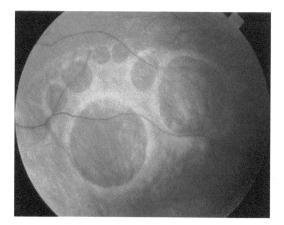

A. Nothing, this is a normal finding.

B. Presence of an inner hole.

C. Presence of high myopia.

D. Presence of an outer retinal hole.

127. A 4-year-old boy presents to your clinic with nystagmus. Examination shows findings similar to the following image. What is true regarding this patient's condition?

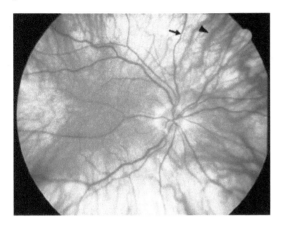

A. Ocular albinism is usually autosomal recessive.

B. Female carriers of ocular albinism have detectable ocular abnormalities.

C. Patients with ocular albinism often have nystagmus but normal visual acuity.

D. Chediak–Higashi syndrome is associated with fatal episodes of abnormal bleeding.

128. You are consulted on a 58-year-old male hospitalized with a history of small-cell lung carcinoma. He complains of seeing lights he knows is not there, and decreased vision in dim light. These symptoms have been progressive. His acuity is 20/40 OU. On exam, he has minimal to trace cataracts. The arterioles are thin and his optic nerves appear mildly pale. Select the most correct statement about his most likely condition.

A. The time course of visual loss progression is not distinguishable from retinitis pigmentosa.

B. The condition never results in clinical visual loss without a known primary having been discovered.

C. Steroids do not play a therapeutic role.

D. Anti-recoverin antibodies are sometimes found.

129. Upon returning to clinic from the operating room at the county hospital, your attending tells you to "go do this laser" for the right eye of a patient. Which of the following pigments is NOT considered a primary target for retinal laser photocoagulation?

A. Oxidized reduced hemoglobin

B. Xanthophyll

C. Melanin

D. Lipofuscin

130. A patient present with proliferative diabetic retinopathy and is consented for panretinal photocoagulation (PRP). Which of the following is *not* a complication of laser photocoagulation?

A. Permanent loss of corneal sensation

B. Pupillary abnormalities

C. Exudative retinal detachment

D. Choroidal detachment

131. A 42-year-old investment banker, recently divorced, is referred to your office from a local ophthalmologist due to new visual distortion and 20/30 vision. On exam, there is a pigment epithelial detachment at the fovea without any hemorrhage or evidence of neovascularization. Spectral-domain optical coherence tomography shows some focal thickening of the choroid. You discuss options with him including monitoring, and he would like a quick treatment now. Which statement is *incorrect* regarding photodynamic therapy (PDT)?

A. Back pain and chest pain occur in 2.5% of the patients after PDT.

B. Patients should avoid direct sunlight exposure for 48 hours after PDT.

C. Pain is not related to infusion of verteporfin.

D. 0.7 to 2.2% of the patients may experience severe visual loss after PDT.

132. A patient is referred for an epiretinal membrane and desires restoration of her vision as quickly as possible. She heard that you are "the BEST minimally-invasive, retinal surgeon." After thoroughly explaining the risks, benefits, alternatives, and details of the surgery in layman's terms, she wishes to proceed with a vitrectomy and membrane peel. Which of the following is a considered the most significant intraoperative advantage of small-gauge vitrectomy?

A. Increased postoperative patient comfort

B. Faster visual recovery

C. Preserving conjunctiva for possible glaucoma surgeries

D. Lower rate of retinal tears

133. A 47-year-old patient at the county hospital has history of bilateral proliferative diabetic retinopathy and vitreous hemorrhages that are beginning to clear. Her HbA1c is 14.2%. In addition to intravitreal anti-VEGF therapy, she elects to proceed with panretinal photocoagulation (PRP). Which of the following lenses used for photocoagulation can result in a doubling of the laser spot?

A. Volk Area Centralis lens

B. Ocular Widefield lens

C. Goldmann 3-mirror lens

D. Ocular Mainster PRP 165 lens

134. Which of the following is an indication for performing retinal laser photocoagulation?

A. To ablate ischemic retina

B. To create chorioretinal adhesion

C. To destroy intraocular tumors

D. All of the above

135. Which of the statements is correct?

A. Melanin poorly absorbs the visible spectrum of light.

B. Xanthophyll absorbs infrared light best.

C. Hemoglobin minimally absorbs red and infrared wavelengths.

D. None of the above.

136. A 54-year-old woman presents for follow-up with bilateral nonclearing vitreous hemorrhage (due to proliferative diabetic retinopathy) and moderate nuclear sclerosing cataracts. The view is beginning to improve and you think you can get adequate panretinal photocoagulation treatment. Which laser would be the best choice?

A. Double-frequency YAG

B. Argon green

C. Argon red

D. Diode infrared

137. A 72-year-old woman presents a day early from her postoperative week 1 visit following cataract surgery because of excruciating eye pain, purulence, and worsening vision of her surgical eye. She had noticed her vision improve day 1 and then "all of a sudden" it became worse on day 5. Her external examination photo is shown in the figure. Which of the following is NOT a conclusion of the Endophthalmitis Vitrectomy Study (EVS)?

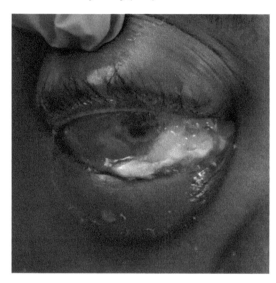

A. Systemic antibiotic treatment with amikacin and ceftazidime does not improve final visual acuity.

B. There is no difference in outcomes between vitrectomy and immediate tap/inject if visual acuity is better than light perception.

C. Vitrectomy and intravitreal amikacin/ceftazidime injection results in better visual acuity if presenting vision is light perception or worse.

D. Vitrectomy and intravitreal amikacin/ceftazidime injection results in better visual acuity regardless of the initial visual acuity.

138. Your internal medicine colleague pages you at 11 pm on Sunday night regarding a 35-year-old immunocompromised patient at the local hospital with a new "white plaque in front of the pupil." You immediately drive across the city to the hospital thinking it might be endophthalmitis. Examination of the patient reveals the findings in the above photograph. Which "endophthalmitis type" and "most common causative organism" pair below is INCORRECT?

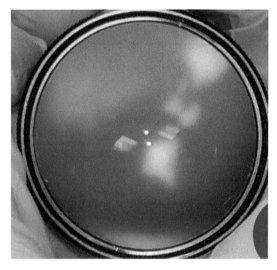

A. Chronic endophthalmitis–*Propionibacterium acnes*

B. Traumatic exogeneous endophthalmitis–*Candida species*

C. Bleb-associated endophthalmitis–*Streptococcus* and *Haemophilus* species

D. Post-cataract surgery–coagulase-negative *Staphylococci*

139. You are examining a 38-year-old man in your clinic who has a characteristic "port wine stain" on the side of his face. Which of the following is INCORRECT regarding his probable condition?

A. Diffuse choroidal hemangioma is usually part of the condition and is usually found on the side ipsilateral to a facial nevus flammeus.

B. Elevated intraocular pressure can be seen in eyes with circumscribed choroidal hemangiomas due to elevated episcleral venous pressure and/or angle malformation.

C. B-scan ultrasound of a choroidal hemangioma typically shows a lesion with low internal reflectively.

D. Photodynamic therapy is considered the treatment of choice for clinically symptomatic small- to medium-sized circumscribed choroidal hemangiomas.

140. What is the most common source of choroidal metastasis in men and women, respectively?

A. Prostate, kidney

B. Prostate, lung

C. Lung, breast

D. Gastrointestinal tract, breast

141. A 53-year-old male presents with decreased vision in the left eye. He has a poorly controlled vasculopathy. His examination reveals normal anterior segment findings but numerous retinal hemorrhages with mild vascular tortuosity. What is most helpful to differentiate ocular ischemic syndrome from central retinal vein occlusion (CRVO)?

A. Location of the hemorrhages

B. Ophthalmodynamometry

C. Fluorescein angiography

D. Optical coherence tomography

142. A 54-year-old poorly controlled man with long-standing diabetes and hypertension presents for his regular screening examination. On dilated fundus examination, you notice the following lesions. What is the most common cause of these lesions?

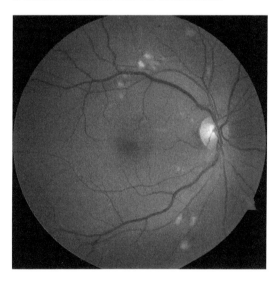

A. Diabetic retinopathy

B. Hypertension

C. HIV retinopathy

D. Interferon retinopathy

267

143. With regards to central artery occlusions, which statement is false?

A. Thirty-two percent of the eyes have a cilioretinal artery.

B. Cilioretinal artery occlusion mostly occurs with central retinal artery occlusion (CRAO).

C. Giant cell arteritis (GCA) should be considered with isolated cilioretinal artery occlusion.

D. Cilioretinal arteries arise from short posterior ciliary vessels.

144. Your last patient of the day is a 79-year-old woman with sudden onset decrease vision in the left eye. She is a well-controlled hypertensive and diabetic. Her visual acuity is NLP on the affected side. The rest of her examination is normal except for the following. What does this clinical picture bring to mind?

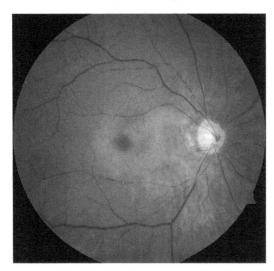

A. Likely malingering

B. Cilioretinal artery occlusion

C. The need for anti-VEGF treatment

D. Involvement of the ophthalmic artery

145. A new patient presents to your clinic for diabetic retinopathy screening after he was diagnosed with diabetes 2 months ago. Which statement regarding diabetic retinopathy (DR) is correct?

A. It is present in 99% of type 2 diabetics at 20 years from time of diagnosis.

B. It is the leading cause of blindness in adults aged 20 to 64 years in the United States.

C. It is diagnosed primarily with fluorescein angiography.

D. It can be classified as mild, moderate, or severe proliferative DR.

146. Which of the following is not a finding of the Diabetes Control and Complications Trial (DCCT) trial?

A. Sulfonylureas did not increase the risk of heart disease.

B. Pregnancy can exacerbate diabetic retinopathy.

C. Intensive blood sugar control reduces the progression of nonproliferative diabetic retinopathy (NPDR) to proliferative diabetic retinopathy (PDR).

D. Intensive blood pressure control can slow progression of retinopathy.

147. A 54-year-old patient presents to clinic for his diabetic screening test. His exam shows the following findings. Which study defined the characteristics of this entity?

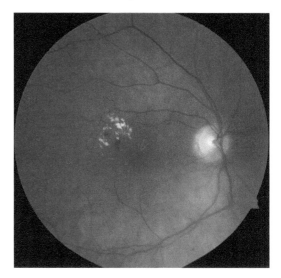

A. Diabetes Control and Complications Trial (DCCT)

B. United Kingdom Prospective Diabetes Study (UKPDS)

C. ETDRS

D. RISE and RIDE

148. A 56-year-old long-standing diabetic patient presents to clinic for his diabetic screening test. You look in the chart and find that a scribble was made to the side mentioning "4:2:1." What does the 4:2:1 rule refer to in this case?

A. A grading system for clinically significant macular edema (CSME)

B. The definition of high-risk proliferative diabetic retinopathy (PDR)

C. The risk of progression to high-risk PDR

D. Criteria for diagnosing severe non-proliferative diabetic retinopathy (NPDR)

149. Which of the following is a finding of the Early Treatment Diabetic Retinopathy Study (ETDRS)?

A. Angiotensin-converting enzyme (ACE) inhibitors or beta blockers are effective in lowering blood pressure to reduce diabetic retinopathy.

B. Panretinal photocoagulation is ineffective in type 2 diabetes.

C. Anti-VEGF medications are effective in treatment of clinically significant macular edema.

D. Focal laser therapy decreased the risk of moderate vision loss in diabetic macular edema.

150. A 54-year-old long-standing diabetic patient presents to clinic for his diabetic screening test. You look in the chart and find that he was diagnosed with clinically significant diabetic macular edema (CSDME). You are about to perform focal laser therapy. Complications of focal laser therapy include which of the following?

A. Choroidal neovascularization

B. Enlarged blind spot

C. Serous choroidal detachment

D. Elevated intraocular pressure

151. A patient has nonproliferative diabetic retinopathy (NPDR) with four quadrants of diffuse intraretinal hemorrhages and venous beading in two quadrants. This patient:

A. Would benefit from panretinal photocoagulation according to the RISE and RIDE trials.

B. Has a 45% chance of progression to proliferative diabetic retinopathy (PDR) in 1 year according to the Early Treatment Diabetic Retinopathy Study (ETDRS).

C. Could experience improvement in diabetic retinopathy with intensive blood pressure and glucose control according to the Diabetic Retinopathy Clinical Research (DRCR) protocol I.

D. Should receive a grid laser pattern of 50 to 100 µm spot size in the macular region.

152. Which is not an option in the treatment of a patient who has type 2 diabetes with this fundus photo?

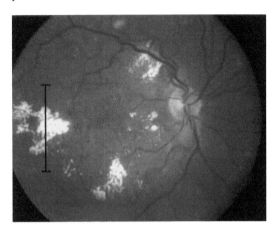

A. Intravitreal anti-VEGF agents

B. Intravitreal corticosteroid

C. Focal laser therapy

D. Photodynamic therapy

153. A 56-year-old patient with decreased vision in the left eye tests positive for the histoplasmin skin test. Which of the following statements is false regarding the pathogen in question?

A. It is endemic along the Mississippi and Ohio river valleys.

B. The fungus is carried within the dropping of the infected bats.

C. Humans are infected by direct skin contact.

D. Systemic infection by the organism results in ocular scarring.

154. A 40-year-old female presents for an annual check. She mentions that she was diagnosed with a subtle ocular finding and was advised to seek a dermatology evaluation. She never followed-up on that recommendation; however, now she complains of vision loss in her left eye and her fundus exam appears as shown below.

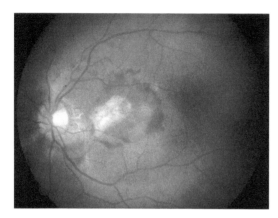

In what retinal layer were the initial ocular findings found?

A. Internal limiting membrane

B. Inner retina

C. Outer plexiform layer

D. Bruch's membrane

155. Which one of these statements is *false* regarding the disease this patient has?

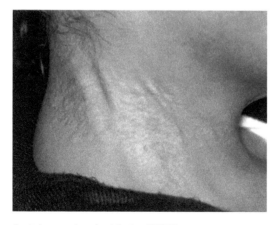

A. It is associated with the ABCC6 gene.

B. Ocular findings of angioid streaks may also be seen in patients with thalassemia.

C. It can be associated with optic nerve head drusen.

D. Retinal findings may mimic Bietti crystalline dystrophy.

156. What is the best course of action upon seeing a 33-year-old man with angioid streaks crossing the fovea with subretinal blood?

A. Observation and use of safety glasses

B. Perform laser photocoagulation

C. Administer an anti-VEGF injection

D. Order a fluorescein angiogram

157. A patient with known reactivity to the histoplasmin skin test come in for an exam. Which one of the following is NOT part of the "4 signs of presumed ocular histoplasmosis syndrome (POHS)"?

A. Punched-out chorioretinal lesions

B. Juxtapapillary pigmented atrophic scars

C. Choroidal neovascularization

D. Vascular sheathing

158. A patient with −9.00 spectacle prescription presents for his annual exam. He asks about the probability of complications associated with his refractive error. What is the prevalence of choroidal neovascularization (CNV) in pathologic/degeneration myopia?

A. 1 to 2%

B. 5 to 10%

C. 10 to 15%

D. 15 to 20%

159. Which statement regarding the treatment of choroidal neovascularization (CNV) secondary to presumed ocular histoplasmosis syndrome (POHS) is false?

A. Photocoagulation reduces the risk of severe vision loss (< 6 lines) compared to observation.

B. Surgical removal of the neovascular complex is beneficial if visual acuity is worse than 20/100.

C. Anti-VEGF agents are the mainstay of treatment for CNV secondary to POHS.

D. POHS patients with subfoveal CNV cannot benefit from laser treatment.

160. Which statement accurately describes pathologic myopia?

A. It affects 25% of the US population.

B. The incidence is higher in African Americans.

C. The spherical equivalent is more than −6.0 D.

D. The axial length greater than 32.5 mm.

161. A 34-year-old man with previously diagnosed pathologic myopia presents for his regular follow-up. On exam, you find multiple isolated round deep hemorrhages. Which statement is true regarding these lesions in this patient?

A. They indicate ingrowth of choroidal neovascularization.
B. They need to be lasered immediately.
C. Anti-VEGF treatment is required.
D. They result from rupture of Bruch's membrane and may require fluorescein angiography.

162. You are consulted to perform a retinopathy of prematurity (ROP) screen on a baby born at 28 weeks with the following fundus findings.

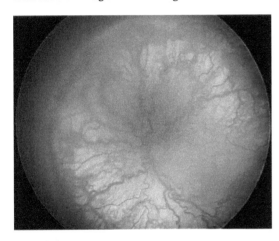

Which of the following most accurately describes the zone of ROP in this patient?
A. Zone 1
B. Zone 2
C. Zone 3
D. Indeterminate

163. Which of the following best describes stage 2 retinopathy of prematurity (ROP)?

A. Retinal detachment, not involving the macula
B. Neovascularization with fibrovascular tissue
C. Tortuous arterioles and dilated venules
D. Elevated ridge

164. Which of the following is recognized as a risk factor for retinopathy of prematurity (ROP)?

A. Birth weight > 2100 g
B. Gestational age > 35 weeks
C. High exposure to supplemental oxygen
D. Maternal alcohol abuse

165. Which of the following management options is most appropriate for this retinopathy of prematurity (ROP) baby?

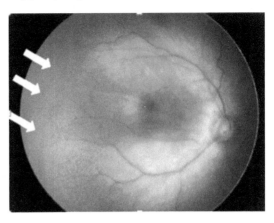

A. Laser treatment is indicated according to the early treatment ROP (ET-ROP) study.
B. Cryotherapy is indicated according to the CRYO-ROP study.
C. Anti-VEGF therapy is indicated according to the BEAT-ROP study.
D. No treatment is indicated at this time.

166. How would you follow a retinopathy of prematurity (ROP) baby with stage 2, zone II, no plus disease?

A. Next day for laser therapy
B. Two weeks
C. Four weeks
D. Six months

167. The fundus photos of a prematurely born neonate are shown here. Which of the following is true regarding this patient's future visual prognosis?

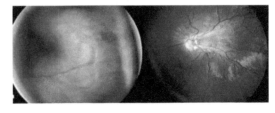

A. Increased risk of hyperopia
B. Increased risk of angle-closure glaucoma
C. Decreased risk of cataract
D. Decreased risk of retinal detachment

168. You see a premature baby with retinopathy of prematurity and recommend laser treatment. When consenting the parents, you discuss risks of treatment. Which of these is not a potential complication of laser treatment for this condition?

A. Vitreous hemorrhage

B. Anterior segment ischemia

C. Endophthalmitis

D. Increased myopia

169. Which of the following best describes type 2 retinopathy of prematurity (ROP)?

A. Zone 1, stage 3 without plus disease

B. Zone 1, stage 2 with plus disease

C. Zone 2, stage 2 with plus disease

D. Zone 2, stage 3 without plus disease

170. A 32-year-old well-appearing female presents for long-standing bilateral photopsias. She was diagnosed with posterior uveitis by another specialist who mentioned that she has no inflammatory cells in her vitreous cavities. Which one of the below diagnoses fits her description?

A. Acute posterior multifocal placoid pigment epitheliopathy (APMPPE)

B. Serpiginous choroiditis

C. Multiple evanescent white dot syndrome (MEWDS)

D. Punctate inner choroidopathy (PIC)

171. A 35-year-old well-appearing female presents for long-standing photopsia in her left eye. She was seen by another specialist who mentioned to her that the condition rarely affects both eyes. Which diagnosis is the specialist referring to?

A. Acute zonal occult outer retinopathy (AZOOR)

B. Multiple evanescent white dot syndrome (MEWDS)

C. Acute posterior multifocal placoid pigment epitheliopathy (APMPPE)

D. Punctate inner choroidopathy (PIC)

172. What is the treatment of choice for the majority of patients with acute posterior multifocal placoid pigment epitheliopathy (APMPPE) in the acute phase?

A. Observation

B. Steroids

C. Anti-VEGF agents

D. Immunomodulators

173. A 40-year-old man presents with geographic patch of grayish yellow placoid lesion in the peripapillary area, at the level of the choroid. He received a systemic work-up which was negative. What is the treatment for this patient's inflammatory condition?

A. Steroids

B. Acyclovir

C. Combination immunosuppressives and steroids

D. Photodynamic therapy

174. Subretinal choroidal neovascularization (CNV) is seen in 20% of which white dot syndrome?

A. Punctate inner choroidopathy (PIC)

B. Acute zonal occult outer retinopathy (AZOOR)

C. Multifocal choroiditis (MFC)

D. Multiple evanescent white dot syndrome (MEWDS)

175. A 40-year-old patient of Mediterranean descent presents with the following finding, and has a positive cutaneous pathergy test as well as new skin lesions.

What is the classic triad found in the disease you suspect?

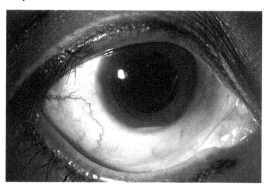

A. Recurrent aphthous ulcers, genital ulcers, and iritis with hypopyon

B. Arteritis of retinal vessels, retinal necrosis, and vitritis

C. Arthritis, conjunctivitis, and urethritis

D. Epiphora, photophobia, and blepharospasm

176. Which human leukocyte antigen (HLA) type is associated with Behcet's disease?

A. HLA-B27

B. HLA-A29

C. HLA-DR2

D. HLA-B5101

177. Which laboratory test would confirm the diagnosis of Behcet's disease?

A. Human leukocyte antigen (HLA) testing

B. Diagnostic paracentesis

C. Kveim–Siltzbach test (KST)

D. None

178. You have been following a 78-year-old patient for idiopathic vitritis that has not responded to topical or systemic steroids and is now starting to become bilateral. Fundus picture shows the following:

What is the next step in this patient's management?

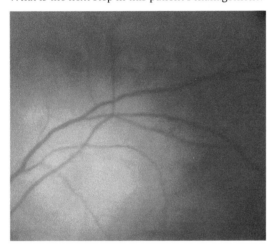

A. Start immunosuppressive treatment

B. Obtain magnetic resonance imaging (MRI)

C. Combine immunomodulators and steroids

D. Vitreous biopsy

179. Which of these uveitic conditions typically has the worst visual prognosis?

A. Acute posterior multifocal placoid pigment epitheliopathy (APMPPE)

B. Serpiginous choroiditis

C. Multiple evanescent white dot syndrome (MEWDS)

D. Punctate inner choroidopathy (PIC)

180. A 50-year-old male presents with blurred vision in the left eye. He admits to macropsia and metamorphopsia in the same eye. His fundus photo, fluorescein angiogram, and optical coherence tomography (OCT) are shown. The thickness of choroid on OCT is 455 μm. What is the diagnosis?

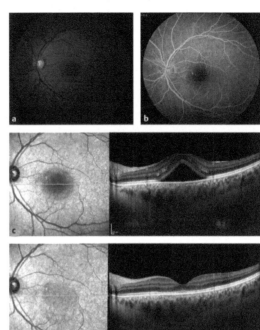

A. Central serous chorioretinopathy (CSR)

B. Age-related macular degeneration (AMD)

C. Vogt–Koyanagi–Harada (VKH) syndrome

D. Idiopathic polypoidal choroidal vasculopathy (IPCV)

181. A 56-year-old African American patient with lung-involving sarcoidosis has been referred to your clinic for an "ocular sarcoidosis rule-out exam." He denies any recent ocular symptoms but thinks he may have had some mild photophobia 3 weeks prior. What percent of patients with sarcoidosis have ocular manifestations?

A. 10%

B. 20%

C. 50%

D. 60%

182. Full-field electroretinography in a patient with MEWDS demonstrates reduced a-wave amplitudes. What part of the retina is assessed by the a-wave?

A. Muller cells and bipolar cells

B. Retinal pigment epithelium

C. Rod and cone cells

D. None of the above

183. Which of these diseases manifest with granulomatous uveitis?

A. Vogt–Koyanagi–Harada (VKH) syndrome

B. Sarcoidosis

C. Syphilis

D. All of the above

184. A 67-year-old woman with vitreomacular traction diagnosed by another specialist is referred to your clinic for surgical evaluation. Which statement is false regarding the management of this and similar pathologies?

A. Macular hole closure rates with vitrectomy is at around 95%.

B. After membrane peeling of macular pucker, 60 to 80% of the patients see two or more lines better.

C. Vitrectomy must be offered to patients with vitreomacular adhesion.

D. Vitrectomy should not be offered to patients with stage 1 macular hole.

185. A poorly controlled diabetic is referred to your surgical clinic for vitrectomy evaluation. He has had multiple injections for recurrent non-clearing vitreous hemorrhages in the setting of proliferative diabetic retinopathy. Which of the following is NOT a strong indication for vitrectomy in diabetes?

A. Tractional retinal detachment involving or threatening the macula

B. Diabetic macular edema that does not respond to intravitreal anti-VEGF and dexamethasone treatment

C. Vitreous hemorrhage that occurred a week ago

D. Development of a peripheral tear within an extrafoveal tractional retinal detachment and increasing amounts of subretinal fluid

186. Which "disease–most common causative agent" pairing is incorrect?

A. Coagulase-negative staphylococci–post-cataract endophthalmitis

B. Nocardia–post-intravitreal anti-VEGF injection endophthalmitis

C. Bacillus cereus–post-traumatic endophthalmitis

D. Streptococci and Hemophilus–Bleb-associated endophthalmitis

187. You see a 70-year-old patient with long-standing inflammation in the left eye. He received cataract surgery 2 years ago. His most recent complaint is related to ongoing photophobia with new-onset floaters. His cataract surgeon noted thickened posterior capsule deposits. What is the most common causative organism for delayed-onset endophthalmitis?

A. Propionibacterium acnes

B. Streptococcus viridans

C. Streptococcus mitis

D. Haemophilus influenzae

188. Which of the following is a risk factor for intraoperative suprachoroidal hemorrhage?

A. Advanced age

B. Glaucoma

C. Aphakia

D. All of the above

8.2 Answers and Explanations

Easy	Medium	Hard

1. Correct: Area of Martegiani (C)

Vitreous is a clear gel-like structure with a volume of 4 cm³. It is 98% water with collagen being the main protein constituent. The outermost part of the gel consists of condensed collagen fibers called the vitreous cortex. The vitreous base is a three-dimensional ring that extends 2 mm anterior and 3 mm posterior to the ora serrata (**B**). Weigert's ligament is an 8-mm disc of condensed vitreous that connects the vitreous gel to the posterior lens with a small retrolental space in its center referred to as Berger space (**A**). A similar space in front of the optic nerve is called the area of Martegiani (**C**). The human vitreous undergoes three stages of development. The primary vitreous consists of the hyaloid artery that extends from the optic nerve to the lens. This is replaced by the secondary vitreous around 10th week of gestation. Cloquet's canal is an S-shaped channel in the vitreous that extends from the optic nerve to the lens and is a remnant of the hyaloid vasculature (**D**). Other remnants of the primary vitreous that sometimes remain present after birth are small opacities at the optic nerve and the posterior lens, known as Bergmeister's papilla and Mittendorf dot, respectively. Tertiary vitreous consists of the zonules that hold crystalline lens in its place.

2. Correct: An area ~5.5 mm in diameter bordered by the disc and temporal vascular arcades (C)

The macula measures 5.5 mm in diameter and is centered at the fovea located 4 mm temporal and 0.8 mm inferior to the optic nerve (**D**). Histologically, the macula consists of two or more ganglion cell layers. The fovea is a 1.5 mm (one disc diameter) area with a central floor of 0.35 mm called the foveola and a central 0.5 mm capillary-free or avascular zone (B). Foveola lacks the ganglion cell and inner nuclear layers, consisting of only cone photoreceptors (**A**), and has a central concavity called the umbo. Surrounding the fovea is a 0.5-mm wide annular zone called the parafovea, where the ganglion cell layer, inner nuclear layer, and outer nuclear layer are the thickest. The parafovea, in turn, is surrounded by a 1.5-mm wide ring referred to as the perifovea.

3. Correct: Retinal pigment epithelium (RPE) (A)

HCQ is an anti-inflammatory drug used mainly in dermatology and rheumatology. Its ocular side effects include corneal deposition, reduced accommodation, and retinopathy that mainly manifests in the macula. HCQ binds to melanin and accumulates in the RPE cells causing a decline in RPE function (A). Over time, shed photoreceptor outer segments accumulate and lead to RPE degeneration. Vision loss may progress even after stopping HCQ as it has a long half-life. As per American Academy of Ophthalmology's 2016 Update, a dose of > 5 mg/kg based on real body weight is recommended. A baseline evaluation at initiation of HCQ treatment is obtained followed by annual examinations after 5 years on treatment. A 10–2 automated visual field and spectral domain optical coherence tomography is recommended to screen for toxicity. As toxicity in Asians can manifest outside of the macula, a 24–2 automated visual field is recommended in this population. Multifocal electroretinography and fundus autofluorescence can also be used.

4. Correct: Fluorescein angiography (FA) (C)

The history and color fundus photograph of this patient is consistent with a branch retinal vein occlusion (BRVO). In BRVO, the extent of capillary nonperfusion is the most important indicator of visual prognosis. For example, eyes with < 5 disc areas of nonperfusion on FA (**C**) have a 40% risk of developing neovascularization. Of the given options, only FA would demonstrate the severity of foveal ischemia as well as capillary nonperfusion. OCT would be helpful in determining the presence of macular edema and need for treatment with intravitreal anti-VEGF injection (**B**). Fundus autofluorescence (**A**) and ICG angiography (**D**) are helpful imaging modalities but do not predict of the likelihood of visual acuity recovery retinal vein occlusions.

5. Correct: Nausea (D)

In fluorescein angiography, a white light in the camera is passed through a blue filter that allows only blue wavelength (465–490 nm) to enter the eye. This blue light excites unbound fluorescein in the retinal and choroidal vessels, which emits photons of green wavelength (520–530 nm). This is then passed through a green filter that only allows green light to exit. Approximately 10% of the patients suffer from nausea and vomiting (**D**), whereas hives (**B**) and anaphylaxis (**C**) occur in 1% and 0.001% (1/100,000) patients.

6. Correct: OCT angiography (B)

Pregnancy is a contraindication to fluorescein angiography (C). In this pregnant patient, the best way to confirm the presence of retinal neovascularization is OCT angiography (**B**). There is no radiation exposure or use of dye in OCT angiography, and it can highlight areas of neovascularization at the vitreoretinal interface (see the given figure ii). In addition, most ophthalmic drops fall under the Food and Drug Administration's use-in-pregnancy category C, meaning these drugs have uncertain safety profile in pregnancy. Anti-VEGF agents are also contraindicated.

7. Correct: Retinal pigment epithelium (RPE) layer (D)

The image shown above is fundus autofluorescence (FAF) showing dark areas in the center correlating with RPE atrophy due to age-related macular degeneration. FAF is a noninvasive imaging modality that is often used to assess the status of the RPE (**D**). FAF signal originates predominantly from lipofuscin and melanolipofuscin inclusion bodies within the RPE and is modulated by presence of other fluorophores found in the adjacent tissues. Various characteristic FAF patterns have been described which may inform the diagnosis of genetic, degenerative, and inflammatory retinal diseases. In addition, the status of the neurosensory retina can be indirectly evaluated with FAF, as reduced photopigment density due to transient or permanent outer retinal disruption can unmask the FAF of healthy RPE producing focal or zonal areas of hyperautofluorescence.

8. Correct: Fluorescein optimally fluoresces at a shorter wavelength than ICG (A)

In FA, a white light is used from a camera which passes through a blue filter that allows only blue wavelength (465–490 nm) to enter the eye. This blue light excites unbound fluorescein in the retinal and choroidal vasculature which emit photons of green wavelength (520–530 nm). This is then passed through a green filter that only allows green light to exit. ICG angiography is used to image the choroidal vasculature as ICG is 98% protein-bound and is therefore retained in choroidal circulation (**C**). Compared to fluorescein, ICG fluoresces at a longer wavelength in the infrared range (790–805 nm) (**A**). In addition, fluorescence efficacy of ICG is only 4% that of fluorescein dye (**B**).

9. Correct: PED that exhibits leakage on fluorescein angiography (D)

The characteristic features of nonexudative AMD include drusen, macular pigmentary alterations (**A**), PEDs (**B**), and atrophy of the RPE and choroid. All of the above listed choices, except (**D**), are pertinent clinical features of dry, i.e., nonexudative, AMD. Exudative AMD is defined by the presence of choroidal neovascularization that leads to serous or hemorrhagic detachments of the retina and/or the RPE and would display leakage on fluorescein angiography (**D**).

10. Correct: 62-year-old man with geographic atrophy in one eye (C)

The original AREDS consisted of 500 mg vitamin C, 400 IU vitamin E, 15 mg beta carotene, 80 mg zinc, and 2 mg copper. The study found that AREDS regimen reduced the risk of progression to advanced age-related macular degeneration (AMD; subfoveal geographic atrophy or choroidal neovascularization) in eyes with unilateral or bilateral intermediate AMD (i.e., one large druse, multiple intermediate drusen, or non-subfoveal geographic atrophy). In addition, patients with advanced AMD in only one eye benefit from AREDS to protect their fellow eye (**C**). Given the higher incidence of lung cancer in smokers with beta carotene, the AREDS2 study suggested substituting beta carotene with a combination of lutein and zeaxanthin. The 40-year-old man with multiple large drusen (**A**) is too young to have AMD and likely has drusen related to another etiology. The AREDS studies did not evaluate effect of vitamins in patients with Stargardt disease (**B**). A patient with bilateral advanced AMD does not qualify for protection from AREDS vitamins as both eyes have already reached advanced state (**D**).

11. Correct: Deposits accumulate between Bruch's membrane and the choriocapillaris (C)

Accumulation of deposits under the retina, though not always classified as age-related macular degeneration, is typically not considered normal with aging. Accumulation of granular material between the RPE and its basement membrane is referred to as the basal laminar deposits. On the other hand, basal linear deposits accumulate between the outer collagenous layer of Bruch's membrane and choriocapillaris. Photoreceptors are reduced in density over time (**A**). Lipofuscin is a byproduct of the visual cycle and continues to accumulate in the RPE throughout life (**B**). Lastly, choroidal thickness reduces with age due to involutional changes in choriocapillaris (**D**).

12. Correct: Subretinal fluid (A)

The characteristic features of nonexudative AMD include drusen (**C**), macular pigmentary alterations (**D**), pigment epithelial detachments, and atrophy of the RPE (**B**) and choroid. The near-infrared and the accompanying OCT show a central area of RPE atrophy also known as geographic atrophy. All of the above listed choices except (**A**) are pertinent clinical features of dry, i.e., nonexudative AMD. Neovascular AMD on the other hand is defined by the presence of choroidal neovascularization that leads to serous or hemorrhagic detachments of the retina and/or the RPE.

13. Correct: Soft (D)

Drusen, a hallmark finding in age-related macular degeneration (AMD), consist of lipoprotein debris and are situated between the retinal pigment epithelium and Bruch's membrane. Drusen are classified as small (>64 μm) (**C**), intermediate (64–124 μm), and large (<124 μm). When adjacent drusen coalesce to a size greater than 350 μm, the term drusenoid pigment epithelial detachment is used. Both the number and size of the drusen impact risk for advanced AMD. In addition, drusen are classified as soft (**C**), hard (**B**), and cuticular (**A**) based on their appearance. Soft, confluent drusen are more likely to progress to choroidal neovascularization.

14. Correct: A complete fundus examination (A)

Despite significant advances in ophthalmic imaging, a complete fundus examination (**A**) remains the most important part of evaluation of any retina patient. It allows the examiner to evaluate for various features of AMD, such as the number, size, distribution and type of drusen, pigmentary changes, hemorrhage, and elevated lesions such as pigment epithelial detachments. In addition, other important incidental findings, for example, retinal breaks, lattice degeneration, and choroidal nevi, can be missed if relying solely on imaging such as fluorescein angiography (**B**) or OCT (**C**).

15. Correct: Cholesterol (B)

The picture above shows an embolus lodged at the arteriolar bifurcation. There are three main types of emboli: cholesterol, calcium, and platelet-fibrin. The embolus demonstrated in this question stem is the so-called Hollenhorst plaque—a bright, yellow, retractile embolus—that typically originates from an atheromatous plaque in the internal carotid artery and consists of cholesterol (**B**). Calcium (**C**) emboli arise from cardiac valves, appear white, and cause distal retinal infarction. Platelet-fibrin (**A**) emboli are dull white and also arise from atheromas in carotid arteries. Whether symptomatic or not, evaluation for carotid occlusive disease with carotid ultrasonography is warranted for patients who are found to have a Hollenhorst plaque.

16. Correct: The cilioretinal arteries provide circulation to the fovea and are not affected (C)

CRAO usually has a devastating effect on central visual acuity as the central retinal artery is typically solely responsible for supplying blood to the inner retinal layers. However, in 15 to 30% of the eyes, part of the macula is supplied by a cilioretinal artery which is derived from a posterior ciliary artery (rather than central retina artery) and is therefore unaffected by a CRAO. Most CRAO cases that maintain good central vision are those with a cilioretinal artery (C). Anti-VEGF agents are not effective against CRAO (D).

17. Correct: Erythrocyte sedimentation rate (ESR)/C-reactive protein (CRP) (D)

Approximately 2% of cases of CRAO are caused by giant cell arteritis (GCA). It is therefore essential to rule out GCA in patients older than 50 years of age, especially when presenting with a history and symptoms suggestive of GCA. A complete blood count should be ordered to evaluate for thrombocytosis along with ESR and CRP (D). A fluorescein angiogram shows profound choroidal ischemia in GCA. Intravenous steroids should be instituted immediately to prevent vision loss in the fellow eye if GCA is suspected. Carotid ultrasound (A) and MRI of the brain (B) are appropriate in cases of embolic CRAO. CT of the orbits (C) is not indicated. Patients with CRAO are followed closely for development of neovascularization.

18. Correct: Carotid ultrasound and referral to vascular surgery (C)

Ocular ischemic syndrome is caused by severe and chronic carotid obstruction. Given reduced blood flow to the eye, the intraocular pressure on the ipsilateral side is usually lower and fundus exam shows narrowed retinal arteries, dilated retinal veins, and midperipheral intraretinal hemorrhages. The profound retinal ischemia can lead to neovascularization requiring treatment with panretinal photocoagulation (A) and/or intravitreal anti-VEGF therapy (B) to reduce the VEGF burden. The definitive treatment, however, requires potential carotid endarterectomy and these patients therefore need carotid ultrasound and referral to vascular surgery (C).

19. Correct: Neuroectoderm (D)

The arrow is pointing to the retinal pigment epithelium (RPE), which is derived from the neuroectoderm (D). The RPE is the only pigmented tissue in the body that is not derived from the neural crest cells. Neuroectoderm also gives rise to the neurosensory retina, optic nerve, axons, and glia. Surface ectoderm (A) is responsible for formation of the lens, lacrimal gland and drainage system, corneal and conjunctival epithelium, as well as various structures of the eyelids and caruncle. Neural crest cells (B) give rise to the sclera, choroid, trabecular meshwork, corneal stroma, and corneal endothelium. Mesoderm (C) is mainly responsible for extraocular and iris muscles as well as temporal portion of the sclera.

20. Correct: It significantly increases the rate of vitrectomy for nonclearing vitreous hemorrhage (D)

ETDRS was a randomized, multicenter trial that compared focal laser photocoagulation against observation in patients with clinically significant diabetic macular edema (CSDME). The study showed that focal laser reduced the risk of visual loss by 50%, thus establishing focal laser as the standard treatment before the arrival of anti-VEGF injections. The same study also showed that aspirin has no effect on diabetic retinopathy (D).

21. Correct: An area of retinal thickening <= one disc area, any part of which lies within one disc diameter of the center of the macula (D)

ETDRS defined CSME based on contact lens slit lamp biomicroscopy. The following criteria were used: (i) retinal thickening within 500 µm of the macular center, (ii) hard exudates within 500 µm of the macular center with adjacent retinal thickening, and (iii) one or more disc diameters of retinal thickening, part of which is within one disc diameter of the macular center (D).

22. Correct: The ETDRS concluded that panretinal photocoagulation (PRP) reduces the risk of severe visual loss in patients with high-risk proliferative diabetic retinopathy (PDR) (A)

Choice A refers to the Diabetic Retinopathy Study (DRS) which randomized PDR or bilateral, severe non-proliferative diabetic retinopathy (NPDR) to PRP versus no PRP. This study found that PRP reduced the risk of severe vision loss in high-risk PDR from 44 to 20%. The laser parameters used for PRP in DRS were 1200 or more 500-µm burns, separated by one-half to one burn width apart at 0.1-second duration. The ETDRS study established the famous "4:2:1" rule for classifying NPDR. Any one feature in the absence of neovascularization from four quadrants with microaneurysms/hemorrhages, two quadrants with venous beading, or one quadrant with intraretinal microvascular abnormalities was classified as severe NPDR. Presence of two of these features was classified as very severe NPDR. ETDRS defined CSME (C) based on contact lens slit lamp biomicroscopy. Aspirin was not shown to affect disease progression in ETDRS (D).

23. Correct: Only if symptomatic (A)

As per American Academy of Ophthalmology Preferred Practice Patterns, nondiabetic women who develop gestational diabetes do not require an eye examination during pregnancy, and do not appear to be at increased risk for developing diabetic retinopathy during pregnancy. However, diabetics who become pregnant should be examined soon after conception and early in the first trimester of the pregnancy. The recommended follow-up is every 3 to 12 months for no retinopathy or moderate non-proliferative diabetic retinopathy (NPDR), or every 1 to 3 months for severe NPDR.

24. Correct: None of the above (D)

Coats disease was originally described as an idiopathic, non-hereditary (**D**), unilateral disorder characterized by retinal telangiectasia, microaneurysms, lipid exudation, and ischemia that predominantly affects young men. If left untreated, severe Coats disease can progress to retinal detachment, neovascular glaucoma, and phthisis bulbi. When occurring in the setting of Facioscapulohumeral muscular dystrophy (FSHD), an autosomal dominant disease, Coats disease is bilateral with equal gender predilection and is referred to as Coats syndrome.

25. Correct: Diabetes mellitus (A)

Known risk factors for branch retinal vein occlusion (BRVO) include age, hypertension (**B**), increased BMI (**C**), hyperlipidemia (**D**), and high intraocular pressure. The Beaver Dam Eye Study showed that BRVO was significantly associated with hypertension. This is thought to be due to the vascular changes induced by uncontrolled changes such as focal arteriolar narrowing and arteriovenous nicking. The hardened arterioles can compress venules at sites of arteriovenous nicking and lead to BRVO. A large meta-analysis showed a significant association of hypertension and hyperlipidemia with BRVO. However, there was no association of diabetes mellitus (**A**) with BRVO. Other factors that are significantly associated with BRVO are BMI, especially in patients younger than 50 years.

26. Correct: Sea fan (D)

The color fundus photography above shows a sea fan (**D**) in the far periphery of this sickle cell disease patient. Corresponding ultra-widefield fluorescein angiography demonstrates leakage around the sea fan, arteriovenous anastomoses, and peripheral drop-out. Sickle cell retinopathy is classified as non-proliferative or proliferative based on the presence or absence of neovascularization. Common findings of nonproliferative retinopathy include salmon patch hemorrhages (**B**), iridescent spots (**A**), and black sunburst lesions (**C**). Salmon patch hemorrhages are pink to orange hemorrhages located between the internal limiting membrane (ILM) and the retina and may represent progressive hemolysis of blood from a blown-out occluded arteriole. Iridescent spots represent the development of a small schisis

cavity after an intraretinal hemorrhage resolves, and glisten with hemosiderin-laden macrophages. Black sunburst lesions represent hyperpigmentation that may represent focal hypertrophy of the retinal pigment epithelium, focal choroidal damage, or intraretinal hemorrhage that tracks down to the subretinal space. Sea fan is a sign of proliferative sickle cell retinopathy.

27. Correct: Applying cryopexy around the peripheral retina (D)

Sickled red blood cells are prone to hemolysis and cause vascular occlusion given their fragile membranes and rigid structure, respectively. Patients with sickle cell disease are therefore prone to ischemia intraoperatively and care must be taken to minimize any maneuvers that would further compromise blood flow. Many argue that scleral buckling (**A**) should be avoided in these patients, but if a buckle is employed then the subretinal blood should be drained first to avoid an increase in intraocular pressure. Epinephrine (**B**) can constrict blood vessels and reduce blood flow that is already compromised. As anterior ciliary arteries run with the extraocular muscles, it is best to avoid removing extraocular muscles in sickle cell patients during surgery (**C**). Cryopexy may be required to seal the causative breaks in retinal detachment (**D**).

28. Correct: Macular edema for 3 months with vision 20/40 (B)

According to Branch Retinal Vein Occlusion Study (BVOS), grid laser is recommended for chronic macular edema with a vision of 20/40 or worse 3 months after initial presentation in the presence of intact macular perfusion (**B**). Although more than five disc areas of nonperfusion (**D**) conferred a high risk for developing neovascularization, the study recommended that sectoral panretinal photocoagulation be performed only once neovascularization develops.

29. Correct: May resolve spontaneously without evidence of choroidal neovascularization (CNV) (A)

The fundus photograph here shows brown, jagged radiations deep to the neurosensory retina which is classic for angioid streaks. The arrow points to a retinal hemorrhage. A break in the Bruch's membrane can be seen in the area of hemorrhage on the corresponding OCT. Angioid streaks can have a varied natural course and can remain asymptomatic and stationary for many years; however, they can also spontaneously progress to develop breaks in the retinal pigment epithelium causing damage to outer photoreceptor layers. Bleeding that occurs in this process in the absence of CNV can resolve spontaneously over time (**A**). However, angioid streaks can also progress to form CNV membranes that result in retinal hemorrhage, edema, and fibrovascular scar with permanent loss of visual potential. CNV-related subretinal hemorrhage that can be identified on fluorescein angiography are treated with intravitreal anti-VEGF.

30. Correct: Wash-out pattern on indocyanine green (ICG) angiography (D)

Choroidal hemangiomas can be either circumscribed or diffuse. A diffuse choroidal hemangioma manifests as widespread red-orange discoloration of the fundus (i.e., a "tomato ketchup fundus") and has a well-known association with Sturge–Weber syndrome. Circumscribed choroidal hemangioma (CCH) usually presents as a unilateral solitary tumor posterior to the equator with no systemic associations. The distinctive angiographic signature of CCH is seen on ICGA as a rapid onset of intense hyperfluorescence seen earlier in the study (more than 30 seconds) compared to other choroidal tumors, followed by a characteristic loss of dye or "wash out" phenomenon (D, see figures ii and iii). On ultrasonography, high internal reflectivity (C) from multiple vascular channels as well as a high initial A-scan spike from the anterior tumor surface helps distinguish CCH from choroidal melanoma, which has low to medium internal reflectivity and is acoustically hollow.

31. Correct: All of the above (D)

Shown above is a prepapillary vascular loop that is a congenital variant and is usually unilateral in asymptomatic patients. In rare cases, they can bleed into the vitreous or cause a retinal vein or artery occlusion (D).

32. Correct: 8 to 15% (C)

Certain clinical features can help in stratifying the risk of a retinal break in the setting of an acute posterior vitreous detachment (PVD) presenting with flashes and floaters. There is an 8 to 15% risk of a retinal break in patients presenting with acute symptomatic PVD (C). The risk increases to almost 50 to 70% when vitreous hemorrhage accompanies acute PVD. Even when no break is identified on the initial exam in the presence of vitreous hemorrhage, there is a 20% risk of a beak within 6 weeks. Shafer sign, denoted by presence of pigment in the anterior vitreous, confers a 90% risk of a retinal break in a phakic patient. A retinal break can be present even in the absence of a Weiss ring indicating a PVD occurred. Therefore, all patients presenting with flashes and floaters must undergo thorough indirect ophthalmoscopy with scleral indentation as needed. A B-scan should be performed when media opacities such as dense cataract or vitreous hemorrhage preclude complete ophthalmoscopy to the ora serrata.

33. Correct: All of the above (D)

Family history, history of intraocular surgery, and history of RD are all risk factors for retinal detachment in a patient with asymptomatic retinal breaks (D). Prophylactic laser retinopexy is therefore often recommended upon discovery of retinal breaks in these patients even when they are asymptomatic.

34. Correct: Meridional fold, lattice degeneration, cystic tuft with peripheral retinal excavation, white-without-pressure (B)

It is important to be able to recognize peripheral retinal findings and know which carry an increased risk of retinal tear and subsequent detachment. Retinal pathologies with increased risk of break and detachment include lattice degeneration, cystic and zonular tractional tufts, meridional folds, enclosed ora bays, peripheral retinal excavations. Meridional folds are pleats of redundant retina commonly aligned with a dentate process and found in superonasal quadrant. Tears may occur at the posterior border of these folds. Lattice retinal degeneration is a thinning of neurosensory retina that can also be associated with retinal tears at the posterior or lateral margin. Cystic retinal tufts are focal areas of elevated glial hyperplasia associated with vitreous or zonular attachment and traction. Peripheral retinal excavation may represent a mild form of lattice degeneration. Retinal lesions that do not predispose to increased risk of retinal breaks include retinal pigment epithelium hyperplasia and hypertrophy, noncystic tufts, peripheral cystoid degeneration, and cobblestone degeneration.

35. Correct: B and C (D)

Hyperfluorescence in fluorescein angiography (FA) can be categorized into four major patterns: staining, pooling, leakage, and transmission (or window) defect. Staining occurs due to uptake of the fluorescein dye into structures such as drusen, peripapillary atrophy, and the optic disc. This type of hyperfluorescence is fixed in size and maintains its intensity in late phases of the FA. Pooling (C) is defined as an increase in fluorescence over time as fluorescein dye accumulates in a closed space, such as a retinal pigmental epithelial detachment, but then reaches a certain size, as it is a fixed space with defined borders. This is in contrast to leakage (B), in which the area of hyperfluorescence has fuzzy borders and continues to increase over time. Transmission or window defect (A) occurs due to a defect in the overlying retinal pigment epithelium that allows normal choroidal fluorescence to be more visible. This pattern of hyperfluorescence reaches its peak intensity in early phases of the FA and fades in the late phases.

around 5% in patients aged 40 years and above. Two histological subtypes exist: typical and reticular. Both subtypes are usually found inferotemporally with the reticular subtype more likely to extend toward the pre-equatorial retina. Although rare, reticular retinoschisis is more likely to result in rhegmatogenous retinal detachments than typical retinoschisis. The cleavage plane in reticular retinoschisis is found in the nerve fiber layer, while it is found in the outer plexiform layer in the typical subtype.

126. Correct: Presence of an outer retinal hole (D)

Retinoschisis is characterized by the abnormal splitting of the neurosensory retina without involvement of the subretinal space. The presence of a demarcation line indicates the presence of subretinal fluid and secondary retinal pigment epithelium changes, which are not normal retinoschisis findings (**A**). Inner retinal holes, though uncommon, are smaller in size and multiple (**B**). The outer retinal holes are more common, usually bigger in size with rolled posterior edges, and less in number (just one or two). Retinoschisis with just outer retinal holes is known as "schisis-detachment" and needs to be observed; however, retinal holes in both outer and inner retinal layer result in "rhegmatogenous retinal detachment" and need early surgical intervention. Hence, the presence of a retinal demarcation line indicates the presence of an outer retinal hole (**D**). The rate of retinal detachment in cases of retinoschisis is low, estimated to be about 3% or less. Retinoschisis is usually present in patients with hyperopic, not myopic, refraction (**C**).

127. Correct: Female carriers of ocular albinism have detectable ocular abnormalities (B)

Albinism refers to a group of different genetic abnormalities with absent or reduce melanin production. Ocular albinism is typically inherited in an x-linked pattern (**A**). Female carriers of ocular albinism may show partial iris transillumination defects and fundus pigment mosaicism, described as "mud-splatter" (**B**). Patients with ocular albinism and nystagmus would usually have subnormal visual acuity (20/100–20/400) (**C**). Chediak–Higashi syndrome describes oculocutaneous albinism (autosomal recessive) combined with extreme susceptibility to infections (**D**). Hermansky–Pudlak syndrome is another type of oculocutaneous albinism, additionally characterized by bleeding susceptibility from platelet dysfunction and is more commonly found in people from Puerto Rico.

128. Correct: Anti-recoverin antibodies are sometimes found (D)

Cancer-associated retinopathy (CAR) is a paraneoplastic syndrome characteristic by retinal degeneration related to a systemic malignancy. It is usually distinguished from RP by rapid progression (**A**). Patients with CAR often present with progressive visual loss before a primary cancer has been diagnosed—and if there is no known neoplasm, a search for one should be undertaken (**B**). Steroids and/or immunosuppressive therapy may halt and sometimes reverse the vision loss in patients with CAR (**C**). Anti-recoverin antibodies (23-kDa protein) were the first antibodies found in CAR (**D**). Anti-enolase antibodies in the setting of CAR are characterized by cone dysfunction. In melanoma-associated retinopathy (MAR), the antibodies are directed toward undefined retinal bipolar cells antigens, and the rods are primarily affected.

129. Correct: Lipofuscin (D)

The effectiveness of any photocoagulator depends on how light is transmitted by the ocular tissue and how well that light is absorbed by pigment in the target tissue. Melanin is an excellent absorber of green, yellow, red, and infrared wavelengths (**C**). Hemoglobin easily absorbs blue, green, and yellow with minimal absorption of red wavelengths (**A**). Macular xanthophyll readily absorbs blue light but minimally absorbs yellow or red wavelengths (**B**). Lipofuscin is not a target for photocoagulation (**D**).

130. Correct: Permanent loss of corneal sensation (A)

Laser photocoagulation is a common office-based procedure to treat a variety of retinal pathologies. Potential side effects should be discussed with the patients prior to the procedure. Pain during the laser treatment is a frequent side effect. Hence, PRP treatments (usually over 1200 spots) may be divided into several sessions. In addition, heavy laser during one sitting has been found to be associated with exudative retinal detachments and choroidal effusions (**C and D**). Pupillary abnormalities have been found if heavy laser is applied along the horizontal meridians (**B**). Though some case reports describe a transient loss of corneal sensation after PRP, no definitive evidence of permanent loss of corneal sensation related to PRP has been found. Loss of corneal sensation in diabetic patients receiving PRP is likely secondary to underlying peripheral neuropathy rather than direct effects of PRP.

131. Correct: Pain is not related to infusion of verteporfin (C)

The use of verteporfin in photodynamic therapy has a number of side effects due to the photosensitizing properties of the molecule. It is important to discuss these potential side effects with patients prior to the procedure: (1) Back pain (2.5% incidence) is common in patients receiving verteporfin injections

(**A**). Other sites of pain include leg, groin, chest, buttock, arm, and shoulder. The infusion of verteporfin is directly related to the pain (**C**). Body pain should subside after cessation of the infusion. (2) Patients should avoid direct sunlight exposure for 48 to 72 hours after PDT (**B**). (3) A minority of patients lose vision with PDT treatment, likely due to PDT-related impairment of the choroidal circulation.

132. Correct: Lower rate of retinal tears (D)

Small-gauge vitrectomy has revolutionized the field of retinal surgery and facilitated surgical intervention with minimal trauma. While all of the answer choices above (**A, B, and C**) are correct, the most significant in terms of outcomes is likely related to the lower rate of intraoperative iatrogenic retinal tears/breaks associated with the small-gauge instruments (**D**).

133. Correct: Ocular Mainster PRP 165 lens (D)

Many lenses are used to assist in laser photocoagulation of the retina. Each lens has its own magnification power, which results in particular image and laser spot sizes. See the table below for the image magnification and laser spot size for the lenses listed above:

Lens	Image magnification	Laser spot magnification	Field of View (°)
Goldmann 3-mirror	0.93x	1.08x	140
Volk Area Centralis	1.06x	0.94x	70–84
Mainster PRP 165	0.51x	1.96x	165–180
Mainster Widefield	0.68x	1.5x	118–127

134. Correct: All of the above (D)

Laser photocoagulation is a common outpatient procedure that could be used for multiple indications. Panretinal photocoagulation is commonly used in the management of diabetic retinopathy as per investigated in the Diabetic Retinopathy Study (**A**). In addition, laser therapy can be used to manage peripheral holes and tears of the retina (**B**). Small retinal capillary hemangioblastoma lesions in the setting of Von Hippel–Lindau can be treated with laser photocoagulation (**C**).

135. Correct: Hemoglobin minimally absorbs red and infrared wavelengths (C)

Melanin is an excellent absorber of green, yellow, red, and infrared wavelengths (**A**). Xanthophyll absorbs blue but it minimally absorbs yellow and red wavelengths (**B**). Hemoglobin easily absorbs blue, green, and yellow with minimal absorption of red wavelength (**C**).

136. Correct: Argon red (C)

Red laser offers good penetration through moderate nuclear sclerosis and moderate vitreous hemorrhage, as it has minimal hemoglobin absorption (**C**). Laser choice is dependent on the specific goals of treatment and certain patient factors. Double-frequency YAG lasers are not commonly used in the setting of panretinal photocoagulation as the mechanisms of action is related to photodisruption rather than photocoagulation (**A**). Green lasers are well absorbed by melanin and hemoglobin. Hence, it may not be an ideal choice for patients with proliferative diabetic retinopathy and vitreous hemorrhage (**B**). Infrared lasers have similar characteristics to red lasers but offer deeper penetration and may cause more discomfort than argon red lasers (**D**).

137. Correct: Vitrectomy and intravitreal amikacin/ceftazidime injection results in better visual acuity regardless of the initial visual acuity (D)

EVS was designed to evaluate the best protocol in dealing with acute endophthalmitis after cataract surgery. The EVS findings showed no benefit in systemic antibiotic therapy (**A**). The EVS showed no difference in outcomes between the vitrectomy or immediate tap/inject groups in patients presenting with hand motion or better visual acuity (**B**). However, patients presenting with visual acuity of light perception or worse did better with vitrectomy and intravitreal amikacin/ceftazidime injection (**C**).

138. Correct: Traumatic exogenous endophthalmitis–*Candida species* (B)

Pictured on indirect ophthalmoscopy here are classic intravitreal "fluff balls" with vitreous haze associated with probable *Candida* endophthalmitis in an immunocompromised patient. All matched answers are correct except for (**B**). The rate of postvitrectomy endophthalmitis is lowest among all postsurgical cases (0.03–0.046%). The most common organisms responsible for postcataract surgery endophthalmitis is coagulase-negative *Staphylococcus* and *Staphylococcus aureus* (**D**). *Streptococcus* and *Haemophilus*, relatively common pathogens following trabeculectomy surgery, can be particularly devastating (**C**). *Propionibacterium acnes* classically presents months to years after an uncomplicated cataract surgery (**A**). *Bacillus cereus* is a typical associated organism of traumatic endophthalmitis, not *Candida*. *Candida* and other fungal species would be expected in endogenous endophthalmitis in immunocompromised patients, as in this case.

139. Correct: B-scan ultrasound of a choroidal hemangioma typically shows a lesion with low internal reflectively (C)

Diffuse choroidal hemangioma is part of the Sturge–Weber syndrome and is usually ipsilateral to the skin findings (A). Elevated intraocular pressure is a common feature in cases with diffuse choroidal hemangiomas due to elevated outflow pressure, angle malformation, or both (B). B-scan ultrasonography findings include high internal reflectivity, choroidal thickening, and may show overlying subretinal fluid (C). Many treatment modalities have been suggested, including low-dose radiation (external beam photon radiotherapy, plaque radiotherapy, proton beam irradiation, gamma knife radiotherapy, and stereotactic radiotherapy) but photodynamic therapy is the treatment of choice in small- to medium-sized circumscribed choroidal hemangiomas (D).

140. Correct: Lung, breast (C)

Ocular metastasis has been estimated to be the most common intraocular tumor in adults. The uvea is the most common site for ocular metastasis. The most common primary cancer sites for uveal metastasis in males are lung (40%), gastrointestinal tract (9%, D), and kidney (8%, A). In females, the most common sites included breast (68%), lung (12%, B), and other (4%). Of note, breast cancer is the most common cancer to metastasize to the choroid in overall population studies (47%). Within a population of patients with uveal metastases from breast cancer, 62% of subjects presented with unilateral metastasis. The same population had a survival rate of 65% at 1 year, 35% at 3 years, and 24% at 5 years.

141. Correct: Ophthalmodynamometry (B)

The finding of low arterial perfusion on ophthalmodynamometry is the most helpful diagnostic test to help make the diagnosis. Another useful tip is to gently press (digital pressure) on the upper eye lid while examining the fundus to look for retina arterial pulsations that are visible in ocular ischemic syndrome (OIS). Hemorrhages located mid-peripherally are not always found in OIS; hemorrhages are usually less numerous in OIS compared to CRVO (A). In OIS, the retinal veins are mostly dilated, but not tortuous; on the other hand, in CRVO, veins are both dilated and tortuous. Fluorescein angiography shows delayed and patchy choroidal filling defects and delayed arm-to-choroid/retina circulation time in OIS (C). The optical coherence tomography shows decreased choroidal thickness in OIS (D).

142. Correct: Diabetic retinopathy (A)

Diabetic retinopathy is the most common cause of cotton wool spots and is caused by focal arteriolar infarcts of capillaries within the nerve fiber layer. Hypertension is the second most common cause (B). HIV and interferon retinopathy are less common causes of cotton wool spots (C, D).

143. Correct: Cilioretinal artery occlusion mostly occurs with central retinal artery occlusion (CRAO) (B)

Cilioretinal artery occlusion mostly occurs with central retinal vein occlusion (CRVO), rather than CRAO, and is postulated to be due to increased vascular hydrostatic pressure associated with a CRVO. Cilioretinal arteries arise from the short posterior ciliary vessels (D). They are found in 32% of eyes (A). GCA can present with an isolated cilioretinal artery occlusion (C).

144. Correct: Involvement of the ophthalmic artery (D)

NLP vision raises the possibility of an ophthalmic artery occlusion, particularly in an elderly individual, because of the simultaneous ischemia of the both choroidal and retinal circulation. A diagnosis of malingering is usually a diagnosis of exclusion and should only be reached once all investigations are complete and there are no alternative explanations (A). Cilioretinal artery occlusion may impact macular function but would not cause NLP vision (B). Anti-VEGF treatment is not indicated in the standard management of acute central retinal artery occlusion (CRAO) but maybe used in cases with secondary neovascularization (C).

145. Correct: It is the leading cause of blindness in adults aged 20 to 64 years in the United States (B)

DR is the leading cause of blindness in patients aged 20 to 64 years in the United States (B). The Wisconsin Epidemiology Study of Diabetic Retinopathy showed that 99% of type 1 diabetics and 60% of type 2 diabetics show evidence of DR 20 years after the diagnosis of diabetes (A). The diagnosis of DR is made by the combination of clinical examination, systemic metabolic derangements, and tests such as fluorescein angiography and optical coherence tomography (C). DR is classified as nonproliferative (mild, moderate, severe) and proliferative (with high-risk characteristics) (D).

146. Correct: Pregnancy can exacerbate diabetic retinopathy (B)

The DCCT found that sulfonylureas did not increase the risk of heart disease, intensive blood sugar control reduces the risk of progression of NPDR to PDR, and intensive blood pressure control can slow the progression of retinopathy (A, C, and D). Pregnancy can significantly exacerbate diabetic retinopathy, but this was not a finding of the DCCT (B). It is usually recommended that pregnant patients with diabetes undergo an ophthalmic examination in their first trimester. Pregnant patients with severe NPDR/DME should be reviewed every 1 to 3 months. For those with no retinopathy, mild or moderate NPDR, follow-up could be individualized.

147. Correct: ETDRS (C)

The photograph shows clinically significant macular edema (CSME). CSME is a clinical diagnosis and is defined as: retinal thickening within 500 μm of the macular center; hard exudates within 500 μm of the macular center with adjacent retinal thickening; or one or more disc diameters of retinal thickening, part of which is within one disc diameter of the macular center. The Early Treatment Diabetic Retinopathy Study (ETDRS) defined CSME and found that focal laser therapy was a beneficial treatment modality. The DCCT and UKPDS explored the effects of intensified sugar control on progression of diabetic retinopathy (**A, B**). RISE/RIDE (Ranibizumab for Diabetic Macular Edema) showed the beneficial effects of ranibizumab in the management of center-involving DME (**D**).

148. Correct: Criteria for diagnosing severe non-proliferative diabetic retinopathy (NPDR) (D)

The 4:2:1 rule was defined by the Early Treatment Diabetic Retinopathy Study (ETDRS) to help clinicians identify patients at higher risk to progress to proliferative diabetic retinopathy. Severe NPDR was characterized by any one of the following: diffuse intraretinal hemorrhages and microaneurysms in four quadrants, venous beading in two quadrants or intraretinal microvascular abnormalities (IRMA) in one quadrant (**D**). The ETDRS defined the criteria for CSME (**A**) and high-risk PDR (**B**) but this was not the purpose of the 4:2:1 rule. The definition of high-risk PDR included new vessels on or within one disc diameter of the optic disc (NVD) with or without vitreous or preretinal hemorrhage; or vitreous and/or preretinal hemorrhage accompanied by new vessels, either NVD or NVE ≥ 1/4 disc area.

149. Correct: Focal laser therapy decreased the risk of moderate vision loss in diabetic macular edema (D)

The ETDRS study demonstrated conclusively the benefit of focal macular laser in the treatment of diabetic macular edema (**D**). The ETDRS study was also crucial in determining that scatter laser PRP reduces the risk of disease progression and vision loss in severe nonproliferative and early proliferative stage retinopathy (**B**). ACE inhibitors (**A**) and anti-VEGF (**C**) therapy were not part of the ETDRS study.

150. Correct: Choroidal neovascularization (A)

Focal laser therapy is an important modality in the treatment of CSDME as per the Early Treatment Diabetic Retinopathy Study. Some of the complications include foveal burn, secondary choroidal neovascularization, and inadvertent scotoma. The other complications (**B, C, and D**) are not known to occur with focal laser therapy.

151. Correct: Has a 45% chance of progression to proliferative diabetic retinopathy (PDR) in 1 year according to the Early Treatment Diabetic Retinopathy Study (ETDRS) (B)

The patient described satisfies two criteria within the 4:2:1 rule (diffuse intraretinal hemorrhages and microaneurysms in four quadrants, venous beading in two quadrants, or intraretinal microvascular abnormality [IRMA] in one quadrant). This would classify the patient as having very severe NPDR. The ETDRS found that such patients had a 45% chance of progression to PDR in 1 year (**B**). The ETDRS did not find any benefit to grid laser in patients with very severe NDPR (**D**). The RISE and RIDE trials investigated the use of ranibizumab in diabetic macular edema (DME) (**A**). The DRCR protocol I compared the use of intravitreal ranibizumab (0.5 mg) plus prompt or deferred focal/grid laser; or intravitreal triamcinolone (4 mg) combined with focal/grid laser versus focal/grid laser alone in the management of DME (**C**).

152. Correct: Photodynamic therapy (D)

Photodynamic therapy has not been shown to be of benefit in diabetic macular edema. All other answer choices have been found to benefit diabetic macular edema in different trials: RISE and RIDE trials (**A**), DRCR Protocol I (**B**), ETDRS (**C**).

153. Correct: Humans are infected by direct skin contact (C)

Human infection usually happens through inhaling the fungus, which then passes into the blood stream (**C**). Histoplasma capsulatum is an endemic fungus to the Mississippi and the Ohio River valleys (**A**). It is carried on the feathers of birds as well as the droppings of infected bats (**B**). Ocular scarring usually results once the systemic infection resolves (**D**).

154. Correct: Bruch's membrane (D)

Angioid streaks appear as bilateral, narrow, jagged lines, deep to the retina. They represent crack-like breaks in a structurally abnormal and highly calcified Bruch's membrane. Angioid streaks can be associated with numerous systemic diseases, the most common being pseudoxanthoma elasticum as well as Ehlers–Danlos syndrome, Paget's disease of bone, sickle cell disease, and other hemoglobinopathies.

155. Correct: Retinal findings may mimic Bietti crystalline dystrophy (D)

This patient has pseudoxanthoma elasticum, a disease caused by mutation in the ABCC6 gene (**A**). Similar findings of angioid streaks may be found in patients with sickle cell disease or thalassemia, Paget's disease, Ehlers–Danlos, or they can also be idiopathic (**B**). Pseudoxanthoma elasticum is sometimes associated with optic nerve head drusen (**C**). Bietti crystalline dystrophy is associated with characteristic crystalline deposits not seen in pseudoxanthoma elasticum (**D**).

156. Correct: Order a fluorescein angiogram (D)

Angioid streaks can cause subretinal hemorrhages from choroidal fibrovascular ingrowth. These hemorrhages can resolve spontaneously or can lead to choroidal neovascularization which can be recurrent and lead to progressive visual loss. A fluorescein angiogram would help in ruling out an underlying choroidal neovascularization and clarify the source of the blood. Observation and use of safety glasses will not be helpful in this case (**A**). Laser photocoagulation has not been shown to help in case with subretinal blood secondary to angioid streaks (**B**). Anti-VEGF therapy could be used in the treatment of choroidal neovascularization but a fluorescein angiogram would be the next best step to ensure appropriate use of anti-VEGF (**C**).

157. Correct: Vascular sheathing (D)

POHS is a clinical syndrome that is considered a consequence of a presumed infection with the yeast form of *Histoplasma capsulatum*. It is defined by four clinical signs: (1) Punched-out chorioretinal lesions (**A**), (2) lack of vitritis, (3) juxtapapillary pigmented atrophic scars (**B**), and (4) choroidal neovascularization (**C**).

158. Correct: 5 to 10% (B)

High myopia is defined as a having a spherical equivalent of greater than –6.00 D or an axial length of more than 26.5 mm. While the definition of pathologic myopia is one that is evolving, it can be thought of as high myopia in addition to pathologic changes associated with the myopic status, such as posterior staphyloma, Forster–Fuchs spots or chorioretinal degeneration. One of the most serious complications of pathologic myopia is CNV, which often leads to sudden-onset decrease in vision. The prevalence of CNV is estimated at 5 to 10% in eyes with an axial length greater than 26.5 mm.

159. Correct: Surgical removal of the neovascular complex is beneficial if visual acuity is worse than 20/100 (B)

The Macular Photocoagulation Study (MPS) enrolled patients with choroidal neovascular membranes from age-related macular degeneration (AMD) as well as POHS. The trial showed that untreated eyes with POHS and extrafoveal CNV had a 44% risk of severe vision loss at 5 years versus 9% in the treatment group (**A**). Submacular surgery showed some mild visual benefit but recurrence rates remained unacceptably high after surgery (**B**). Anti-VEGF

agents are the mainstay of treatment for CNV secondary to POHS (**C**). The MPS study showed that unlike AMD, subfoveal CNV in patients with POHS did not benefit from laser photocoagulation (**D**).

160. Correct: The axial length greater than 32.5 mm (D)

Pathologic myopia is defined as high myopia with any posterior myopia-specific pathology from axial elongation. Myopia, not pathologic myopia, affects 25% of the US population (**A**). The incidence is highest in Asians and lowest in African Americans (**B**). The spherical equivalent is usually higher than –8.00 D (**C**) and the axial length is equal to or greater than 32.5 mm (**D**).

161. Correct: They result from rupture of Bruch's membrane and may require fluorescein angiography (D)

Isolated round deep hemorrhages are common in pathological myopia. They are related to rupture of Bruch's membrane and may require fluorescein angiography for further analysis (**D**). The use of fluorescein angiography could help to distinguish this entity from an underlying choroidal neovascular membrane (**A**) which would benefit from anti-VEGF therapy (**C**).

162. Correct: Zone 2 (B)

ROP is categorized by the severity of the disease in zones of the retina. It is categorized by involvement of the lowest number (most posterior) zone and the highest stage observed in each eye. Zone I is a circle, the radius of which extends from the center of the optic disc to twice the distance from the center of the optic disc to the center of the macula (**A**). Zone II extends centrifugally from the edge of zone I to the nasal ora serrata, and temporally it corresponds to the anatomic equator (**B**). Zone III is the residual temporal crescent of retina anterior to zone II (**C**). This patient has ROP stage 3, zone II, plus disease, note dilated and tortuous vessels in all quadrants (**B**).

163. Correct: Elevated ridge (D)

Accurate staging is of vital importance in the evaluation and management of patients with ROP. Stage 1 describes a thin, flat demarcation line that separates the avascular retina anteriorly from the vascularized retina posteriorly. Stage 2 describes an elevated ridge with height and width, which extends above the plane of the retina. Small isolated tufts of neovascular tissue, commonly called "popcorn," may be seen posterior to the ridge. Stage 3 describes extraretinal fibrovascular neovascularization extending from the ridge into the vitreous (**B**). Stage 4 describes a partial retinal detachment, which can be classified as extrafoveal (stage 4A) (**A**) and foveal (stage 4B). Stage

5 describes a total funnel-shaped retinal detachment and can be further subdivided depending upon whether the anterior and posterior portions of funnel are open or narrowed. Plus disease includes abnormal arteriolar tortuosity and venous dilation (**C**) along with iris vascular engorgement, pupillary rigidity, and vitreous haze.

164. Correct: High exposure to supplemental oxygen (C)

A number of factors have been consistently associated with increased risk for the development of ROP and include low birthweight (less than 1500 g) (**A**), gestational age (> 32 weeks) (**B**), and extended supplemental oxygen (C). Maternal alcohol abuse is an important consideration in developmental anomalies in newborns (especially fetal alcohol syndrome), but no association with ROP incidence has been found (**D**).

165. Correct: No treatment is indicated at this time (D)

The image shows an eye with an elevated ridge temporally (stage 2) in zone 2 of the right eye. No evidence of plus disease is seen. As per the ET-ROP study, neonates with this stage fall into type 2 of the trial who benefited from close follow-up. Ablative laser applies in certain criteria (type 1 ROP: zone 1, any stage ROP with plus disease; zone II, stage 2 or 3 ROP with plus disease; and eyes with threshold ROP: at least 5 contiguous or 8 cumulative clock hours of stage 3 ROP in zone I or II, in the presence of plus disease).

166. Correct: Two weeks (B)

Stage 2 ROP within zone II with no evidence of plus disease does not fit the treatment criteria for the early treatment ROP (ET-ROP) study (**A**). The following follow-up schedule is usually recommended for ROP patients: **1-week or less follow-up:** Immature vascularization: zone I—no ROP Immature retina extends into posterior zone II, near the boundary of zone I Stage 1 or 2 ROP: zone I Stage 3 ROP: zone II The presence or suspected presence of aggressive posterior ROP **1- to 2-week follow-up:** Immature vascularization; posterior zone II Stage 2 ROP: zone II Unequivocally regressing ROP: zone I **2-week follow-up:** Stage 1 ROP: zone II Immature vascularization: zone II—no ROP Unequivocally regressing ROP: zone II **2- to 3-week follow-up:** Stage 1 or 2 ROP: zone III Regressing ROP: zone II

167. Correct: Increased risk of angle-closure glaucoma (B)

Patients with retinopathy of prematurity (ROP) are known to encounter multiple anatomical complications related to their underlying prematurity as well as potential treatment. Neonates with ROP are known to have increased risk of myopia (A), increased risk of cataract (C) and retinal detachment (**D**). On the other hand, they are at increased risk of angle-closure glaucoma (**B**) due to steeper corneas, shallower anterior chambers, and larger lens-to-axial length ratios than normal eyes. In addition, secondary forms of angle-closure glaucoma could be found in this population secondary to anterior segment neovascularization and secondary ciliary body effusion post-laser retinopexy.

168. Correct: Endophthalmitis (C)

Laser ablation is considered the mainstay treatment for patients with type 2 retinopathy of prematurity (ROP) as per the early treatment ROP (ET-ROP) study. A number of treatment-related complications have been reported and include vitreous hemorrhage (**A**), anterior segment ischemia (**B**), posttreatment transient myopia and long-term myopia (**D**). Endophthalmitis is not a potential complication of laser treatment (**C**).

169. Correct: Zone 2, stage 3 without plus disease (D)

The early treatment ROP (ETROP) study was able to refine the use of retinal laser ablation in ROP patients. Based on the results of the study, patients are now classified into two groups with different treatment recommendations. Type 1 (Treat): zone I, plus disease and stage 1, 2, or 3; zone I, no plus disease and stage 3; zone II, plus disease with stage 2 or 3. Type 2 (watch and wait): Zone I, stage 1 or 2 without plus disease; Zone II, stage 3 without plus disease.

170. Correct: Punctate inner choroidopathy (PIC) (D)

PIC is a bilateral idiopathic inflammatory disorder of the choroid which is known to affect young myopic females. Vitritis is not considered part of this disease entity (**D**). APMPPE is a bilateral inflammatory chorioretinopathy known to affect both men and women equally. Mild vitreal inflammation is noted in 50% of cases (**A**). Serpiginous choroiditis is a rare inflammatory entity that accounts for less than 5% of posterior uveitis. It has a higher prevalence in men and affects young- to middle-aged adults. Mild vitritis is seen in 30% of active cases (**B**). MEWDS is an inflammatory posterior uveitis which primarily affects people between the ages of 20 and 45 years. The syndrome has a greater predilection for females than males and usually presents unilaterally and with mild vitritis (**C**).

171. Correct: Multiple evanescent white dot syndrome (MEWDS) (B)

MEWDS is an inflammatory posterior uveitis which primarily affects people between the ages of 20 and 45 years. The syndrome has a greater predilection for females than males, and presents usually unilaterally and with mild vitritis (although it can rarely can be bilateral). AZOOR is an inflammatory posterior uveitis characterized by rapid loss of one or more large zones of outer retinal function, minimal fundus changes, electroretinographic abnormalities, and permanent visual field loss that is associated with delayed development of visible atrophic changes in the pigment epithelium. The majority of patients progress to bilateral involvement with long-term follow-up (**A**). APMPPE is a bilateral inflammatory chorioretinopathy known to affect both men and women equally. Mild vitreal inflammation is noted in 50% of cases (**C**). PIC is a bilateral idiopathic inflammatory disorder of the choroid which typically affects young myopic females (**D**).

172. Correct: Observation (A)

APMPPE is a bilateral inflammatory chorioretinopathy. It presents with yellow, creamy, placoid lesions in the macula at the level of the retinal pigment epithelium. Recovery is usually spontaneous within 1 to 2 weeks. Visual acuity usually takes weeks to recover with an overall good long-term prognosis. There is no evidence that corticosteroids or any other treatment modality is beneficial (**B, C, and D**).

173. Correct: Combination immunosuppressives and steroids (C)

Serpiginous choroiditis is a rare inflammatory entity that accounts for less than 5% of posterior uveitis. It shows a higher prevalence in men and affects young- to middle-aged adults. Mild vitritis is seen in 30% of active cases. Treatment with systemic steroids (**A**) or acyclovir (**B**) has been attempted but the results are generally poor. Combination immunosuppressives (including mycophenolate, cyclosporine, azathioprine) with prednisone appear to halt disease activity (**C**) in patients and should be initiated immediately after the diagnosis is suspected.

174. Correct: Multifocal choroiditis (MFC) (C)

In cases of MFC, almost 20% of patients suffer from subfoveal CNV; this complication is the leading cause of vision loss in that subpopulation. Subretinal CNV can be seen in cases secondary to inflammatory choroiditis. It has been reported to occur in 30% of eyes with PIC at areas of previous scars (A). CNV is not commonly associated with MEWDS or AZOOR (**B and D**).

175. Correct: Recurrent aphthous ulcers, genital ulcers, and iritis with hypopyon (A)

This patient likely has Behcet's disease. Behcet's disease is a chronic recurrent systemic inflammatory disease, and consists of a triad of recurrent aphthous oral ulcers, genital ulcers, and acute iritis with hypopyon.

The combination of arteritis, retinal necrosis, and vitritis is usually consistent with a diagnosis of acute retinal necrosis which is usually related to a virus from the herpes family (**B**). The triad of arthritis, conjunctivitis, and urethritis usually describes reactive arthritis ("Reiter's syndrome"). The syndrome most frequently follows genitourinary infection with *Chlamydia trachomatis*, but other organisms have also been implicated (**C**). The triad of epiphora, photophobia, and blepharospasm is usually related to a diagnosis of congenital glaucoma (**D**).

176. Correct: HLA-B5101 (D)

Behcet's disease is a chronic recurrent systemic inflammatory disease, and consists of a triad of recurrent aphthous oral ulcers, genital ulcers and acute iritis with hypopyon. The HLA type associated with Behcet's disease is HLA-B5101 (**D**). HLA-B27 associated uveitis is a distinct entity characterized by a male predominance and frequent association with seronegative arthritic syndromes, such as ankylosing spondylitis, reactive arthritis, psoriatic arthritis, and inflammatory bowel disease (**A**). HLA-A29 is associated with birdshot choroiditis (**B**). Pars planitis and multiple sclerosis-related uveitis is associated with HLA-DR2 (**C**).

177. Correct: None (D)

Behcet's disease is a chronic recurrent systemic inflammatory disease which consists of a triad of recurrent aphthous oral ulcers, genital ulcers, and acute iritis with hypopyon. Systemic occlusive vasculitis manifestations usually predominate the clinical picture and precede the ocular involvement. HLA-B5101 is associated with Behcet's disease but it is not a diagnostic test (**A**). Behcet's disease has noninfectious etiology, so no role of paracentesis (**B**). KST consists of injecting the Kveim reagent, a particulate suspension prepared from granulomatous splenic tissue of a patient with sarcoidosis, into the skin of a person with suspected sarcoidosis (**C**). No single laboratory test is diagnostic for Behcet's disease (**D**).

178. Correct: Vitreous biopsy (D)

Intraocular lymphoma usually presents as a bilateral iritis, vitritis, retinal vasculitis, and creamy yellow subretinal/retinal pigment epithelium infiltrates. The diagnosis of intraocular lymphoma should always be considered in elderly patients with minimal response to topical and systemic steroids in the setting of chronic bilateral uveitis with negative systemic work-up. A vitreous biopsy through pars plana vitrectomy and cytological examination by an experienced cytopathologist is indicated to rule out intraocular lymphoma. Immunosuppression is usually used as a long-term steroid sparing measure, rather than an escalatory measure in cases of steroid-resistant uveitis (**A**). A combination of immunosuppression and

297

steroids is equally not indicated in similar cases (C). Obtaining an MRI would be beneficial as many cases of intraocular lymphoma would manifest central nervous system findings and may further help in the systemic management of the patient (**B**).

179. Correct: Serpiginous choroiditis (B)

Serpiginous choroiditis is an aggressive inflammatory entity that accounts for less than 5% of posterior uveitis cases. Combination immunosuppressives (e.g., mycophenolate, cyclosporine, azathioprine) with prednisone appear to halt disease activity in patients and should be initiated immediately once the diagnosis is suspected (**B**). APMPPE and MEWDS are both self-limited entities with good long-term visual prognosis (**A, C**). PIC usually affects young myopic females, and in these cases choroidal neovascularization is a common cause of vision loss. Anti-vascular endothelial growth factor therapy is commonly used as a treatment modality with good outcomes (**D**).

180. Correct: Central serous chorioretinopathy (CSR) (A)

Increased choroidal thickness has been associated with a number of clinical conditions including central serous chorioretinopathy (**A**), VKH syndrome (**C**), and sympathetic ophthalmia. Neither exudative nor dry AMD is associated with increased choroidal thickness (**B**). VKH syndrome is a bilateral granulomatous panuveitis associated with extraocular manifestations such as meningismus (malaise, fever, headache, neck stiffness, and abdominal pain) and skin findings (alopecia, poliosis, and vitiligo) (**C**). This patient has features of CSR: fluorescein angiogram shows a smokestack leak, and OCT shows neurosensory macular detachment and thickened choroid (**A**). IPCV is characterized by orange-red elevated lesions, often visible as nodular elevation of retinal pigment epithelium along with neurosensory detachment, and often associated with serous exudation and/or hemorrhage, and these polypoidal lesions are best seen as nodular hyperfluorescence on indocyanine green angiography (**D**).

181. Correct: 50% (C)

Patients with sarcoidosis may have a variety of ocular manifestations including anterior segment findings (e.g., mutton-fat keratic precipitates, iris nodules, and posterior synechiae). In addition, patients can have intermediate uveitis, retinal periphlebitis with the characteristic "candlewax drippings," multifocal choroiditis, and optic nerve swelling. Up to 50% of patients with sarcoidosis have ocular manifestations (**C**).

182. Correct: Rod and cone cells (C)

The electroretinogram (ERG) is a diagnostic test that measures the electrical activity generated by neural and nonneuronal cells in the retina in response to a light stimulus. The a-wave is the initial negative deflection, derived from the cones and rods of the outer photoreceptor layers. The b-wave, which follows the a-wave temporally, is derived from the inner retina, predominantly Muller and ON-bipolar cells (**A**). The c-wave, which follows the b-wave, is derived from the retinal pigment epithelium and photoreceptors (**B**).

183. Correct: All of the above (D)

Manifestations of granulomatous uveitis include: conjunctival granulomas, mutton-fat keratic precipitates, iris nodules, and choroidal granulomas. A limited number of entities present with granulomatous inflammation and include sarcoidosis (**B**), tuberculous infection, syphilis (**C**), VKH syndrome (A) and sympathetic ophthalmia.

184. Correct: Vitrectomy must be offered to patients with vitreomacular adhesion (C)

Vitreomacular adhesion is a benign entity that is clearly visualized in patients using optical coherence tomography. It usually has no deleterious effects on visual acuity (**C**). The management of macular holes was revolutionized with the advent of pars plana vitrectomy. Furthermore, the inclusion of internal limiting membrane peeling increased the closure rates to around 95% (A). In 60 to 80% of cases, patients with epiretinal membranes (macular puckers) improved by two Snellen acuity lines after vitrectomy with membrane peeling (**B**). Stage 1 macular holes resolve spontaneously in 50% of cases and hence surgical intervention is not indicated; rather, observation is the recommended management (**D**).

185. Correct: Vitreous hemorrhage that occurred a week ago (C)

Acute vitreous hemorrhage is generally not an indication for surgical intervention in diabetic retinopathy. New vitreous hemorrhage in the setting of diabetic retinopathy may be closely observed, or may be managed with panretinal photocoagulation and anti-VEGF therapy. Surgical indications in the setting of vitreous hemorrhage include: monocular status, underlying macular-threatening tractional detachment, ghost-cell glaucoma and lack of improvement over a period of weeks to months. Vitrectomy in the setting of diabetic retinopathy is indicated in a number of other situations, including macula-threatening/involving tractional retinal detachment (**A**), diabetic macular edema that does not improve with intravitreal anti-VEGF and steroid therapy if a tractional component is present (**B**), and development of a progressive combined rhegmatogenous-tractional retinal detachment (**D**).

186. Correct: Nocardia–post-intravitreal anti-VEGF injection endophthalmitis (B)

Coagulase-negative staphylococcus and streptococcus are responsible for most cases of post-intravitreal anti-VEGF injection endophthalmitis, not *Nocardia*. As per the endophthalmitis vitrectomy study (EVS), coagulase-negative staphylococcus was the most prevalent organism in cases of post-cataract endophthalmitis (**A**). Similarly, Bacillus cereus is usually found in the setting of post-traumatic endophthalmitis (**C**), whereas *Streptococci* and *Haemophilus* species are found in bleb-associated endophthalmitis (**D**).

187. Correct: Propionibacterium acnes (A)

Delayed-onset endophthalmitis is characterized by chronic low-grade anterior and/or posterior inflammation, mild decrease in vision, and classically thickened lens capsule deposits. The most common organism responsible for this presentation is Propionibacterium acnes (**A**).

188. Correct: All of the above (D)

Suprachoroidal hemorrhage is a devastating intraoperative complication with a guarded prognosis. It is usually related to significant alterations in intraoperative pressure. Classical risk factors include: Advanced age (**A**), glaucoma (**B**), myopia, aphakia (**C**), arteriosclerotic cardiovascular disease, hypertension, choroidal hemangiomas associated with Sturge–Weber syndrome, and intraoperative tachycardia.

Chapter 9

Uveitis

Richard M. France, Stephanie M. Llop Santiago

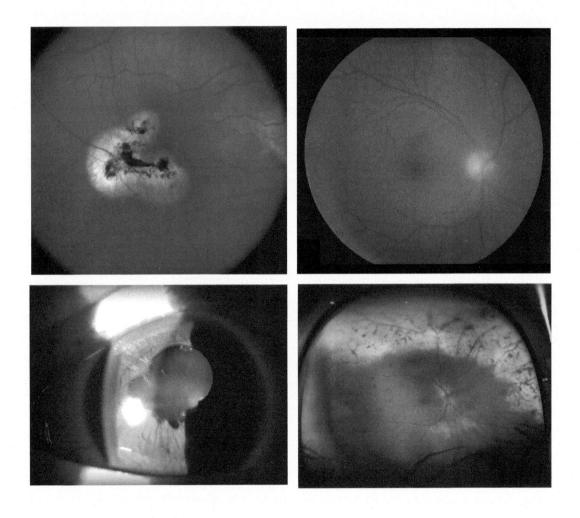

9.1 Questions

Easy | Medium | Hard

Consider the following case for questions 1 and 2:

1. A 32-year-old male patient presents with a 3-day history of pain, photophobia, and decreased vision in the left eye. The patient denies any prior medical history. On slit lamp examination, there is evidence of nongranulomatous keratic precipitates, 3+ cell in the anterior chamber, and moderate-to-severe vitritis in the left eye. Work-up shows a positive rapid plasma reagin (RPR) and fluorescent treponemal antibody absorption test (FTA-ABS). What other test would be imperative to order based on this diagnosis?

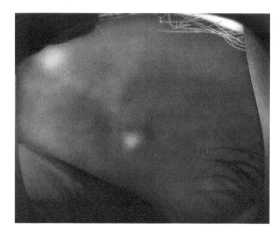

A. Human immunodeficiency virus (HIV) testing

B. Angiotensin-converting enzyme (ACE) and lysozyme

C. Human leukocyte antigen B27 (HLA-B27)

D. Herpes simplex virus (HSV) 1 and 2 and varicella-zoster virus (VZV) titers

2. What is the best treatment recommended for a patient with syphilitic uveitis?

A. Intramuscular ceftriaxone for 10 days followed by oral prednisone

B. Aqueous crystalline penicillin G IV for 10 to 14 days with topical corticosteroids

C. Benzathine penicillin G single dose and topical corticosteroids

D. Benzathine penicillin G daily with probenecid for 10 to 14 days

3. A 27-year-old female patient with history of multiple sclerosis presents to you as a consult for the management of her uveitis. She was diagnosed with intermediate uveitis in both eyes 9 months ago and has been unable to taper oral prednisone below 20 mg without having recurrence of inflammation. When considering immunosuppression therapy, which of the following drugs should be avoided?

A. Mycophenolate mofetil

B. Adalimumab

C. Methotrexate

D. Azathioprine

4. Which of the following has the strongest human leukocyte antigen (HLA) association with ocular disease?

A. HLA-B27 and psoriatic arthritis

B. HLA-B7 and ocular histoplasmosis

C. HLA-B51 and Behcet's disease

D. HLA-A29 and birdshot chorioretinopathy

5. A 26-year-old woman presents for evaluation after coming back from a cruise and reporting vision changes in her right eye for the past 3 days. She describes her vision as blurry with a central area where she sees many dots. Her left eye is asymptomatic. Two weeks prior to the trip, she experienced cold symptoms, including a runny nose. On examination, her vision is 20/50 OD and 20/20 OS. There is no anterior chamber or vitreous cell. On follow-up 2 weeks after the initial examination, the vision improves to 20/30 OD, and fundus examination only shows perifoveal granularity. Optical coherence tomography (OCT) is shown. Given the most likely diagnosis, what would you tell this young patient about the prognosis?

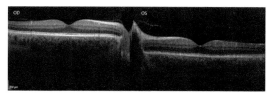

A. Aggressive treatment with steroids and immunomodulatory therapy is mandatory to avoid blindness.

B. The disease is known to cause multiple relapses.

C. The disease course is typically self-limiting, and prognosis is excellent.

D. She should have regular examinations to check for involvement of the other eye, which is common.

6. A 36-year-old myopic woman with a prescription of −3.00 OU presents due to acute vision loss of her left eye and metamorphopsia. On examination, her best corrected visual acuity is 20/200 OD and 20/20 OS. Slit lamp examination is unremarkable OU. Posterior examination shows clear vitreous and multiple deep yellow-white lesions of about 100 to 200 μm in size in both eyes. The right eye also has a grayish perifoveal elevation, confirmed to be a choroidal neovascular membrane on optical coherence tomography (OCT). What is the most common presumed diagnosis?

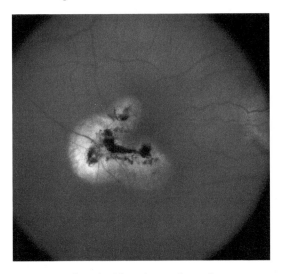

A. Presumed ocular histoplasmosis syndrome
B. Multifocal choroiditis with panuveitis
C. Punctate inner choroidopathy (PIC)
D. Birdshot chorioretinopathy

7. A 16-year-old adolescent girl with a history of juvenile idiopathic arthritis (JIA) comes to have her regular eye examination. She is currently asymptomatic. On slit lamp examination, she has 5 cells/high-power field (hpf) in the anterior chamber of her right eye with faint haze and 26 cells/hpf in her left eye with a hazy view of the iris and lens details. The rest of the anterior and posterior examination is within normal limits. How would you grade the patient's degree of anterior-chamber cell and flare using the Standardization of Uveitis Nomenclature (SUN) criteria?

A. 0.5+ cell and 1+ flare OD/3+ cell and 3+ flare OS
B. 0.5+ cell and 0.5+ flare OD/3+ cell and 3+ flare OS
C. 1+ cell and 1+ flare OD/2+ cell and 2+ flare OS
D. 1+ cell and 1+ flare OD/3+ cell and 2+ flare OS

8. A 25-year-old woman is diagnosed with chronic anterior uveitis OU and has been unable to taper off topical steroids, so immunosuppression therapy is recommended to control her disease. After discussing risks versus benefits of the possible therapies, methotrexate (MTX) is decided to be adequate as a first-line treatment. When she is about to leave the room, the patient asks you if she is going to be able to have kids in the future. Which of the following is the best way to approach this question?

A. Tell the patient she needs to avoid sexual intercourse for the duration of the treatment since there's always a risk of pregnancy.
B. Educate the patient about the risk of pregnancy while on immunomodulatory therapy (IMT) and consult your OB/GYN colleague to further discuss contraception options.
C. Start the treatment and tell the patient that her concerns will be discussed at the next visit.
D. Tell the patient that IMT needs to be started to avoid vision loss and complications associated with topical steroids and that it may permanently affect her ability to conceive in the future.

9. A 76-year-old male patient, who had uncomplicated cataract surgery 1 year ago in his right eye and 3 months ago in his left eye, presents due to chronic inflammation in his left eye that worsened after a YAG capsulotomy done 1 month postoperatively. Inflammation improves with topical steroids but recurs every time he tries to discontinue them. On examination, his best-corrected visual acuity is 20/20 OD and 20/40 OS; he has granulomatous inflammation OS with anterior chamber and vitreous cell. No hypopyon is identified. Posterior examination shows a slightly hazy view of the retina but no focal areas of retinitis. Examination of the right eye is within normal limits. What is the next best step in the management of this patient?

A. Increase the dose of topical steroids to every 1 hour, and follow up in 1 week.
B. Pars plana vitrectomy (PPV) with injection of intravitreal antibiotics.
C. Intraocular lens (IOL) explantation with complete capsulectomy and intravitreal vancomycin.
D. Obtain aerobic, anaerobic, and fungal cultures, Gram and Giemsa stain, and inject intravitreal antibiotics.

10. A 71-year-old female pseudophakic patient with a past medical history of hypertension reports floaters in both eyes for the past 6 months. An initial infectious work-up that included syphilis, tuberculosis (TB), and Lyme testing was negative. She was treated with topical steroids and later periocular steroids, but her inflammation returned once the effect of the injection was gone. She was scheduled for a vitrectomy in her left eye; the vitreous specimen is shown. Based on the findings, which of the following tests would you order next?

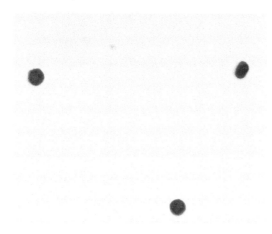

A. Erythrocyte sedimentation rate (ESR) and temporal artery biopsy

B. Complete blood count (CBC) and lymph node biopsy

C. MRI brain/lumbar puncture

D. CT head and orbits

11. A 14-year-old adolescent boy with no prior medical history presents due to decreased vision in his left eye. He denies pain, redness OS, or any symptoms in the right eye. On examination, his vision is 20/25 OD and 20/400 OS. Slit lamp examination is unremarkable OU. There is evidence of an afferent pupillary defect (APD) in the left eye, and fundus examination shows arteriolar narrowing with diffuse retinal pigment epithelium (RPE) degeneration and optic nerve atrophy OS. The right eye is within normal limits. What is the next step in establishing a diagnosis?

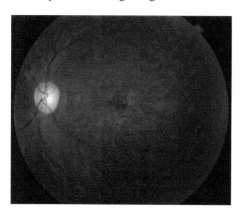

A. Fluorescein angiography and indocyanine green (ICG) angiography

B. Electroretinogram (ERG)

C. Examine the fundus of his siblings and/or parents

D. Genetic testing

12. A 25-year-old male patient with no prior medical or ocular history presented to an ophthalmologist complaining of blurry vision, floaters, pain, and light sensitivity in the left eye. His vision was 20/20 OD and 20/50 OS. He had a normal anterior examination OD, but 3+ cell OS with 2+ flare OS. The patient deferred dilation at the time; he was started on topical steroids every 1-hour OS with an appointment to return in 1 week. When he returns to his follow-up, he reports that his vision has decreased significantly and is now CF OS. On examination, the patient has 2+ cell with 2+ flare OS, and on dilation, there is evidence of dense vitritis with 3+ haze and large areas of retinal necrosis coalescing in the periphery. The patient sees you for a second opinion and asks how it is possible that his vision deteriorated so much if he was evaluated only a week before. How would you best approach this possible diagnostic error with your patient?

A. "Tell the patient that he should sue the previous doctor for failing to diagnose acute retinal necrosis on his first visit."

B. "Start treatment with intravitreal foscarnet, do an a/c tap for viral polymerase chain reaction (PCR), and tell the patient that he needs to forget about the past."

C. "Send him to the prior ophthalmologist to start treatment for possible acute retinal necrosis."

D. "Start treatment right away and explain to the patient that infections in the eye tend to progress quickly and it is possible that the retinal findings were not present on the first visit, although dilation should always be performed in new cases of uveitis."

13. A 43-year-old Hispanic patient with no past medical history presents to the urgent care due to sudden-onset pain, redness, and light sensitivity in the left eye for 2 days. He also reports blurry vision and floaters. He denies any symptoms in the right eye. Fundus examination and fluorescein angiography OS is demonstrated. Which of the following is false based on the most likely diagnosis?

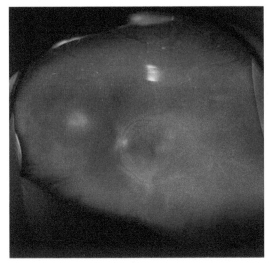

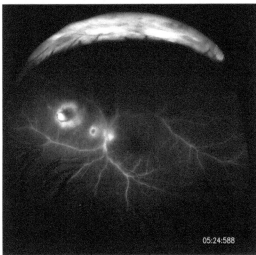

A. It is the most common cause of infectious posterior uveitis.

B. Neuroimaging is warranted for all patients with bilateral disease.

C. It usually reactivates adjacent to a previous scar, but there could be multiple lesions or bilateral involvement.

D. Segmental arterial plaques, known as Kyrieleis' arteriolitis, could be seen.

14. What is the mechanism of action of nonsteroidal anti-inflammatory drugs (NSAIDs)?

A. Inhibition of phospholipase A2

B. Inhibition of inosine monophosphate dehydrogenase

C. Inhibition of cyclooxygenase (COX-1 and -2) resulting in reduced synthesis of prostaglandins

D. Inhibition of neutrophil migration and T-lymphocyte activation

15. Juvenile idiopathic arthritis (JIA)-associated uveitis is most common in which of the following?

A. Early-onset pauciarticular disease

B. Late-onset pauciarticular disease

C. Still's disease

D. Early-onset polyarticular disease

16. Which medication has been associated with a sterile hypopyon anterior uveitis?

A. Indinavir

B. Cidofovir

C. Pentamidine

D. Entecavir

17. A 48-year-old male patient presents for evaluation due to pain, tenderness, and marked redness in both eyes for the past 2 weeks. He also has had recent breathing problems and has been diagnosed with an atypical reactive airway disease. On examination, there are signs of scleritis in both eyes. Laboratory evaluation shows negative antinuclear antibody (ANA), anti–double-stranded DNA (anti-dsDNA) and perinuclear antineutrophil cytoplasmic antibody (p-ANCA) studies but positive cytoplasmic ANCA (c-ANCA). What is the pathophysiology of the suspected diagnosis?

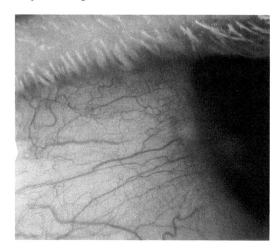

A. Necrotizing granulomatous vasculitis of the upper and lower respiratory tract and of small arteries and veins

B. Arterial occlusive disease with no venous involvement

C. Formation of noncaseating granulomas with Langerhans' multinucleated cells

D. Immune complex deposition in the basement membrane

18. A 32-year-old male patient with history of recurrent anterior uveitis OS presents for evaluation due to a possible new flare-up. His past medical history is positive for ankylosing spondylitis. On examination, his vision is 20/20 and 20/50 with normal intraocular pressure. Slit lamp examination is unremarkable OD but demonstrates 4+ cell with 4+ flare OS with early posterior synechiae. With regard to the most likely diagnosis, what other area may be inflamed apart from the eye and lumbosacral spine?

A. Heart

B. Brain

C. Kidneys

D. Liver

19. A 35-year-old man with no prior medical history developed a diarrheal illness 2 weeks ago. He went to urgent care because he is also having pain in his knees and is having discomfort with urination. From urgent care he was referred to you because his eyes are red and irritated. Which one of the following concerning the most likely diagnosis is false?

A. Almost 90% of cases are in men.

B. It may follow a bout of urethritis.

C. Skin lesions may be present.

D. The most common finding is anterior uveitis.

20. A 45-year-old woman from Mississippi presents for her initial evaluation after noticing that her vision is not as good in her left eye. She has never been diagnosed with any medical or ocular conditions. On examination, her vision is 20/20 and 20/80 and on Amsler's grid, she notices a central distortion in her left eye. Slit lamp examination shows a quiet anterior-chamber OU with clear vitreous. Fundus examination shows bilateral peripapillary atrophy and multiple small, white, atrophic chorioretinal scars in both eyes. Her left eye also has a macular scar with an adjacent area of subretinal discoloration. Which of the following concerning the presumed diagnosis is true?

A. Maculopathy generally precedes the formation of punched-out lesions.

B. The vitritis associated with the condition may decrease vision.

C. Fundus lesions in their acute phase represent a retinitis with a secondary choroidal reaction.

D. A patient with a macular histoplasmosis spot has about one-in-four chance of active maculopathy over the next 3 years.

21. Potential adverse effects of the pharmacologic management of toxoplasmosis include all of the following except which one?

A. Pseudomembranous colitis

B. Stevens–Johnson syndrome

C. Microcystic anemia

D. Aggravation of diabetes mellitus

22. A 38-year-old male patient presents due to pain, redness, and decreased vision in the right eye for 2 days. He denies any prior medical history. Review of systems is remarkable for occasional oral ulcers in the gums and tongue. He also had a genital ulcer once. His vision is 20/400 OD and 20/20 OS. On slit lamp examination, there is a 1.5-mm hypopyon with 4+ anterior-chamber cell and posterior synechiae. The fluorescein angiography OD is shown. Based on the most likely diagnosis, which of the following is true?

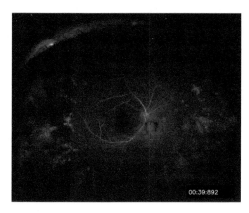

A. Ocular disease is bilateral in only 30% of cases.

B. Steroids are always required and are generally used as long-term therapy.

C. The pathophysiology is a nongranulomatous necrotizing obliterative vasculitis.

D. There are no cardiovascular risks associated with the presumed diagnosis.

23. A 23-year-old African American male patient presents to urgent care complaining of pain, redness, light sensitivity, and blurry vision in both eyes. He has no prior medical history or history of trauma. Review of systems is positive for tinnitus and headaches. His vision was 20/40 OU but distorted. Slit lamp examination shows 3+ cell and 2+ flare in the anterior chamber with early posterior synechiae formation. Fundus examination shows vitritis and multiple areas of retinal elevation with serous retinal detachments. What is the typical fluorescein angiography pattern seen in the most likely diagnosis?

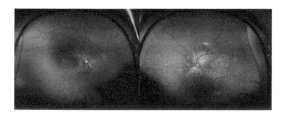

A. A smoke stack of leakage into subretinal space

B. Multiple pinpoint areas of fluorescein into the subretinal space

C. Diffuse retinal venous staining and leakage

D. Well-defined lacy hyperfluorescence with late leakage

24. Early findings in Vogt-Koyanagi-Harada (VKH) syndrome include all the following except which one?

A. Serous retinal detachments

B. Tinnitus

C. Granulomatous anterior segment inflammation

D. Vitiligo

25. A 55-year-old female patient with sympathetic ophthalmia was treated with high-dose oral prednisone and had resolution of her serous retinal detachments. The dose has been gradually decreased, and 4 months into therapy, she is on prednisone 20 mg daily without major side effects. She is on topical prednisolone acetate 1% four times a day and her visual acuity is 20/30 OD and HM OS. There are 2+ cells in the anterior chamber of both eyes with no vitritis, cystoid macular edema, or subretinal fluid. What is the most appropriate next step?

A. Start steroid-sparing immunotherapy.

B. Increase prednisone to 40 mg followed by slower taper.

C. Periocular injections of triamcinolone.

D. Increase topical steroids to every 2 hours and continue to taper oral prednisone.

26. A 22-year-old man from New York presents with redness, pain, and photophobia in both eyes. He also notices floaters and blurry vision. On review of systems (ROS), he denies any previous illness, sick contacts, tick bites, or travel abroad. He did go on a hiking trip a few weeks ago. He mentioned that he had a rash in his thigh but it disappeared. On examination, he has evidence of anterior and intermediate uveitis with no retinal involvement. Which of the following is true regarding the most likely diagnosis and uveitis?

A. The recommended treatment for this type of uveitis with severe posterior segment manifestations requires intravenous antibiotic therapy.

B. Laboratory criteria for the diagnosis of the underlying pathology only consists of the isolation of *borrelia Burgdorferi*.

C. Ocular involvement has not been reported in stage 1 manifestations.

D. It is transmitted to humans through the bite of infected *Ixodes burgdorferi*.

27. A 36-year-old female patient is referred from optometry due to her fundus findings. Patient reports minimal pain and redness in the right eye for the last 2 weeks. On initial evaluation, her vision is 20/20 OU and her fundus examination is seen in the figure. What would you expect to see in this patient's fluorescein angiography?

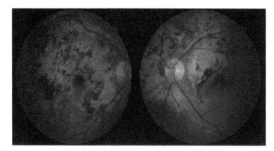

A. Early hyperfluorescence with late leakage of the lesions

B. Early hypofluorescence due to blockage of choroidal staining and late staining of the active edge

C. Early hypofluorescence with late staining of acute active lesions

D. Early hyperfluorescence that fades in the late phases

28. A 48-year-old female patient presents for a second opinion due to lack of improvement of her eye redness and severe tenderness that has been present for the past 3 weeks. She has no prior medical history and no known drug allergies. Patient was prescribed loteprednol drops four times a day OU, which the patient admits is using regularly but has not seen any improvement. Which of the following is false regarding the treatment of scleritis?

A. If initial nonsteroidal anti-inflammatory drug (NSAID) fails, a second should be tried before switching to corticosteroids.

B. Systemic corticosteroids remain the mainstay of noninfectious scleritis.

C. Subconjunctival injection of corticosteroids is indicated on severe cases concerning for necrosis.

D. Scleral reinforcement surgery may be needed to avoid globe rupture.

29. A 37-year-old male patient arrives to your office with 1-day history of pain, redness, and photophobia in the left eye. He admits he had a previous episode of "eye inflammation" 10 years ago in the same eye. He denies any past medical history, and review of systems (ROS) is positive for chronic low back pain, but he admits he does a lot of heavy lifting. On examination, there are 4+ cell in the anterior-chamber OS with fibrin and multiple posterior synechiae. What would be the most appropriate test to determine the possible diagnosis based on this patient's history?

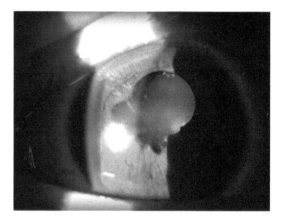

A. Spine CT Scan

B. Anterior-chamber paracentesis

C. Fluorescein angiography and OCT macula

D. Sacroiliac plain X-ray

30. A 21-year-old female patient with no prior medical history goes to the university medical center with history of arthralgia, fever, fatigue, and loss of appetite. Upon questioning, she also admits her eyes have been red and blurry. Upon evaluation by ophthalmology, she has KPs, 2+ anterior chamber cells OU, and posterior synechiae OU. Fundus examination is within normal limits. Laboratory results ordered in the walk-in clinic showed elevated erythrocyte sedimentation rate (ESR), proteinuria, and white cell casts. Which of the following is not part of the criteria for a clinical diagnosis of this syndrome?

A. Associated systemic illness with possible elevated ESR and eosinophilia

B. Abnormal urinalysis with increased B2 microglobulin, proteinuria, and presence of eosinophils, pyuria or hematuria, white cell casts, and glucosuria

C. Abnormal serum creatinine level or decreased creatinine clearance

D. Renal biopsy

31. A 35-year-old woman from the Midwest region of the United States experienced loss of vision in the left eye to a level of 20/400. Examination revealed multiple discrete choroidal scars. The vision subsequently improved to 20/30, but a relapse occurred, and the visual acuity OS declined to count fingers. The funduscopic findings in the left eye are illustrated in the figure . Cells were present in the posterior vitreous. Fluorescein angiography revealed staining of the retinal pigment epithelial (RPE) lesions in the right eye. Which of the following clinical entities is most consistent with this clinical presentation?

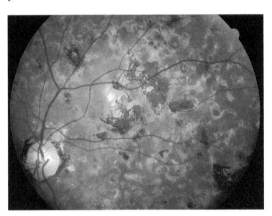

A. Multifocal choroiditis with panuveitis (MCP)

B. Acute posterior multifocal placoid pigment epitheliopathy (APMPPE)

C. Birdshot chorioretinopathy

D. Presumed ocular histoplasmosis (POHS)

32. Which of the following is the most appropriate instruction to a patient beginning oral cyclophosphamide therapy?

A. The patient should take 1 mg of folic acid daily.

B. The patient should get the live influenza vaccine every year.

C. The patient should maintain adequate hydration.

D. The medication should be taken on an empty stomach and should avoid dairy products.

33. Which of the following findings is least likely manifestation of systemic lupus erythematosus (SLE)?

A. Cotton wool spots with intraretinal hemorrhages

B. Scleritis

C. Chronic anterior uveitis

D. Serous retinal detachment

34. A 57-year-old female patient presented to the emergency room with acute vision loss of her right eye with pain and photophobia for the past 3 days. She has past medical history of coronary artery disease (CAD) and hypertension (HTN). No prior ocular history. On examination, she has nongranulomatous keratic precipitates, 3+ anterior chamber cell, and moderate vitritis with retinal examination OD seen in the figure. Right eye examination is unremarkable. Intraocular pressure is 32 mm Hg OD and 16 mm Hg OS. Which of the following is true regarding the most likely diagnosis?

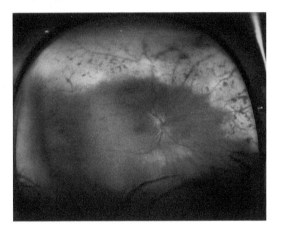

A. The posterior pole is typically involved early in the disease.

B. Polymerase chain reaction (PCR) is the most sensitive, specific, and rapid diagnostic method for detecting the causative organism.

C. Pathophysiology is occlusive vasculopathy of venous system only.

D. The most common causative organism is herpes simplex virus 2 (HSV-2).

35. A 23-year-old college student presents for evaluation due to decreased vision in the right eye with mild redness. She denies any trauma or previous medical conditions, and has not traveled recently, though she did move in with a new roommate and her cat. A review of systems (ROS) is positive for malaise but no fever, joint pain, skin rash, cough, or any other symptoms. On examination, her vision is 20/70 OD and 20/20 OS. Intraocular pressure is 19 mm Hg OD and 17 mm Hg OS. Anterior segment is unremarkable, but a slight afferent pupillary defect (APD) is noticed in the right eye. Fundus examination shows optic nerve head edema OD extending to the macula with a few exudates. Left eye is normal. What is the most common uveitic manifestation of this disease process?

A. Neuroretinitis

B. Focal retinochoroiditis

C. Intermediate uveitis

D. Optic nerve infiltration

36. A 40-year-old Black male patient is referred for evaluation due to possible uveitis. The patient has had fever for the past week, with droopiness of the left side of the face, incomplete blink, and associated redness, pain, and photophobia of both eyes. On review of systems (ROS), he admits having bilateral facial swelling but no cough or breathing problems and no skin rashes. His vision is 20/50 and 20/70 with evidence of mutton-fat keratic precipitates (KP), iris nodules, and 3+ anterior chamber cell. Fundus examination is normal OU. A chest X-ray done showed hilar adenopathy. What is the most likely diagnosis based on this patient's findings?

A. Taches de bougie syndrome

B. Neurosarcoidosis

C. Lofgren's syndrome

D. Heerfordt's syndrome

37. A 53-year-old male patient presents as a consult due to history of multiple episodes of inflammation in his right eye. He tells you that every time he develops pain and redness in his eye, he goes to the local ophthalmologist, and they find anterior-chamber cell and a very high intraocular pressure (IOP). Previous treatment has consisted of topical steroids and IOP-lowering drops. He is always able to taper off the drops and remains quiet without inflammation and normal IOP for months and sometimes years before the next episode develops. What viral organism has been linked to the most likely diagnosis?

A. Cytomegalovirus (CMV)

B. Herpes simplex virus (HSV) 1 and 2

C. Rubella

D. Varicella-zoster virus (VZV)

38. A 28-year-old male patient with no prior medical history was referred for ophthalmology evaluation due to changes in his vision. He describes his vision as "not normal" with "central areas that are distorted." Mild redness and photophobia are noted. On review of systems (ROS) he explains that he is having headaches and feels "like I'm not myself" for 3 weeks. He also had malaise and myalgia. On examination, his vision was 20/60 OU with trace cell in the anterior-chamber OU and 1+ cell vitreous cell. Amsler's grid shows paracentral scotomas. Fundus examination and fluorescein angiography (FA) are seen in the images. Work-up including rapid plasma reagin (RPR), fluorescent treponemal antibody absorption (FTA-ABS), chest X-ray (CXR), and Lyme titers was negative. Which of the patient's symptoms would need further work-up and possibly treatment for this condition?

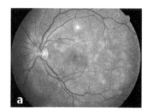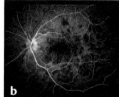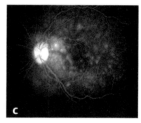

A. Paracentral scotomas

B. History of malaise and myalgia

C. Headaches and "not feeling like myself"

D. Eye redness and photophobia

39. A 38-year-old male patient with history of HIV, CD4 100, and unknown viral load is sent for a screening evaluation. The patient is asymptomatic, though he admits he also has history of Kaposi's sarcoma treated with chemotherapy. No prior ocular history. What is the most common fundus finding expected in this patient?

A. Cytomegalovirus (CMV) retinopathy

B. HIV retinopathy

C. Progressive outer retinal necrosis (PORN)

D. *Cryptococcus* choroiditis

40. Which of the following is not true regarding glaucoma management in uveitis?

A. Most cases of uveitic glaucoma, especially if pseudophakic or aphakic, require aqueous drainage devices.

B. Cyclodestructive procedures may worsen ocular inflammation and could lead to hypotony and phthisis.

C. When medical management with drops is not enough to achieve good intraocular pressure (IOP), a laser trabeculoplasty is a good option before proceeding to surgery.

D. Meticulous control of inflammation using immunomodulatory therapy (IMT) and steroids improves visual acuity outcomes and overall success of glaucoma surgery.

Consider the following case for questions 41 and 42:

41. A 65-year-old female patient with prior medical history of diabetes mellitus (DM) and hypertension (HTN) presents for evaluation due to 3 days history of a painful rash in the right side of her forehead with associated vesicles that extend into the tip of the nose. She also has conjunctival injection and reports her vision is slightly blurry. On examination, her vision is 20/50 OD and 20/20 OS; intraocular pressure (IOP) is 30 and 21 mm Hg. Slit lamp examination shows multiple vesicles in the upper and lower lid, and fluorescein delineates a dendritiform lesion with negative staining. There are fine keratic precipitates (KP) and 1+ cell in the anterior-chamber OD. Left eye is unremarkable. Dilated fundus examination OU shows few microaneurysms and dot blot hemorrhages but no signs of retinitis, neovascularization of the disc (NVD) or neovascularization elsewhere (NVE). Which of the following best explains the pathogenesis of this condition?

A. Cell-mediated immunity and not direct viral infection.

B. The virus remains latent in B lymphocytes and mucosal epithelial cells throughout life spreading through saliva.

C. Live virus spreading from the skin via sensory nerve axons.

D. Endogenous reactivation of latent virus.

42. What is the recommended treatment for this patient?

A. Oral valacyclovir 1 g three times a day × 7 to 10 days

B. Oral acyclovir 400 mg five times a day for 7 to 10 days

C. Oral famciclovir 250 mg three times a day for 7 to 10 days

D. Topical trifluridine every 3 hours for 14 days

43. A 75-year-old female patient with history of cataracts OU presents due to redness, pain, and light sensitivity in her left eye that started after trauma 3 days prior to presentation under unclear circumstances. Her vision is 20/100 OD and counting fingers (CF) OS. On slit lamp examination, right eye was only remarkable for a 3+ nuclear sclerotic (NS) cataract. Left eye has evidence of ciliary flush, corneal edema, with a self-sealed 1-mm corneal laceration, multiple keratic precipitates (KP), 3+ cell and flare, posterior synechiae, and an intumescent cataract with a small violation of the anterior capsule. No posterior view but B scan showed an attached retina with clear vitreous. What histologic finding would you expect to see in this patient?

A. Engorged macrophages and lens protein clogging the trabecular meshwork

B. Neutrophils around the lens material with surrounding lymphocytes, plasma cells, epithelioid cells, and occasional giant cells forming a zonal granuloma

C. Presence of immunoglobulin E (IgE), mast cells, and basophils in the anterior chamber

D. Refractile bodies in the aqueous representing lipid-laden macrophages

44. A 50-year-old male patient with long-standing blindness in his right eye due to trauma presents with vision loss in his left eye. Patient's last eye examination was a year ago with visual acuity of no light perception OD and 20/30 OS. On current presentation, his vision decreased to 20/100 OS and slit lamp examination of the left eye shows 2+ cell with 1+ flare, keratic precipitates (KP), 2+ vitreous cell with 1+ haze, and a serous retinal detachment OS. Which of the following is true regarding the histopathologic features of the suspected diagnosis?

A. Diffuse necrotizing infiltration of the choroid with predominance of neutrophils.

B. Nodular clusters of epithelioid cells containing pigment, located in the retina.

C. Dalen–Fuchs nodules are pathognomonic of sympathetic ophthalmia (SO).

D. Absence of inflammatory involvement of the choriocapillaris and retina.

45. A 30-year-old male from India presents for evaluation of vision loss and floaters in the left eye for 3 days. He has no prior medical history but recalls having previous episodes of vision loss and floaters in the same eye. On examination, there is evidence of a vitreous hemorrhage with no evidence of retinal breaks. When you obtain previous records, there is evidence of multiple episodes of retinal and vitreous hemorrhage with a fluorescein angiography that shows periphlebitis in the periphery and vasculitis with neovascularization. What should be included in this patient's work-up of vasculitis with recurrent hemorrhages?

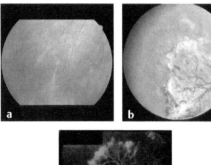
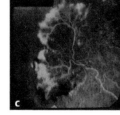

A. Herpes simplex virus (HSV) 1 and 2 titers

B. Toxoplasma gondii IgM titers

C. Interferon gamma release assay

D. Erythrocyte sedimentation rate (ESR) and C-reactive protein (CRP)

46. A 51-year-old female patient presents for evaluation as a second opinion due to blurry vision in her right eye for the past 3 years. She also mentions that people tell her that the color of her eyes is different. She denies any prior ocular history including any trauma. On examination, best-corrected vision is 20/50 OD and 20/25 OS, and there is evidence of diffuse stellate keratic precipitates (KP) over the entire endothelium with 2+ anterior chamber cell and few cells in the anterior vitreous. No synechiae but there is diffuse stromal atrophy. She also has evidence of a visually significant cataract OD. Posterior examination is unremarkable. The patient is interested in cataract surgery. What would you tell this patient in this regard?

A. Cataract surgery can be performed, but there is an increased risk of postoperative hyphema.

B. Aggressive treatment with topical corticosteroids is necessary to control inflammation before cataract surgery.

C. Cataract surgery is indicated but an intraocular lens cannot be implanted at the time of surgery.

D. Prophylaxis with oral valganciclovir is recommended prior to surgery.

47. A 17-year-old adolescent girl complains of blurred vision and floaters which have increased over several months. Her visual acuity last year was 20/20 OU, but now is 20/60 OD, 20/50 OS. Examination shows bilateral anterior-chamber cells, a mild peripheral cortical cataract, 1+ vitreous cells and 1+ haze, a few snowball vitreous opacities, and small snowbanks at the ora serrata OU. What is the most likely cause of her decreased vision?

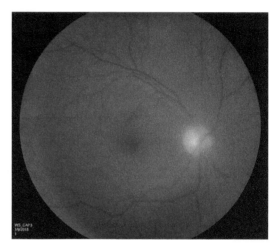

A. Vitritis

B. Cystoid macular edema (CME)

C. Cortical cataracts

D. Peripheral retinal vasculitis

48. An 8-year-old girl with history of juvenile idiopathic arthritis (JIA) presents for evaluation of a corneal scar. The mother reports her daughter has a white mark in her right eye that has been noticed on previous examinations but never addressed. On examination, her best-corrected visual acuity (BCVA) is 20/100 and 20/25. Corneal examination shows a band-shaped, horizontal, gray-white subepithelial corneal opacity, more evident in the interpalpebral fissure involving the visual axis OD. In the left eye, there are similar findings at 3 and 9 o'clock not involving the visual axis. She has trace cell OU, and there is also evidence of cataracts. What is the recommended treatment for her corneal pathology?

A. Bandage contact lenses

B. Alcohol epithelial debridement

C. Phototherapeutic keratectomy (PTK)

D. Manual superficial keratectomy with sodium ethylenediaminetetraacetic acid (EDTA)

cultures of the aqueous or undiluted vitreous and sending for Gram/Giemsa staining, immediately followed by injection of intravitreal antibiotics. (**B**) PPV and injection of antibiotics is therapeutic in some patients, but with this patient's relatively good vision would not be preferred without a confirmed diagnosis. (**C**) Some patients might need to undergo capsulectomy and IOL explantation despite treatment with PPV and antibiotics, but it would not be the next best step in this case. (**A**) Topical steroids can be increased to control inflammation, but this does not bypass the need for cultures.

10. Correct: MRI brain/lumbar puncture (C)

Any patient with chronic vitreous inflammation that does not respond to treatment as expected warrants additional investigation. Primary central nervous system lymphomas (PCNSLs) mainly affect patients in the fifth to seventh decade of life with 25% developing ocular involvement; in 15% of patients, ocular involvement is the only manifestation. MRI studies show isointense lesions on T1 and isointense to hyperintense lesions on T2. Cerebrospinal fluid analysis shows lymphoma cells in one-third of patients. (**A**) ESR and temporal artery biopsy are recommended in cases of suspected giant cell arteritis (GCA), (**B**) CBC and lymph node biopsy would be part of the work-up for systemic lymphoma, and (**D**) CT of the head might show periventricular lesions in PCNSL, but orbital CT is not indicated.

11. Correct: Electroretinogram (ERG) (B)

Diffuse unilateral subacute neuroretinitis (DUSN) in an uncommon disease caused by a nematode infection that should always be in the differential diagnosis of young, otherwise healthy patients with posterior uveitis, since early recognition could prevent permanent vision loss. It is characterized by the insidious onset of unilateral vision loss, and early stages are characterized by moderate to severe vitritis, optic disc swelling, and multiple focal lesions in the postequatorial fundus that vary in size (1200–1500 μm). A serous retinal detachment (RD) may be seen. The later stages are typified by arteriolar narrowing, optic atrophy, and diffuse RPE degeneration. Electroretinographic testing is important since abnormalities can be evident even when it is performed early in the disease. (**A**) Fluorescein angiography (FA) and ICG can be performed, but findings are typically nonspecific and does not contribute as much as an ERG to the diagnosis. (**C**) This condition is infectious, unilateral, and not hereditary, so examining the fundus of close relatives would not be as important nor (**D**) genetic testing indicated.

12. Correct: "Start treatment right away and explain to the patient that infections in the eye tend to progress quickly and it is possible that the retinal findings were not present on the first visit, although dilation should always be performed in new cases of uveitis" (D)

Patients should always make informed decisions about their care, and this includes understanding the potential benefits or risks for the treatments or procedures proposed. On his first visit he deferred dilation, perhaps because he didn't understand the importance of the dilated examination in his condition. It is important to always communicate information to the patient, including potential errors that might have occurred, to maintain a trustworthy patient–physician relationship. (**A**) Recommending legal action against a colleague would be unprofessional; communicating with the previous physician as colleague will allow him or her to be aware of the new diagnosis. (**B**) Starting treatment right away is of utmost importance in this rapidly progressive disease, but ignoring the patient's concerns is never recommended. (**C**) Delaying treatment in this condition could potentially result in blindness.

13. Correct: Neuroimaging is warranted for all patients with bilateral disease (B)

Toxoplasma chorioretinitis is (**A**) the most common cause of infectious posterior uveitis caused by the parasite *Toxoplasma gondii*. Human infection may be congenital or acquired, and presenting symptoms frequently include unilateral pain, floaters, and hazy vision. The classic presentation is a focal white retinitis with overlying vitritis ("headlight in the fog") (**C**), often near a previous scar. (**D**) Retinal vessels may show perivasculitis with segmental arterial plaques known as Kyrieleis' arteriolitis. Neuroimaging is warranted only for immunocompromised patients with HIV/AIDS given the frequent association of ocular disease and cerebral involvement in these patients (up to 56%).

14. Correct: Inhibits cyclooxygenase (COX-1 and -2) resulting in reduced synthesis of prostaglandins (C)

NSAIDs work by inhibiting COX-1 and -2, reducing the synthesis of prostaglandins that mediate inflammation. COX-1 is present in almost all cells and COX-2 seems to be related to inflammation. Specific COX-2 inhibitors were developed, but some had to be removed from the market due to severe cardiovascular events. (**A**) One of the mechanisms by which corticosteroids decrease inflammation is believed to be through inhibition of phospholipase A2. (**B**) Mycophenolate mofetil is an antimetabolite that works by inhibiting inosine monophosphate dehydrogenase. (**D**) Cyclosporine and tacrolimus are calcineurin inhibitors that eliminate T-cell receptor signal transduction and downregulate interleukin-2.

15. Correct: Early-onset pauciarticular disease (A)

JIA is usually classified based on presenting factors, including the number of joints involved. The majority (80–90%) of patients with JIA that have uveitis have pauciarticular onset (four or fewer joints). This group is further subdivided into girls that develop the disease before age 5 and are antinuclear antibody (ANA) positive, and older boys (75% are human leukocyte antigen B27 [HLA-B27] positive) in whom the uveitis tends to be acute and recurrent rather than chronic. (**B**) Early onset has a higher risk than late-onset pauciarticular disease. (**C**) Still's disease, or systemic onset, rarely is associated with uveitis and (**D**) patients with polyarticular onset only present with uveitis in about 10% of cases.

16. Correct: Cidofovir (B)

Multiple systemic and topical medications have been associated with uveitis. These include rifabutin, bisphosphonates, sulfonamides, diethylcarbamazine, metipranolol, and anticholinesterase inhibitors, among others. One that could incite uveitis development with the presence of a hypopyon is cidofovir, a cytosine analogue effective against cytomegalovirus (CMV). Treatment is with aggressive topical steroids and cycloplegics; stopping the medication is not necessarily required unless hypotony develops. (**A**) Indinavir and (**D**) entecavir are antiretroviral medications that have not been particularly associated with uveitis nor is (**C**) pentamidine, an antimicrobial used for the treatment and prevention of Pneumocystis pneumonia.

17. Correct: Necrotizing granulomatous vasculitis of the upper and lower respiratory tract and of small arteries and veins (A)

Granulomatosis with polyangiitis (formerly known as Wegener's granulomatosis) is a multisystem autoimmune disorder characterized by necrotizing granulomatous vasculitis of the upper and lower respiratory tract and of small arteries and veins with associated focal segmental glomerulonephritis. Involvement of the sinuses is a very characteristic feature, followed by pulmonary and renal disease. Ocular involvement is seen in up to 50% of patient throughout the course of the disease (orbital involvement, scleritis, rarely uveitis). Diagnosis is confirmed with tissue biopsy. Patients have to be treated with steroids and immunomodulatory therapy (IMT), since without therapy, mortality can be up to 90% in 1 year. (**B**) Involvement is of both arteries and veins. (**C**) Sarcoidosis is characterized by formation of noncaseating granulomas with Langerhans' multinucleated cells. (**D**) Immune complex deposition in the basement membrane of the kidney tubules is seen in tubulointerstitial injury in lupus nephritis.

18. Correct: Heart (A)

About 5% of patients with human leukocyte antigen B27 (HLA-B27) spondyloarthropathies could have aortitis with aortic insufficiency. Other associations include arthritis, colitis, and rarely lung involvement (pulmonary apical fibrosis). When ocular involvement develops, it is typically acute, recurrent episodes of anterior uveitis. The mainstay of treatment is nonsteroidal anti-inflammatory drugs (NSAIDs). (**B**) No brain, (**C**) kidney, or (**D**) liver disease is particularly associated with the presence of HLA-B27.

19. Correct: The most common finding is anterior uveitis (D)

Reactive arthritis consists of the classic triad of urethritis, polyarthritis, and conjunctivitis. Conjunctivitis is the most common eye manifestation. Nongranulomatous iritis may occur in up to 10% of patients. Human leukocyte antigen B27 (HLA-B27) is found in up to 95% of patients and occurs most frequently in men (**A**). Although the typical presentation is associated with urethritis (**B**), it can also follow an episode of diarrhea or dysentery. Two other skin conditions (**C**) that are considered major criteria are keratoderma blenorrhagicum (affecting the palms and soles) and circinate balanitis.

20. Correct: A patient with a macular histoplasmosis spot has about one-in-four chance of active maculopathy over the next 3 years (D)

Ocular histoplasmosis syndrome is a multifocal choroiditis believed to be caused by infection with *Histoplasma capsulatum*, usually found in endemic areas of the United States (Ohio and Mississippi River valleys). There is a classic triad of findings: multiple white, atrophic choroidal scars, peripapillary pigmentation, and maculopathy, in the absence of vitreous cells (**B**). The pathogenesis is thought to involve initial infection causing choroiditis that subsides and leaves atrophic scars (**C**). This may result in the disruption of the Bruch membrane with subsequent proliferation of subretinal vessels, so maculopathy follows the formation of histoplasmosis spots (**A**).

21. Correct: Microcystic anemia (C)

None of the treatments for toxoplasmosis is characterized by causing microcystic anemia. Clindamycin has been effective in managing acute lesions, but the development of pseudomembranous colitis is a possible complication (**A**). The classic regimen includes the use of sulfadiazine, and sulfa drugs can cause Stevens–Johnson syndrome (**B**). The use of prednisone as part of the treatment may aggravate diabetes in patients at risk (**D**).

22. Correct: The pathophysiology is a non-granulomatous necrotizing obliterative vasculitis (C)

Behcet's disease is a chronic, relapsing, occlusive systemic vasculitis of unknown etiology. Ocular manifestations occur in up to 70% of patients and are characterized by nongranulomatous necrotizing obliterative vasculitis that can affect one or multiple areas of the uveal tract. Ocular manifestations appear to be more severe in men, and up to 80% of cases are bilateral (**A**). Oral aphthae are the most frequent finding in Behcet's disease, but cardiac involvement can include endocarditis, myocarditis, endomyocardial fibrosis, coronary arteritis, and pericarditis, seen in up to 17% of patients (**D**). Treatment with steroids is extremely useful to control the explosive acute phase of the disease, but given the side effect profile and the frequency of patients becoming steroid-resistant, almost all cases require long-term immunomodulatory therapy (IMT) (**B**).

23. Correct: Multiple pinpoint areas of fluorescein into the subretinal space (B)

Vogt-Koyanagi-Harada syndrome is characterized by chronic, bilateral, diffuse, granulomatous panuveitis. There are four stages: prodromal, acute uveitic, convalescent, and chronic recurrent. During the acute phase, fluorescein angiography (FA) typically reveals numerous punctate hyperfluorescent foci at the level of the retinal pigment epithelium (RPE), followed by pooling of the fluid. A smoke stack of leakage is typically seen in central serous chorioretinopathy (**A**). Diffuse retinal venous staining and leakage is a nonspecific description that can be seen when there is retinal vasculitis (**C**). Finally, well-defined lacy hyperfluorescence with late leakage can be seen in multiple evanescent white dot syndrome (MEWDS) (**D**).

24. Correct: Vitiligo (D)

The prodromal stage of VKH is marked by flu-like symptoms, and patients may present with headaches, tinnitus (**B**), nausea, and fever, among other symptoms. During the acute uveitic phase, diffuse, granulomatous anterior uveitis is present (**C**), with a variable degree of vitritis, disc hyperemia and swelling, and multiple serous retinal detachments (**A**). The convalescent stage occurs weeks later and some of the integumentary changes include vitiligo, poliosis, and alopecia. The chronic recurrent phase is characterized by repeated bouts of granulomatous anterior uveitis.

25. Correct: Start steroid-sparing immunotherapy (A)

This patient with sympathetic ophthalmia has active disease despite the high dose of oral prednisone (20 mg). This is an indication to start immunosuppressive therapy. Increasing topical steroids is appropriate to control anterior-chamber inflammation, but further tapering of oral prednisone will put this patient at risk for worsening inflammation resulting in loss of vision due to chronic inflammation with frequent exacerbations that characterize this disease (**D**). Increasing prednisone to 40 mg can be done to control inflammation in the short term, but this must be followed by immunosuppressive therapy to achieve the goal of tapering the prednisone to 7.5 mg or less and avoiding the multiple side effects seen with long-term prednisone therapy (**B**). A periocular injection of triamcinolone might be considered in special circumstances in which systemic treatment is contraindicated for cystoid macular edema, but this patient has been on oral prednisone for 4 months without major side effects, so she should be a good candidate for immunomodulatory therapy (**C**).

26. Correct: The recommended treatment for this type of uveitis with severe posterior segment manifestations requires intravenous antibiotic therapy (A)

The treatment recommendations for Lyme disease vary depending on the clinical manifestation. Like syphilitic uveitis, intraocular inflammation in Lyme disease is treated as a central nervous system (CNS) manifestation and warrants neurologic evaluation, including lumbar puncture. If there are severe posterior segment manifestations or confirmed CNS involvement, the treatment should be intravenous as well as for patients with mild disease who relapse when oral antibiotics are discontinued. After starting the appropriate antibiotic regimen, topical steroids/cycloplegics may be started to treat anterior uveitis. The Centers for Disease Control and Prevention (CDC) recommends a two-step protocol for the diagnosis of Lyme disease: IgM and IgG by enzyme-linked immunosorbent assay (ELISA) followed by western blot testing. Polymerase chain reaction (PCR)-based assays have been used successfully but (**B**) are not the only laboratory criteria. (**C**) Ocular involvement has been seen in all stages, and the most common ocular finding of early stage 1 is follicular conjunctivitis. (**D**) Lyme disease is the most common tick-borne illness in the United States caused by the spirochete *Borrelia burgdorferi* transmitted by the tick *Ixodes scapularis* in the northeast and mid-Atlantic and *Ixodes pacificus* in the western United States.

27. Correct: Early hypofluorescence due to blockage of choroidal staining and late staining of the active edge (B)

Serpiginous choroiditis is an uncommon, chronic, progressive inflammatory condition of unknown etiology that usually presents with paracentral scotomata and decreased vision. Classically, fundus examination shows gray-white lesions at the level of the retinal pigment epithelium (RPE) that extend from the optic nerve in a pseudopodial manner. Disease activity is typically confined to the borders or leading edges of the advancing lesion seen in F/A as late staining. (**A**) Early hyperfluorescence with late leakage indicates the presence of choroidal neovascularization (CNV). (**C**) Early hypofluorescence with late staining of acute active lesions is seen in multifocal choroiditis with panuveitis, whereas atrophic lesions show (**D**) early hyperfluorescence that fades in the late phases (transmission defect).

28. Correct: Subconjunctival injection of corticosteroids is indicated on severe cases concerning for necrosis (C)

Scleritis is typically a painful condition with a risk of permanent structural damage to the eye and the most common form is noninfectious. Subconjunctival injections of corticosteroids may be effective in anterior scleritis of the nonnecrotizing type, but they should be avoided if there is a concern for necrosis because of potential complication of localized necrotizing disease following injection. Treatment of noninfectious scleritis includes the use of NSAIDs (**A**), and a second agent can be tried if the first one fails before switching to corticosteroids that are (**B**) the mainstay of scleritis therapy. (**D**) Scleral reinforcement may be needed if there is thinning and concern for globe rupture that in these cases could be secondary to minor trauma.

29. Correct: Sacroiliac plain X-ray (D)

Ankylosing spondylitis (AS) symptoms include lower back pain and stiffness after inactivity. Up to 90% of patients with AS are HLA-B27 positive and the ophthalmologist may be the first physician to suspect the disease. Sacroiliac imaging studies should be ordered when history is suggestive of AS, and patients should be referred to rheumatologist and instructed about risk of deformity if untreated. Nonsteroidal anti-inflammatory drugs (NSAIDs) are the mainstay of treatment. (**A**) Spine CT scan may be useful in selected patients, but usually plain films are performed first, and MRI has been shown to be superior to CT scanning. (**B**) HLA-B27 should be ordered but angiotensin-converting enzyme (ACE) levels are not necessary. (**C**) Fluorescein angiography and OCT macula wouldn't help to establish the etiology of the uveitis in this young patient with acute, recurrent anterior uveitis.

30. Correct: Renal biopsy (D)

Tubulointerstitial nephritis and uveitis (TINU) occurs predominantly in adolescent girls and women in their early 20s and 30s. Patients typically present with systemic symptoms like fever, anorexia, fatigue, and arthralgia followed by eye symptoms: redness, pain, photophobia, and blurry vision. The definitive diagnosis can only be made with a renal biopsy but is a very invasive procedure, and usually a reliable clinical diagnosis can be made with the following criteria: (**A**) associated systemic illness consisting of fever, weight loss, anorexia, fatigue, myalgia, and arthralgia with possible elevated ESR, eosinophilia, and abnormal liver function tests (LFTs). (**B**) Abnormal urinalysis with increased B_2 microglobulin, proteinuria and presence of eosinophils, pyuria or hematuria, white cell casts and glucosuria, and (**C**) abnormal serum creatinine level or decreased creatinine clearance. TINU syndrome is very responsive to high-dose oral corticosteroids.

31. Correct: Multifocal choroiditis with panuveitis (MCP) (A)

MCP is an idiopathic inflammatory disorder of unknown etiology affecting the choroid, retina, and vitreous. It is most often seen in young myopic females and classic clinical findings include punched-out white-yellow dots in a peripapillary, midperipheral, and anterior equatorial distribution with varying degrees of anterior segment and vitreous inflammation. The presence of vitritis excludes POHS diagnosis or punctate inner choroidopathy (PIC) (**D**). The lesions in MCP are typically smaller than those seen in birdshot (**C**) or APMPPE (**B**) and usually evolve intro atrophic scars. Birdshot lesions do not become pigmented over time.

32. Correct: The patient should maintain adequate hydration (C)

Cyclophosphamide is an alkylating agent whose active metabolites alkylate DNA and RNA purines, resulting in impaired DNA replication. Myelosuppression and hemorrhagic cystitis are the most common side effects, so when administered orally, patients should be instructed to drink more than 2 L of fluid daily. Weekly complete blood count (CBC) and urinalysis (UA) are monitored, and if there is microscopic hematuria, hydration should be increased; any signs of gross hematuria should be a reason to discontinue the medication. When patients are on methotrexate, an inhibitor of dihydrofolate reductase, (**A**) folic acid is given at a dose of 1 mg/d to reduce side effects. (**B**) Patients in immunosuppressive therapy should not get live vaccination including live influenza vaccine and MMR. Finally, (**C**) mycophenolate mofetil is recommended to be taken on an empty stomach.

33. Correct: Chronic anterior uveitis (C)

Ocular manifestations in SLE occur in 50% of patients and lupus retinopathy is the most well-recognized posterior segment manifestation. (A) Cotton wool spots with or without intraretinal are thought to be due to the underlying microangiopathy of the disease. Other manifestations include severe retinal vascular occlusive disease (both arterial and venous), lesions in the eyelids (discoid lupus), secondary Sjogren's syndrome, (B) scleritis, cranial nerve palsies, optic neuropathy, and in rare cases uveitis. Lupus choroidopathy presents with (D) serous elevations of the retina, retinal pigment epithelium (RPE), or both, and choroidal infarctions might develop.

34. Correct: Polymerase chain reaction (PCR) is the most sensitive, specific, and rapid diagnostic method for detecting the causative organism (B)

Acute retinal necrosis is acute, fulminant disease that may arise without systemic prodrome and usually present with acute unilateral vision loss with associated pain, photophobia, and floaters. Initially panuveitis is observed with heavy vitreous infiltration, and within 2 weeks, if untreated, there is development of occlusive retinal arteriolitis and multifocal yellow-white peripheral retinitis. Early on, lesions have scalloped edges that later coalesce to form 360-degree creamy retinitis that progresses to full-thickness necrosis. (A) The posterior pole is usually spared, and the mechanism involves (C) occlusive vasculopathy with arteriolar involvement. (D) Recent studies with PCR suggest that the most common causative organism is varicella-zoster virus followed by HSV-1, HSV-2, and rarely cytomegalovirus.

35. Correct: Focal retinochoroiditis (B)

Bartonella henselae is a gram-negative rod known to be the principal agent of cat scratch disease (CSD), a feline-associated zoonotic disease with the highest age-specific incidence among children younger than 10 years. The most well-known manifestation of *B. henselae* is neuroretinitis (A); however, focal retinochoroiditis is the most common uveitic manifestation. Ocular involvement occurs in 5 to 10% of patients with CSD and includes Parinaud's oculoglandular syndrome with unilateral granulomatous conjunctivitis and lymphadenopathy. Less common presentations include (C) intermediate uveitis, (D) inflammatory mass of the optic nerve, or isolated nerve swelling among others. The diagnosis is based on clinical features together with confirmatory serologic testing.

36. Correct: Heerfordt's syndrome (D)

Sarcoidosis is a multisystem granulomatous disorder that can affect any ocular tissue (in up to 50% of patients with systemic disease), uveitis being the most frequent manifestation. Uveoparotid fever or Heerfordt's syndrome is one form of acute sarcoidosis that presents with uveitis, parotitis, fever, and facial nerve palsy. Another one is (C) Lofgren's syndrome that consists of acute iritis, erythema nodosum, febrile arthropathy, and bilateral hilar adenopathy. (A) Taches de bougie is another name for the candle wax drippings or irregular nodular granulomas along retinal venules that can be seen when there is posterior segment involvement. (B) Neurosarcoidosis is uncommon and can affect a combination of intracranial structures with or without associated papilledema, the spinal cord, as well as peripheral nerves. Topical, periocular, and systemic corticosteroids are the mainstay of treatment for ocular sarcoidosis.

37. Correct: Cytomegalovirus (CMV) (A)

Glaucomatocyclitic crisis or Posner–Schlossman syndrome usually manifests as recurrent unilateral episodes of anterior-chamber inflammation and elevated IOP. Signs include corneal edema, keratic precipitates (KP), and low-grade cell and flare. Treatment is with topical steroids and IOP-lowering medications. Recent studies have found an association with CMV infection. This is a diagnosis of exclusion and other causes like (B) HSV, (C), Rubella, and (D) VZV need to be ruled out.

38. Correct: Headaches and "not feeling like myself" (C)

Acute posterior multifocal placoid pigment epitheliopathy (APMPPE) is an uncommon condition that usually presents in young healthy adults with (B) initial flu-like symptoms in about half of the cases. They typically present with sudden onset of bilateral although asymmetric vision loss with (A) associated central or paracentral scotomas. They may have a mild to moderate vitreous reaction and in fundus examination, there is evidence of multiple, flat, yellow-white placoid lesions at the level of the retinal pigment epithelium (RPE) throughout the posterior pole. The diagnosis of APMPPE is based on the clinical findings and FA that show early hypofluorescence of the lesions due to blockage with late staining. This condition can be associated to central nervous system vasculitis, so any neurologic symptoms warrant further work-up since the use of systemic corticosteroids might be considered under this scenario. Otherwise, there are no convincing data that treatment with corticosteroids improves visual outcome and the majority of patients regain vision of 20/40 or better. (D) Eye redness and photophobia could be seen in APMPPE and do not warrant additional work-up or treatment.

39. Correct: HIV retinopathy (B)

HIV retinopathy is the most common ocular finding in patients with AIDS and can be seen in up to 70%

331

of patients. Findings include cotton wool spots, retinal hemorrhages, and microaneurysms. (**A**) CMV retinitis was very common before the highly active antiretroviral therapy (HAART) era and is still the most common opportunistic infection in AIDS patients. (**C**) PORN is a rare infection in HIV patients caused by varicella-zoster virus (VZV) or herpes simplex virus (HSV) viruses. It is very characteristic for its lack of significant vitreous inflammation. (**D**) Disseminated Cryptococcus neoformans in patients with AIDS may result in choroiditis or direct invasion of the optic nerve.

---

40.   Correct: When medical management with drops is not enough to achieve good intraocular pressure (IOP), a laser trabeculoplasty is a good option before proceeding to surgery (C)

Laser trabeculoplasty should be avoided in eyes with uveitis as well as (**B**) cyclodestructive procedure due to the risk of worsening inflammation. When medical management fails, filtering surgery is indicated and the standard trabeculectomy has a greater risk of failure in these patients. (A) Most cases of uveitic glaucoma, especially if pseudophakic or aphakic, require aqueous drainage devices with tube shunts that may be placed in the anterior chamber or vitreous cavity in vitrectomized patients. These implants have higher chances than the standard trabeculectomy to success long term. (**D**) As with any other surgical procedure in uveitis patients, meticulous control of perioperative inflammation is key for success and avoids complications that may affect visual outcomes like cystoid macular edema (CME) or hypotony.

---

41.   Correct: Endogenous reactivation of latent virus (D)

Following primary infection, varicella-zoster virus (VZV) becomes latent in sensory neural ganglia; shingles represents endogenous reactivation of latent virus often associated to a waxing level of immunity to infection. Zoster is more common in patients on immunosuppressive therapy, in those with malignancy or debilitating medical conditions. Ocular involvement occurs in greater than 70% of patients with zoster of the ophthalmic division of trigeminal nerve. (**B**) Epstein–Barr virus (EBV) remains latent in B lymphocytes for life, and (**C**) active herpes simplex infection usually spreads from the skin or mucosal surface via sensory nerve axons. (**A**) Cell-mediated immunity might be the pathogenesis of stromal keratitis, but this is not completely understood.

---

42.   Correct: Oral valacyclovir 1 g three times a day × 7 to 10 days (A)

The recommendation for treatment of herpes zoster ophthalmicus (HZO) is either oral valacyclovir 1 g three times a day, (**B**) oral acyclovir but 800 mg five times a day or (**C**) oral famciclovir 500 mg three times a day × 7 to 10 days. IV acyclovir is recommended when there is disseminated infection in immunosuppressed patients. (**D**) Topical antivirals are not effective.

---

43.   Correct: Neutrophils around the lens material with surrounding lymphocytes, plasma cells, epithelioid cells, and occasional giant cells forming a zonal granuloma (B)

Uveitis may result from an immune reaction to lens material that could follow trauma (surgical or accidental) or leakage of the lens protein through an intact capsule in hypermature lenses. Clinically, patients show granulomatous or nongranulomatous anterior uveitis, KP, and may develop posterior synechiae. A hypopyon might be present, and intraocular pressure (IOP) is commonly elevated. Histologically a zonal granulomatous inflammation is centered at the site of the injury. Treatment consist of topical steroids and cycloplegics. If inflammation is severe, systemic steroids might be needed. Surgical removal of all lens material is usually curative. (**A**) Engorged macrophages clogging the trabecular meshwork is the mechanism of IOP elevation in phacolytic glaucoma. (**C**) There are no mast cells or basophils present in lens-induced uveitis, which makes the term phacoanaphylactic a misleading one. (**D**) Swollen macrophages can be seen in the aqueous of a patient with phacolytic glaucoma.

---

44.   Correct: Absence of inflammatory involvement of the choriocapillaris and retina (D)

The histologic features of sympathetic ophthalmia (SO) are similar in the exciting eye and the sympathizing eye. In SO, there is no involvement of the retina or the choriocapillaris. (**A**) There is a diffuse, granulomatous, nonnecrotizing infiltration of the choroid with predominance of lymphocytes. (**B**) Nodular clusters of epithelioid cells containing pigment are called Dalen–Fuchs nodules and are located between the retinal pigment epithelium (RPE) and the Bruch membrane and (**C**) are not pathognomonic of SO. They can also be seen in Vogt-Koyanagi-Harada (VKH) syndrome and sarcoidosis.

---

45.   Correct: Interferon gamma release assay (C)

Eales' disease is a peripheral retinal perivasculitis associated to tuberculosis (TB) that usually present in young otherwise healthy men with recurrent unilateral or bilateral but asymmetric retinal and vitreous hemorrhages. The typical finding is periphlebitis, but they may also develop venous occlusion, peripheral nonperfusion with neovascularization, and possible tractional retinal detachment. In this case, the patient comes from an endemic country, so an interferon gamma release assay could determine if the patient has prior exposure to TB, although the diagnosis would be finally supported by evidence of polymerase chain reaction (PCR)-based assays of *Mycobacterium tuberculosis* DNA from an ocular sample. (**A**) This would be an atypical presentation of herpetic disease without areas of retinitis, and positive serologies do not confirm the diagnosis. (**B**) *Toxoplasma* could cause vasculitis but usually in association with a focal area of chorioretinitis next to a previous scar. (**D**) ESR and CRP are nonspecific markers of inflammation that would not help narrow down the etiology of this patient's condition.

46. Correct: Cataract surgery can be performed but there is an increased risk of postoperative hyphema (A)

Known as Amsler's sign, patients with Fuchs' heterochromic iridocyclitis (FHI) may have abnormal blood vessels that bridge the angle and could bleed during surgery. (**B**) Treatment with topical steroids usually do not resolve inflammation, so this is not indicated. (**C**) Patients with FHI typically have good prognosis and do well with cataract surgery and intraocular lens implantation. The etiology of FHI remains unclear, but it has been associated with cytomegalovirus infection and rubella although (**D**) treatment with valganciclovir is not indicated.

47. Correct: Cystoid macular edema (CME) (B)

Pars planitis refers to those patients with intermediate uveitis where there is snowbank or snowball formation in the absence of an associated systemic condition or infection. It is the most common type of intermediate uveitis and 80% are bilateral. CME often develops after long-standing inflammation and is the major cause of vision loss in these patients. (**A**) The vitreous is the main site of inflammation in intermediate uveitis but with 1+ vitritis is most likely not the main cause of decreased vision in this patient. (**C**) Cataracts are often seen secondary to the use of steroids. (**D**) In up to 10% of patients, peripheral retinal vasculitis, specifically phlebitis, could result in ischemia that can lead to neovascularization and secondary vitreous hemorrhages, peripheral tractional and rhegmatogenous detachments.

48. Correct: Manual superficial keratectomy with sodium ethylenediaminetetraacetic acid (D)

Patients with band keratopathy should be treated with scraping of the epithelium and chelation with EDTA and allowed to heal before cataract surgery is attempted. This is a common presentation in patients with JIA, because they typically are asymptomatic and may have chronic underlying inflammation for months or years at the time of diagnosis. (**A**) Bandage contact lenses are a nonsurgical option when band keratopathy is symptomatic, but this wouldn't be the definitive treatment in this 8-year-old with potential risk for amblyopia. (**B**) Alcohol debridement can be used to remove the epithelium, but this has to be followed

with application of the chelating agent. (**C**) PTK using excimer laser is not advised as a primary treatment, because calcium ablates at a different rate from stroma and could produce a severely irregular surface.

49. Correct: Indocyanine green angiography (ICG) (C)

Birdshot chorioretinopathy or vitiliginous chorioretinitis is an uncommon disease that is predominantly seen past the fourth decade in White women of European descent. Initial symptoms are usually floaters, blurred vision, nyctalopia, or difficulties with color vision. Anterior-segment inflammation might be absent and the degree of vitritis might vary. The classical finding on fundus examination is the presence of multifocal hypopigmented, ovoid cream-colored lesions at the level of the choroid and retinal pigment epithelium (RPE) in the postequatorial fundus, more evident nasally emanating from the disc. These could be very subtle and often missed on initial examination. ICG angiography shows multiple hypofluorescent spots, which are often more numerous than those seen with the indirect ophthalmoscope. (**B**) FA findings are inconsistent and is more useful to look for vasculitis, macular edema, or optic disc inflammation. (**A**) OCT macula is useful to look for cystoid macular edema (CME) and (**D**) vitreous biopsy is relevant when there is a concern for a possible malignancy or an infectious process that is not responding to treatment as expected. Other testing includes electroretinogram (ERG) and visual fields, which are useful to monitor disease progression and response to therapy.

50. Correct: B-scan ultrasonography (A)

Ocular toxocariasis is an uncommon disease of children and young adults that results from tissue invasion by the larvae of *Toxocara canis* or *Toxocara cati*. Patients usually present with unilateral vision loss, pain, strabismus, or leukocoria. Posterior segment findings include three recognizable syndromes: leukocoria secondary to severe vitreous inflammation and chronic endophthalmitis (25% of cases); localized macular granuloma (25% of cases), or peripheral granuloma (50% of cases). The most important differential diagnostic consideration is sporadic unilateral retinoblastoma. A B-scan and CT scan are useful to confirm the absence of calcium that is typically seen in RB. The final diagnosis is based on ocular findings, (**B**) supportive laboratory data and imaging studies. (**C**) An examination under anesthesia is warranted when there's poor cooperation, especially when there is a high concern for RB, but in this instance, a biopsy would be contraindicated. (**D**) Laser photocoagulation may be considered if live larvae are identified or in the rare instance of a copy number variation associated to an inactive granuloma.

51. Correct: Every 3 months (C)

The frequency of ophthalmologic examinations in patients with JIA depend on the presence of ANA titers, the age at onset of diagnosis, and the type of JIA (oligoarthritis, polyarthritis, or systemic disease). In this case with age less than 6 years at onset, involvement of two joints with +ANA and duration of disease of less than 4 years, examinations should be performed every 3 months regardless of the symptoms since in most cases, patients are asymptomatic. (**A**) Patients with systemic disease rarely have ocular involvement and should be examined once a year as well as those with –ANA that have had the disease for over 4 years or the onset was more than 6 years of age. (**B**) Patients with oligo- or polyarthritis, +ANA, and onset less than 6 years of age but who have had the disease for over 4 years could be examined every 6 months, as well as +ANA with onset greater than 6 years of age within 4 years of the diagnosis or –ANA if it was diagnosed at less than 6 years of age and the duration of disease is less than 4 years. (**D**) Follow-ups should never be guided based on symptoms, since most patients are asymptomatic.

52. Correct: Hematogenous (B)

Cytomegalovirus (CMV) retinitis is the most common ophthalmic manifestation of both congenital CMV infection and in the context of HIV/AIDS. There are two variants: classic or fulminant retinitis, granular or indolent and perivascular form. Early CMV retinitis may present as a small retinal infiltrate similar to a cotton wool spot but that progresses without treatment. CMV reaches the eye via hematogenous route, with passage across the blood–ocular barrier, infecting retinal vascular endothelial cells and cell-to-cell transmission within the retina. (**A**) Congenital form is usually associated with systemic manifestations including fever, thrombocytopenia, anemia, and hepatosplenomegaly. (**C**) There is no direct invasion through ocular surface, and (**D**) this is not caused via iatrogenic means.

53. Correct: *Pseudomonas aeruginosa* (D)

Infectious scleritis may occur in the setting of trauma or previous surgery. This patient had recent pterygium surgery and the most common organism seen in this scenario is *P. aeruginosa*, especially if mitomycin C was used or beta-irradiation. It could also be secondary to bacterial infections like (**B**) *Nocardia* or (**C**) *Actinomyces*, mycobacterial infections, (**A**) fungi, and viral like herpes simplex virus and varicella-zoster virus that tend to be chronic. Cultures should always be obtained, and treatment consists of antibiotics with possible debridement of infected tissue and scleral graft patching if there is severe thinning.

54. Correct: Hepatitis panel, antineutrophil cytoplasmic antibodies (ANCA) (A)

The diagnosis of polyarteritis nodosa (PAN) is made by fulfilling 3/10 classification criteria including weight loss; myalgia, weakness, elevated diastolic BP (> 90 mm Hg), positive hepatitis B serology among others. PUK associated with scleritis could be the presenting manifestation of PAN like in this patient. About 10% of patients are positive for hepatitis B, reason why it is part of the diagnostic criteria. Diagnosis is important since without treatment, the mortality rate in 5 years is 90%. Tissue biopsy confirms the diagnosis. (**B**) RPR is ordered in every work-up to rule out syphilis; ANA would be important to rule out systemic lupus erythematosus (SLE) but *Toxoplasma* titers are not indicated. (**C**) Aside from the chest X-ray that helps rule out granulomatous changes associated to sarcoidosis or active pulmonary tuberculosis (TB), CBC, ESR, CRP are nonspecific tests that alone would not help establish the diagnosis. (**D**) Lupus anticoagulans is not indicated.

55. Correct: Retinoblastoma (B)

Diffuse infiltrating retinoblastoma is a rare manifestation of retinoblastoma that could be present as a masquerade syndrome of uveitis. About 1 to 3% of cases may present with unilateral inflammation including chemosis, pseudohypopyon, and vitritis. The pseudohypopyon typically changes with positioning and is whiter than the typical yellowish hypopyon. These cases can be a diagnostic challenge since any sampling (aqueous or vitreous) could have the risk of tumor spread. Most of these patients are treated with topical steroids and IOP-lowering medications initially, but lack of expected improvement has to alert us about the possibility of malignancy. (**A**) *Toxocara* presenting like chronic endophthalmitis is part of the differential diagnosis, but retinoblastoma is by far the most important to rule out. (**C**) Herpetic infections presenting with hypopyon in a 4-year old would be extraordinarily rare, and (**D**) sarcoidosis is a possible etiology of inflammation in children but more serious etiologies have to be discarded first.

56. Correct: Koeppe nodule (B)

Typical slit lamp findings in patients with sarcoidosis include granulomatous or mutton-fat KPs, iris nodules, and snowballs in the inferior anterior vitreous. Nodules that are prominent in the pupillary border are known as Koeppe nodules. (**A**) Busacca nodules are seen in the anterior face of the iris and (**C**) Berlin nodules are seen in the angle. (**D**) Lisch nodules are seen in close to 100% of patients with neurofibromatosis type 1.

57. Correct: Oral corticosteroids along with immunomodulatory therapy (IMT) (C)

The goal for treatment in Behcet's disease is not only to treat the explosive acute episodes, but also to prevent relapses that could result in permanent vision loss, reason why IMT is indicated. Systemic corticosteroids are used to treat the acute inflammation, but they need to be started together with IMT. Antimetabolites like azathioprine, mycophenolate mofetil, or anti-TNFs like infliximab are recommended. (A) Colchicine is used for the treatment of mucocutaneous ulcer but has no value for ocular involvement. (B) Treating with corticosteroids alone will put this patient at risk for vision loss if a relapse develops. (D) Cyclosporine has been used with limited success and is recommended as second-line treatment.

58. Correct: Glaucoma filtration surgery (A)

This patient with visual field defect and uncontrolled IOP needs additional treatment to control glaucoma. From the options listed, filtration surgery has been done successfully in patients with uveitic glaucoma. (B) Laser trabeculoplasty is contraindicated since it can trigger additional inflammation and potentially increase IOP even more. (C) Acetazolamide is contraindicated in this patient with sulfa allergy. (D) Latanoprost has been implicated to cause or worsen intraocular inflammation, but this patient has a quiet anterior chamber and controlling her glaucoma is of utmost importance to avoid permanent visual field loss.

59. Correct: Posterior pole may be involved early (D)

Progressive outer retinal necrosis (PORN) is a variant of herpetic acute necrotizing retinitis occurring in severely immunosuppressed patients. The most common cause is varicella-zoster virus but herpes simplex virus has also been isolated. In contrast to acute retinal necrosis, in PORN the posterior pole tends to be involved early in the disease course and they have (C) minimal or no vitreous inflammation secondary to the profound immunosuppression. (B) Retinal vasculature is minimally involved, and (A) the visual prognosis is very poor with a rate of up to 70% of retinal detachment.

60. Correct: A 26-year-old myopic woman with photopsias in the right eye, mild vitritis, and abnormal ERG (delayed 30-Hz flicker) (B)

AZOOR is characterized by loss of one or more zones of outer retinal function and typically affects young myopic females with photopsias, minimal or no funduscopic changes, and abnormal ERG, specifically a delayed 30-Hz-flicker response. Approximately 50% of cases are associated to mild vitritis and (A) is usually unilateral but both eyes can be affected; it is not associated to the development of CNVM. Visual field defects including enlargement of the blind spot can be seen as well as loss of inner/outer segment line on OCT but (C) not typically on a 50-year-old hyperopic woman. (D) Funduscopic changes could range from subtle retinal pigment epithelium (RPE) changes to vessel attenuation and late pigment migration but no presence of defined hypopigmented lesions is typical of AZOOR. Cancer-associated retinopathy and melanoma-associated retinopathy should be considered as part of the differential diagnosis.

61. Correct: Herpes simplex virus 1 (HSV-1) (C)

Acute anterior uveitis if often associated with herpetic disease. Usually, the iritis is a keratouveitis and may develop stellate keratic precipitates. Ocular hypertension is frequently seen and is a helpful diagnostic hallmark as well as the presence of iris atrophy that can be seen with HSV, VZV, or CMV and can be patchy or sectorial. Based on patient's age and prevalence, the most likely organism in this case is HSV-1. Anterior uveitis with CMV is uncommon but could be seen with same presentation in immunocompetent adults (A). VZV would be the most common culprit in older patients (D). HLA-B27-related uveitis tends to present with recurrent anterior uveitis but is not typically associated with elevated IOP, stellate KPs, or iris atrophy (C).

62. Correct: Prednisolone acetate 1% every 1-hour OD (A)

Mainstay of treatment for acute anterior uveitis is aggressive use of topical steroids every 1 to 2 hours followed by taper once inflammation in controlled. (B) It is preferable to begin therapy with a high dose and taper as the inflammation subsides, rather than beginning with a low dose that may have to be increased. (C) Periocular steroid injections should only be used only when infectious causes of inflammation have been ruled out. (D) Oral steroids have many side effects and should also be avoided until infectious etiologies are discarded or treated with respective antimicrobials.

63. Correct: Varicella-zoster virus (VZV) (D)

Acute anterior uveitis is often associated with herpetic disease. Usually, the iritis is a keratouveitis and may develop stellate keratic precipitates. Ocular hypertension is frequently seen and is a helpful diagnostic hallmark as well as the presence of iris atrophy that can be seen with HSV, VZV, or CMV and can be patchy or sectorial. Based on patient's age and prevalence, the most likely organism in this case is VZV, and it can be seen even if the cutaneous component occurred in the past or was minimal. Anterior uveitis with CMV is uncommon but could be seen with same presentation in immunocompetent adults (A). HLA-B27-related uveitis tends to present with recurrent anterior uveitis, usually in younger patients and is not typically associated with elevated IOP, stellate KPs, or iris atrophy (**B**). HSV would be the most common culprit in younger patients (**C**).

64. Correct: B$_2$ microglobulin (B)

An adolescent girl with this presentation is suggestive of the diagnosis of tubulointerstitial nephritis and uveitis (TINU). As part of the clinical criteria for the diagnosis of TINU, patient have abnormal urinalysis with increased B$_2$ microglobulin, proteinuria, and the presence of eosinophils, pyuria, or hematuria. Abnormal creatinine level or decreased creatinine clearance are often present. ACE levels are ordered when sarcoidosis is suspected but it would be less likely in this 18-year-old with non-granulomatous uveitis without synechiae; ACE levels in the pediatric population are often elevated and could be misleading (**A**). ANA is usually positive in patients with juvenile idiopathic arthritis, which typically presents before 16 years of age, and the most common presentation is chronic anterior uveitis that is asymptomatic (**C**). HLA-B27 related uveitis is usually unilateral and not commonly associated with general malaise and myalgia (**D**).

65. Correct: Sarcoid-related uveitis (C)

This patient has bilateral granulomatous iridocyclitis with mutton-fat KP, occurring in approximately two-thirds of patients with ocular sarcoidosis. She also has bilateral hilar adenopathy on chest X-ray (single best screening test), suggestive of sarcoidosis. Ultimately, the diagnosis is made with biopsy. HLA-B27 is present in approximately 5% of the general population and its presence does not provide an absolute diagnosis, even less in this classical presentation of bilateral granulomatous disease (**A, B**). TB-associated uveitis is part of the differential diagnosis of granulomatous anterior uveitis but work-up did not indicate a positive purified protein derivative (PPD) or serum gamma assay, and chest X-ray findings would be different (**D**).

66. Correct: Previous history of trauma or intraocular surgery (A)

Vogt-Koyanagi-Harada (VKH) and sympathetic ophthalmia (SO) have similar clinical presentation and are both bilateral, diffuse granulomatous panuveitides, but SO patients have history of accidental or surgical trauma to one eye. This is an essential question that may help distinguish between the two entities. Family history of uveitis or autoimmune disease (**B**), history of chronic cough or shortness of breath (**C**) and sexual activity, including high-risk behavior (**D**) should all be questions asked as part of the medical history in any patients with uveitis.

67. Correct: Ocular histoplasmosis syndrome (B)

Ocular histoplasmosis syndrome is a multifocal choroiditis believed to be caused by infection with *Histoplasma capsulatum*; usually found in endemic areas of the United States (Ohio and Mississippi River valleys). The classic triad: multiple white, atrophic choroidal scars, peripapillary pigmentation and maculopathy, in the absence of vitreous cells. The pathogenesis is thought to involve initial infection causing choroiditis that subsides and leaves atrophic scars. This may result in disruption of the Bruch membrane with subsequent proliferation of subretinal vessels and CNVM formation. MCP is accompanied by varying degrees of vitritis (**A**), not seen in this patient. *Toxoplasma* chorioretinitis is the most common cause of infectious retinochoroiditis and classically appears as a focal, white retinitis with overlying vitritis, often next to a pigmented chorioretinal scar (**C**). TB should always be in the differential diagnosis of uveitis and needs to be ruled out, especially if starting treatment with corticosteroids but less likely in this case based on typical presentation (**D**).

68. Correct: Birdshot chorioretinopathy (B)

Also known as vitiliginous chorioretinitis, birdshot is an uncommon disease predominantly seen in White women of northern European descent past the fourth decade of life. Highly correlated with the presence of *HLA-A29* gene. Presenting symptoms are blurry vision, floaters, and sometimes nyctalopia or problems with color vision. Varying degrees of vitritis can be seen, as well as characteristic multifocal hypopigmented, ovoid, cream-colored lesions at the level of the choroid and retinal pigment epithelium (RPE). FA typically does not highlight the lesions, but ICG shows multiple hypofluorescent spots that are often more numerous than those seen on fundus examination or FA. MEWDS usually presents in younger patients, is unilateral, and small perifoveal dots can be seen but disappear (**A**). Sarcoidosis is part of the differential diagnosis and should be ruled out as part of the work-up of these patients (**C**). In multifocal choroiditis, the presence of lesions should be evident on the fundus examination, often in combination with scars or atrophic lesions (**D**).

69. Correct: Increase methotrexate dose since patient had recurrence of cystoid macular edema (CME) on prednisone 15 mg (D)

This patient with pars planitis has active disease despite the use of methotrexate 15 mg and prednisone 15 mg. The goal of treatment is to achieve control of disease and a prednisone dose of 7.5 mg or less. Her dose of methotrexate can still be increased up to 25 mg (depending on side effects) before calling it a failure (**B**) and switching therapy to a different agent. Increasing oral prednisone (**C**) can be done in the short term for fast control of inflammation, but it is not a safe option long term, and steroid-sparing therapy should be optimized. To continue prednisone taper would put this patient at risk for more inflammation, since she has active disease on the current dose that is not a safe dose long term (**A**).

70. Correct: Pulse with IV methylprednisolone daily for 3 days (A)

In cases of explosive onset of severe noninfectious posterior uveitis, panuveitis or risk of corneal perforation, intravenous, high-dose, pulse methylprednisolone (1 g/d) therapy may be administered for 3 days, followed by taper of oral prednisone. Topical steroids should be used with caution and are not the indicated treatment since they can aggravate corneal melt (**B**). The patient showed progression while on prednisone 60 mg and methotrexate takes at least 4 to 6 weeks to start working, so continuing the current dose of prednisone would be inadequate and could put this patient at risk for perforation (**C**). Preparing for a possible emergent procedure is always important but should not be the next step in the management of this patient, since patient has not perforated yet (**D**).

71. Correct: Fill out the papers with her current examination, visual acuity, and assessment (C)

As physicians we will encounter ethical dilemmas in our practice and should be able to know how to approach them. In the case of this patient, the doctor has been clear to the patient about her examination and prognosis, but the patient insists on applying for disability. Ultimately, it is not our decision as the patient's provider to determine disability. We should complete all requested documents without lying or exaggerating the actual findings, since this would be an unlawful action (**B**). After the patient is oriented, it is her right to submit the case, and we should collaborate with documenting the information requested by the disability office (**A**). Referring to social security would be inadequate, since we know this patient does not have any disabilities based solely on her ocular condition (**D**). This decision should be done by the patient and/or any provider that considers she has a condition that might qualify her for disability benefits.

72. Correct: Idiopathic (C)

Episcleritis is a relatively common cause of eye redness. Most cases are idiopathic, but it can be associated with systemic condition in up to a quarter of patients. Usually, it is seen in one eye at a time without pain and typically does not have discharge or crustiness. In the office, differentiation of episcleritis versus scleritis can be aided by application of phenylephrine 2.5% that blanches conjunctival and episcleral vessels but leaves scleral vessels undisturbed. Scleritis is very often associated with pain and marked tenderness to palpation and does not

clear with instillation of phenylephrine. Herpes is a possible but rare cause of episcleritis (**A**). Rheumatoid arthritis (**D**) and SLE (**B**) are more commonly associated with scleritis, and although they could be associated with episcleritis, it only happens in 25 to 30% of patients.

73. Correct: Discontinue steroid drop and start trifluridine every 2 hours (C)

Most cases of herpes simplex virus (HSV) epithelial keratitis resolve spontaneously, however, treatment shortens the course and might reduce associated neuropathy. Topical trifluridine every 2 hours is efficacious but should be discontinued within 10 to 14 days to avoid toxicity. Oral acyclovir or valacyclovir have been used effectively, but IV treatment is not indicated (**A**). Topical corticosteroids are contraindicated (**B**) in the presence of active epithelial disease. Placing a bandage contact lens is not appropriate, but sometimes minimal debridement can speed up resolution (**D**).

74. Correct: Nephrotoxicity (D)

Tacrolimus is a calcineurin inhibitor that eliminate T-cell receptor signaling and downregulate *IL-2* gene transcription. Its main side effect is nephrotoxicity, but because of its lower dose and increased potency, it is less common than cyclosporine. The most common side effects of cyclosporine are systemic hypertension (**B**) and nephrotoxicity. Diarrhea is a common side effect of mycophenolate mofetil (**A**). Hematuria can be seen with cyclophosphamide (**C**); if micro hematuria is seen, hydration should be increased, but if gross hematuria develops, medication must be discontinued.

75. Correct: Rhabdomyolysis (A)

Combining a statin with cyclosporine may increase statin levels with risk of myopathy and rhabdomyolysis. It may also increase cyclosporine levels which is a risk for toxicity. Reversible hepatotoxicity can occur in up to 15% of patients on methotrexate (**C**). Fatty liver (**B**) and thrombocytopenia (**D**) are not risks of this regimen.

76. Correct: Congenital cytomegalovirus (CMV) (D)

CMV retinitis is the most common ophthalmic manifestation of congenital CMV infection, but it is rare and usually presents with retinal scars that may include the macula and almost never active chorioretinitis. Congenital rubella syndrome could present with unilateral or bilateral pigmentary retinopathy, often described as salt-and-pepper fundus. In patients with posterior uveitis, syphilis should always be part of the differential since ocular manifestations are protean and affect all structures. Posterior segment findings of acquired syphilis include vitritis, chorioretinitis, vasculitis, retinitis, and posterior placoid chorioretinitis (**B**). Serpiginous choroiditis is characterized by the presence of gray-white lesions at the level of the retinal pigment epithelium (RPE) projecting in a geographic manner from the optic nerve in the posterior fundus (**A**). Sarcoidosis can also affect any ocular tissue, and posterior segment involvement can occur in up to 20% of patients although this presentation in the picture would be rare (**C**).

77. Correct: Sarcoidosis (A)

Vasculitis in the setting of sarcoidosis primarily affects the venous system, known as periphlebitis that could be linear or segmental. Occlusive retinal vascular disease (branch retinal vein occlusion [BRVO] or central retinal vein occlusions [CRVO]) can occur. Lupus retinopathy may present with severe retinal vascular occlusive disease that involves both arterial and venous thrombosis (**B**). Posterior segment involvement in Behcet's disease is classically an obliterative, necrotizing retinal vasculitis that affects both arteries and veins (**C**). Susac's syndrome is a rare entity characterized by the triad of encephalopathy, hearing loss, and retinal arterial branch occlusions (**D**).

78. Correct: HLA-B27 (B)

In eyes with active inflammation we can often see low IOP caused by decreased aqueous production from the ciliary body. Typically, patients with HLA-B27 uveitis present with a severe, fibrinous reaction in the anterior chamber with low-to-normal IOP. Posner–Schlossman syndrome, also known as glaucomatocyclitic crisis, is characterized by episodes of acute elevation of IOP on presentation, with associated anterior-chamber inflammation. (**A**) Etiology is unknown. Treatment is focused on controlling inflammation and lowering IOP during the acute episode with most patient being able to discontinue drops between attacks. In ocular toxoplasmosis, up to 20% of patients have acutely elevated IOP (**C**). HSV infection frequently presents with elevated IOP in the involved eye, and its presence is a helpful diagnostic hallmark. Herpetic reactivation may directly cause trabeculitis (**D**).

79. Correct: Cataract surgery should be performed when at least 3 consecutive months of quiescence can be documented (C)

The absence of inflammation for 3 or more consecutive months before surgery should be a prerequisite for any elective intraocular surgery. This is important to decrease complications and for better outcomes along with aggressive control of inflammation in the perioperative period. Telling the patient to have surgery as soon as anterior-chamber cell resolves would not be ideal and could put this patient at risk for worse outcomes (**A**). In general, uveitic eyes could have more complicated surgeries due to the presence of synechiae, zonular instability, among others but although the patient should know these risks, offering cataract surgery now is not recommended (**B**). Treatment with steroids, starting 1 to 2 weeks prior to surgery and continuing during the postoperative period is recommended, but this should be done in addition to waiting 3 or more months of quiet disease (**D**).

80. Correct: A 53-year old with light blue iris OD, unilateral cataract, diffuse fine KP, and 1+ cell. Normal examination OS (D)

Macular edema rarely occurs in patients with Fuchs'. The disease is characterized by the presence of cells in the anterior chamber and anterior vitreous, iris atrophy, and small white stellate KPs distributed diffusely throughout the cornea. Patients with birdshot often develop CME (**A**). The most common cause of vision loss in patients with intermediate uveitis is CME (**B**). Finally, CME after cataract surgery is common even in patients without history of uveitis, more so in patients who develop postoperative inflammation (**C**).

81. Correct: Macrophages and epithelioid cells (C)

Mutton-fat keratic precipitates are seen with granulomatous inflammation like sarcoidosis. They are large, greasy-white deposits in the endothelium formed from macrophages and epithelioid cells.

82. Correct: Use of a checklist that includes the steps to follow before, during, and after administering a medication including verification of two patient identifiers (A)

Patient safety should be a priority in all settings of patient care. When we are performing surgeries, there are mechanisms in place for verification to avoid wrong side surgery. For administration of medications, the same protocols should be in place to prevent medication errors that could be fatal. Using a checklist including two patient identifiers would have prevented this error from happening. A punitive approach is not ideal for the patients or the employees; it doesn't ensure that other personnel are not going to incur in the same mistake (**B**). Changing personnel regularly could be done but would most likely bring other errors, since they don't feel familiar with the tasks performed, having to learn new instructions or protocols every time they are changed (**C**). Finally, some patients are very aware of their treatment and know the name of the medication and dose, but that is not the case for every patient, and this is not a reliable approach to prevent this type of error (**D**).

83. Correct: ACAID represents an attenuated afferent arc (B)

ACAID represents an attenuated effector arc. It is the best studied mechanism of immune privilege (**A**). Immunization with an antigen in the skin provokes a strong delayed-type sensitivity; immunization of the anterior chamber results in a robust antibody response and absence of delayed-type hypersensitivity (**C**). Splenectomy eliminates ACAID, indicating the importance of the spleen for generation of immune deviation (**D**).

84. Correct: 30 months (B)

The sustained-release fluocinolone 0.59-mg implant is effective for a median of 30 months with a mean time of 38 months to first recurrence. There is no consensus on scheduled replacements of the implant to prevent recurrences once the median time of efficacy is over. In the Multicenter Uveitis Steroid Treatment (MUST) trial which followed patients for 7 years, uveitis recurrences and associated vision loss were significant after 5 years of implantation.

85. Correct: Infliximab (A)

Infliximab is a tumor necrosis factor-α (TNF-α) inhibitor used in noninfectious uveitis. Many side effects have been associated to its use including drug-induced lupus, demyelinating disease, and new malignancy including lymphoma. From the options mentioned, infliximab wouldn't be the best option in this patient that has previous history of lymphoma. Mycophenolate mofetil has not been implicated with increased risk of lymphoma in uveitis patients (**B**). Cyclosporine has been associated to increased risk of primary skin cancers in patients with psoriasis but no risk of lymphoma (**C**). Rituximab is used for the treatment of lymphoma as well as autoimmune disorders like rheumatoid arthritis or granulomatosis with polyangiitis (**D**).

86. Correct: This occurs with an increase an increase in the CD4 count of at least 50 to 100 cells/μL (B)

Immune recovery uveitis (IRU) can occur in patient with previous CMV retinitis, whose immune status improves after initiation of HAART and only occurs in eyes infected with CMV (**A**). It is more likely to occur in patients treated with cidofovir. It is defined as an increase in the CD4 count of at least 50 cells/μL to 100 cells/μL. These patients with IRU are more likely to develop macular edema and epiretinal membranes, and macular edema can be resistant to treatment (**C**). Although steroids are used for the treatment, intravitreal injections should be avoided due to the potential risk of CMV infection reactivation (**D**).

87. Correct: Carotid Doppler ultrasonography (B)

Ocular ischemic syndrome is a nonneoplastic masquerade syndrome of uveitis. It results from hypoperfusion of the eye due to carotid artery obstruction. Patients are typically males older than 65 years. Ocular findings could include the presence of anterior-chamber cells and flare that is typically out of proportion to the number of cells. Diagnostic studies should include carotid

Doppler ultrasonography where ipsilateral carotid stenosis greater than 90% would support the diagnosis, although it has been documented in people with less degree of stenosis if they don't have good collateral circulation. Treatment involves endarterectomy. HIV testing wouldn't be indicated just based on the patient's presentation although possible risk factors should be addressed in the medical history (**A**). Chest X-ray is the best screening test for sarcoidosis, but this would be an atypical presentation at this age with the unilateral retinal findings (**C**). Brain MRI is not useful in this case (**D**).

88. Correct: There was no statistically significant difference in visual acuity at 2 years (A)

The MUST trial is a randomized clinical trial that compared the fluocinolone implant to standard systemic therapy in patients with noninfectious intermediate, posterior, and panuveitis. The primary outcome was a change from baseline in best-corrected visual acuity in uveitic eyes. At 2 years, there was no significant difference in visual acuity between the groups. Significantly better control of inflammation with more local adverse events was seen in the fluocinolone implant group (**B**). Most patients in the implant group develop cataract, but this was 90% of phakic eyes (**C**). No increased risk of malignancy was seen in either of the groups (**D**).

89. Correct: No treatment is recommended in most cases, despite the presence of cells (C)

Treatment with topical corticosteroids for Fuchs' heterochromic iridocyclitis typically does not resolve anterior-chamber inflammation, so aggressive treatment is not recommended (**B**). Patient almost never develop synechiae, so cycloplegia is rarely needed (**A**). For the same reasons, immunomodulatory therapy is not recommended for this condition (**D**).

90. Correct: Chest X-ray (CXR) (B)

A chest radiograph is the single best screening test for sarcoidosis, since it may reveal abnormalities in up to 90% of patients. The classic finding is hilar adenopathy. CT scan is more sensitive but also more expensive as a screening test, may be valuable in patients with negative CXR but with high clinical suspicion (**A**). ACE and lysozyme levels are neither diagnostic nor specific (**C**). Tissue biopsy is required for proven diagnosis, since there must be histologic evidence of noncaseating granulomas (**D**).

91. Correct: Vogt-Koyanagi-Harada (VKH) disease (D)

The acute phase of VKH is characterized by blurry vision is both eyes, 1 to 2 days after central nervous system signs, marked bilateral granulomatous anterior uveitis, vitritis, thickening of the posterior choroid, hyperemia of the disc with swelling, and multiple serous retinal detachments. It is more common in Hispanics, Asians, Asian Indians, Native Americans, and Middle Easterners. Sympathetic ophthalmia may have similar presentation, but this patient has no prior ocular history (trauma or surgery) (**C**). Lupus choroidopathy is rare and characterized by serous elevations of the retina, retinal pigment epithelium (RPE) or both with choroidal infarction, and copy number variation in a patient with systemic lupus erythematosus (**B**). Neuroretinitis is usually unilateral with unilateral optic disc swelling and formation of a macular star; typically, it does not have this bilateral presentation of panuveitis (**A**).

92. Correct: *Toxoplasma chorioretinitis* (C)

Toxoplasmosis is the most common cause of infectious chorioretinitis. Classical presentation appears as a focal, white retinitis with overlying vitritis, often adjacent to a pigmented scar. In some patients, especially those immunocompromised and older patients, may present with large, multiple lesions or bilateral disease. Acute retinal necrosis is characterized by panuveitis followed by occlusive retinal vasculitis and peripheral necrotizing retinitis. This patient has evidence of multiple hyperpigmented scars, so less likely ARN (**A**). Fungal endophthalmitis is typically seen in sick patients with recent hospitalization, systemic antibiotic use, indwelling catheters, debilitating disease such as diabetes, history of immunomodulatory therapy (IMT), neutropenia, organ transplantation, and intravenous drug use among others, none of which are mentioned in this patient. It typically starts in the choroid and eventually breaks into the vitreous (**B**). Finally, multifocal choroiditis with panuveitis is commonly a bilateral disease in females, and retinal findings are typically smaller in size and multiple (**D**).

93. Correct: Despite low IOP, serous choroidal detachments are very rare in these patients (B)

Serous choroidal detachments are often seen in hypotony and makes management more complicated. Hypotony is usually caused by temporary aqueous hyposecretion from the ciliary body in acute inflammation, but permanent hypotony is seen from ciliary body atrophy and absence of ciliary processes (**A**). In the acute phase of uveitis, hypotony usually responds to steroid treatment and cycloplegia, but long-standing choroidal effusions may require drainage. Chronic hypotony associated to cyclitic membrane may respond to pars plana vitrectomy and membranectomy (**C**). If ciliary processes are present, vitrectomy with silicone oil may help increase IOP and preserve ocular anatomy (**D**).

94. Correct: Differential diagnosis includes bartonellosis, toxoplasmosis, sarcoidosis, and acute systemic hypertension (D)

The differential diagnosis of neuroretinitis is extensive and includes infectious, noninfectious, and idiopathic causes including *Bartonella henselae*, the most common toxoplasmosis and acute systemic hypertension. The typical constellation of findings includes vision loss, unilateral optic disc swelling, not atrophy, and macular star formation (**A**). This syndrome was formerly known as *Leber's idiopathic stellate neuroretinitis* or *idiopathic stellate maculopathy* (**B**). Most patients with *Bartonella*-associated neuroretinitis present with some degree of anterior-chamber inflammation and vitritis (**C**).

95. Correct: Fluorescein angiography (A)

Treatment of pars planitis is usually started if visual acuity is decreased, the patient is symptomatic or if cystoid macular edema (CME) and retinal vasculitis are present. For this reason, a fluorescein angiography is essential in the evaluation of these patients. ANA testing and HLA typing are usually part of the work-up of pediatric patients with uveitis, but its presence or absence does not guide treatment (**B, D**). ICG is useful to assess choroidal processes and not as much for patient with retinal vasculitis (**C**).

96. Correct: *Bacillus spp.* (C)

Endogenous bacterial endophthalmitis is caused by hematogenous dissemination of bacteria causing intraocular infection. It is uncommon, and immunosuppressed patients are most at risk. The most common gram-positive organisms in intravenous drug users is *Bacillus spp. Streptococcus spp.* are the most common in endocarditis patients (**A**) and *Staphylococcus aureus* in skin infections (**B**). The most common gram-negative bacteria are *Neisseria meningitides*, *Haemophilus influenzae*, and enteric organisms (*Escherichia coli* and *Klebsiella spp.*). The most common cause of fungal endophthalmitis is *Candida* (**D**).

97. Correct: Cryptococcosis (B)

The dissemination of *Cryptococcus neoformans* in patients with AIDS may cause multifocal choroiditis, which appears as solitary of multiple yellow-white lesions associated to vitritis, sheathing, papilledema, and anterior-chamber cell. It typically involves the cerebrospinal fluid and cause optic nerve edema and meningitis. The recommended primary treatment for HIV patients is induction with IV amphotericin B plus flucytosine for at least 2 weeks, followed by oral fluconazole. Cerebral involvement may require longer treatment, and when there is ocular involvement, treatment might be supplemented with intravitreal amphotericin injections. Ocular coccidioidomycosis is very rare, and disseminated disease more commonly causes granulomatous conjunctivitis, scleritis/episcleritis, nerve palsies, and orbital infections; uveal involvement is even rarer (**A**). Aspergillus endophthalmitis presents as a yellow infiltrate, often in the macula, and a hypopyon can develop in the subretinal or subhyaloidal space although retinal necrosis and hemorrhages can be seen (**C**). CMV retinitis affects mainly the retina and would not present with multiple choroidal lesions like this patient (**D**).

98. Correct: Non-Hodgkin's B cell (A)

Primary central nervous system lymphoma (PCNSL) is a type of lymphoma that involves the brain, meninges, and eyes without systemic involvement. The majority (98%) are non-Hodgkin's B-cell lymphoma. Approximately 2% are T-cell lymphomas (**C**). It mainly affects older patients in the fifth to seventh decade of life but can affect younger patients if immunocompromised and rarely can occur in children. Hodgkin's lymphoma and anaplastic large-cell lymphoma are not typically seen intraocularly (**B, D**). Treatment typically requires systemic chemotherapy but can be accompanied by intravitreal injections of methotrexate or rituximab.

99. Correct: Cytotoxic therapy with cyclophosphamide or chlorambucil can induce long drug-free remission (C)

Given the low prevalence of serpiginous choroiditis, there is no consensus or standardized treatment. Cytotoxic therapy with cyclophosphamide or chlorambucil has been shown to induce long drug-free remission. Corticosteroids (systemic, periocular, and intravitreal) can be used to treat active lesions (**A**). The addition of IMT is almost always done since corticosteroids alone are ineffective or patient requires long-term treatment (**B**). Anti–vascular endothelial growth factor therapy (anti-VEGF), focal laser photocoagulation, and photodynamic therapy can be used if CNV membranes develop (**D**).

100. Human leukocyte antigen B27 (HLA-B27) (B)

In patients with HLA-B27-related disease and reactive arthritis, uveitis may be the presenting sign and the ophthalmologist might be the first one to diagnose or suspect this diagnosis. HLA-B27 testing is indicated. HIV testing should be ordered in a case-to-case basis if medical history suggest risk factors and if patient agrees (**A**). ESR and CRP are nonspecific or diagnostic (**C**). Patients with low back pain and stiffness should have sacroiliac joint imaging and be referred to rheumatology due to the association with ankylosing spondylitis and risk of deformity (**D**).

341